EX LIBRIS: JOSEPH STEIN

TEXTBOOK
of
RECEPTOR
PHARMACOLOGY
Second Edition

TEXTBOOK
of
RECEPTOR PHARMACOLOGY
Second Edition

Edited by

John C. Foreman, D.Sc., F.R.C.P.

Department of Pharmacology
University College London
United Kingdom

Torben Johansen, M.D.

Department of Physiology and Pharmacology
University of Southern Denmark
Denmark

CRC PRESS

Boca Raton   London   New York   Washington, D.C.

Library of Congress Cataloging-in-Publication Data

Textbook of receptor pharmacology / edited by John C. Foreman, Torben Johansen. —
2nd ed.
    p.   cm.
    Includes bibliographical references and index.
    ISBN 0-8493-1029-6 (alk. paper)
    1. Drug receptors. I. Foreman, John C. II. Johansen, Torben.

RM301.41 .T486 2002
615'.7—dc21   2002067406

Visit the CRC Press Web site at www.crcpress.com

Preface

For about four decades now, a course in receptor pharmacology has been given at University College London for undergraduate students in their final year of study for the Bachelor of Science degree in pharmacology. More recently, the course has also been taken by students reading for the Bachelor of Science degree in medicinal chemistry. The students following the course have relied for their reading upon a variety of sources, including original papers, reviews, and various textbooks, but no single text brought together the material included in the course. Also, almost continuously since 1993, we have organized courses for graduate students and research workers from the pharmaceutical industry from the Nordic and European countries. In many cases, generous financial support from the Danish Research Academy and the Nordic Research Academy has made this possible. These courses, too, were based on those for students at University College London, and we are grateful for the constructive criticisms of the many students on all of the courses that have shaped this book.

The first edition of the book provided a single text for the students, and the enthusiasm with which it was received encouraged us to work on a second edition. There have been very significant steps forward since the first edition of this book, particularly in the molecular biology of receptors. These advances are reflected in the rewritten chapters for the section of this book that deals with molecular biology. At the same time, we realized that in the first edition we included too much material that was distant from the receptors themselves. To include all the cellular biology that is consequent upon a receptor activation is really beyond the scope of any book. Hence, we have omitted from the second edition the material on intracellular second messengers such as calcium, the cyclic nucleotides, and phospholipids. The second edition now concentrates on cell membrane receptors themselves, together with their immediate signal transducers: ion channels, heterotrimeric G-proteins, and tyrosine kinases.

The writers of the chapters in this book have been actively involved in teaching the various courses, and our joint aim has been to provide a logical introduction to the study of drug receptors. Characterization of drug receptors involves a number of different approaches: quantitative description of the functional studies with agonists and antagonists, quantitative description of the binding of ligands to receptors, the molecular structure of drug receptors, and the elements that transduce the signal from the activated receptor to the intracellular compartment.

The book is intended as an introductory text on receptor pharmacology but further reading has been provided for those who want to follow up on topics. Some problems are also provided for readers to test their grasp of material in some of the chapters.

John C. Foreman
Torben Johansen

The Editors

John C. Foreman, B.Sc., Ph.D., D.Sc., M.B., B.S., F.R.C.P., is Professor of Immunopharmacology at University College London. He has also been a Visiting Professor at the University of Southern Denmark, Odense, Denmark, and the University of Tasmania, Hobart, Australia. Dr. Foreman is Dean of Students at University College London and also Vice-Dean of the Faculty of Life Sciences. He was Senior Tutor of University College London from 1989 to 1996 and Admissions Tutor for Medicine from 1982 to 1993. Dr. Foreman was made a Fellow of University College London in 1993 and received the degree of Doctor of Science from the University of London in the same year. He was elected to the Fellowship of the Royal College of Physicians in 2001. Dr. Foreman initially read medicine at University College London but interrupted his studies in medicine to take the B.Sc. and Ph.D. in pharmacology before returning to complete the medical degrees, M.B., B.S., which he obtained in 1976. After internships at Peterborough District Hospital, he spent two years as Visiting Instructor of Medicine, Division of Clinical Immunology, Johns Hopkins University Schools of Medicine, Baltimore, MD. He then returned to University College London, where he has remained on the permanent staff.

Dr. Foreman is a member of the British Pharmacological Society and the Physiological Society and served as an editor of the *British Journal of Pharmacology* from 1980 to 1987 and again from 1997 to 2000. He has been an associate editor of *Immunopharmacology* and is a member of the editorial boards of *Inflammation Research* and *Pharmacology and Toxicology*. Dr. Foreman has presented over 70 invited lectures around the world. He is co-editor of the *Textbook of Immunopharmacology*, now in its third edition, and has published approximately 170 research papers, as well as reviews and contributions to books. His current major research interests include bradykinin receptors in the human nasal airway, mechanisms of activation of dendritic cells, and the control of microvascular circulation in human skin.

Torben Johansen, M.D., dr. med., is Docent of Pharmacology, Department of Physiology and Pharmacology, Institute of Medical Biology, Faculty of Health Sciences, University of Southern Denmark. Dr. Johansen obtained his M.D. degree in 1970 from the University of Copenhagen, became a research fellow in the Department of Pharmacology of Odense University in 1970, lecturer in 1972, and senior lecturer in 1974. Since 1990, he has been Docent of Pharmacology. In 1979, he was a visiting research fellow for three months at the University Department of Clinical Pharmacology, Oxford University, and in 1998 and 2001 he was a visiting research fellow at the Department of Pharmacology, University College London. In 1980, he did his internship in medicine and surgery at Odense University Hospital. He obtained his Dr. Med. Sci. in 1988 from Odense University.

Dr. Johansen is a member of the British Pharmacological Society, the Physiological Society, the Scandinavian Society for Physiology, the Danish Medical Association, the Danish Pharmacological Society, the Danish Society for Clinical Pharmacology, and the Danish Society for Hypertension. He has published 70 research papers in refereed journals. His current major research interests are NMDA receptors in the substantia nigra in relation to cell death in Parkinson's disease and also ion transport and signaling in mast cells in relation to intracellular pH and volume regulation.

Contributors

Sir James W. Black, Nobel Laureate, F.R.S.
James Black Foundation
London, United Kingdom

David A. Brown, F.R.S.
Department of Pharmacology
University College London
London, United Kingdom

Jan Egebjerg, Ph.D.
Department for Molecular and Structural
  Biology
Aarhus University
Aarhus, Denmark

Steen Gammeltoft, M.D.
Department of Clinical Biochemistry
Glostrup Hospital
Glostrup, Denmark

Alasdair J. Gibb, Ph.D.
Department of Pharmacology
University College London
London, United Kingdom

Dennis G. Haylett, Ph.D.
Department of Pharmacology
University College London
London, United Kingdom

Birgitte Holst
Department of Pharmacology
University of Copenhagen
Panum Institute
Copenhagen, Denmark

Donald H. Jenkinson, Ph.D.
Department of Pharmacology
University College London
London, United Kingdom

IJsbrand Kramer, Ph.D.
Section of Molecular and Cellular Biology
European Institute of Chemistry and Biology
University of Bordeaux 1
Talence, France

Thue W. Schwartz, M.D.
Department of Pharmacology
University of Copenhagen
Panum Institute
Copenhagen, Denmark

Contents

Section V: Receptors as Pharmaceutical Targets

Section I

Drug–Receptor Interactions

1 Classical Approaches to the Study of Drug–Receptor Interactions

Donald H. Jenkinson

CONTENTS

1.1   INTRODUCTION

The term *receptor* is used in pharmacology to denote a class of cellular macromolecules that are concerned specifically and directly with chemical signaling between and within cells. Combination of a hormone, neurotransmitter, or intracellular messenger with its receptor(s) results in a change in cellular activity. Hence, a receptor must not only recognize the particular molecules that activate it, but also, when recognition occurs, alter cell function by causing, for example, a change in membrane permeability or an alteration in gene transcription.

The concept has a long history. Mankind has always been intrigued by the remarkable ability of animals to distinguish different substances by taste and smell. Writing in about 50 B.C., Lucretius (in *De Rerum Natura, Liber* IV) speculated that odors might be conveyed by tiny, invisible "seeds" with distinctive shapes which would have to fit into minute "spaces and passages" in the palate and nostrils. In his words:

> Some of these must be smaller, some greater, they must be three-cornered for some creatures, square for others, many round again, and some of many angles in many ways.

The same principle of complementarity between substances and their recognition sites is implicit in John Locke's prediction in his *Essay Concerning Human Understanding* (1690):

> Did we but know the mechanical affections of the particles of rhubarb, hemlock, opium and a man, as a watchmaker does those of a watch, … we should be able to tell beforehand that rhubarb will purge, hemlock kill and opium make a man sleep.

(Here, *mechanical affections* could be replaced in today's usage by *chemical affinities*.)

Prescient as they were, these early ideas could only be taken further when, in the early 19th century, it became possible to separate and purify the individual components of materials of plant and animal origin. The simple but powerful technique of fractional crystallization allowed plant alkaloids such as nicotine, atropine, pilocarpine, strychnine, and morphine to be obtained in a pure form for the first time. The impact on biology was immediate and far reaching, for these substances proved to be invaluable tools for the unraveling of physiological function. To take a single example, J. N. Langley made great use of the ability of nicotine to first activate and then block nerves originating in the autonomic ganglia. This allowed him to map out the distribution and divisions of the autonomic nervous system.

Langley also studied the actions of atropine and pilocarpine, and in 1878 he published (in the first volume of the *Journal of Physiology*, which he founded) an account of the interactions between pilocarpine (which causes salivation) and atropine (which blocks this action of pilocarpine). Confirming and extending the pioneering work of Heidenhain and Luchsinger, Langley showed that the inhibitory action of atropine could be overcome by increasing the dose of pilocarpine. Moreover, the restored response to pilocarpine could in turn be abolished by further atropine. Commenting on these results, Langley wrote:

> We may, I think, without too much rashness, assume that there is some substance or substances in the nerve endings or [salivary] gland cells with which both atropine and pilocarpine are capable of forming compounds. On this assumption, then, the atropine or pilocarpine compounds are formed according to some law of which their relative mass and chemical affinity for the substance are factors.

If we replace *mass* by *concentration*, the second sentence can serve as well today as when it was written, though the nature of the law which Langley had inferred must exist was not to be formulated (in a pharmacological context) until almost 60 years later. It is considered in Section 1.5.2 below.

J. N. Langley maintained an interest in the action of plant alkaloids throughout his life. Through his work with nicotine (which can contract skeletal muscle) and curare (which abolishes this action of nicotine and also blocks the response of the muscle to nerve stimulation, as first shown by Claude Bernard), he was able to infer in 1905 that the muscle must possess a "receptive substance":

> Since in the normal state both nicotine and curari abolish the effect of nerve stimulation, but do not prevent contraction from being obtained by direct stimulation of the muscle or by a further adequate injection of nicotine, it may be inferred that neither the poison nor the nervous impulse acts directly on the contractile substance of the muscle but on some accessory substance.
>
> Since this accessory substance is the recipient of stimuli which it transfers to the contractile material, we may speak of it as the receptive substance of the muscle.

At the same time, Paul Ehrlich, working in Frankfurt, was reaching similar conclusions, though from evidence of quite a different kind. He was the first to make a thorough and systematic study of the relationship between the chemical structure of organic molecules and their biological actions. This was put to good use in collaboration with the organic chemist A. Bertheim. Together, they prepared and tested more than 600 organometallic compounds incorporating mercury and arsenic. Among the outcomes was the introduction into medicine of drugs such as salvarsan that were toxic to pathogenic microorganisms responsible for syphilis, for example, at doses that had relatively minor side effects in humans. Ehrlich also investigated the selective staining of cells by dyes, as well as the remarkably powerful and specific actions of bacterial toxins. All these studies convinced him that biologically active molecules had to become bound in order to be effective, and after the fashion of the time he expressed this neatly in Latin:

*Corpora non agunt nisi fixata.**

In Ehrlich's words (*Collected Papers*, Vol. III, *Chemotherapy*):

When the poisons and the organs sensitive to it do not come into contact, or when sensitiveness of the organs does not exist, there can be no action.

If we assume that those peculiarities of the toxin which cause their distribution are localized in a special group of the toxin molecules and the power of the organs and tissues to react with the toxin are localized in a special group of the protoplasm, we arrive at the basis of my side chain theory. The distributive groups of the toxin I call the "haptophore group" and the corresponding chemical organs of the protoplasm the 'receptor.' ... Toxic actions can only occur when receptors fitted to anchor the toxins are present.

Today, it is accepted that Langley and Ehrlich deserve comparable recognition for the introduction of the receptor concept. In the same years, biochemists studying the relationship between substrate concentration and enzyme velocity had also come to think that enzyme molecules must possess an "active site" that discriminates among various substrates and inhibitors. As often happens, different strands of evidence had converged to point to a single conclusion.

Finally, a note on the two senses in which present-day pharmacologists and biochemists use the term *receptor*. The first sense, as in the opening sentences of this section, is in reference to the whole receptor macromolecule that carries the binding site for the agonist. This usage has become common as the techniques of molecular biology have revealed the amino-acid sequences of more and more signaling macromolecules. But, pharmacologists still sometimes employ the term *receptor* when they have in mind only the particular regions of the macromolecule that are concerned in the binding of agonist and antagonist molecules. Hence, *receptor occupancy* is often used as convenient shorthand for the fraction of the binding sites occupied by a ligand.**

1.2 MODELING THE RELATIONSHIP BETWEEN AGONIST CONCENTRATION AND TISSUE RESPONSE

With the concept of the receptor established, pharmacologists turned their attention to understanding the quantitative relationship between drug concentration and the response of a tissue. This entailed, first, finding out how the fraction of binding sites occupied and activated by agonist molecules varies with agonist concentration, and, second, understanding the dependence of the magnitude of the observed response on the extent of receptor activation.

Today, the first question can sometimes be studied directly using techniques that are described in later chapters, but this was not an option for the early pharmacologists. Also, the only responses that could then be measured (e.g., the contraction of an intact piece of smooth muscle or a change in the rate of the heart beat) were indirect, in the sense that many cellular events lay between the initial step (activation of the receptors) and the observed response. For these reasons, the early workers had no choice but to devise ingenious indirect approaches, several of which are still important. These are based on "modeling" (i.e., making particular assumptions about) the two

---

* Literally: entities do not act unless attached.
** *Ligand* means here a small molecule that binds to a specific site (or sites) on a receptor macromolecule. The term *drug* is often used in this context, especially in the older literature.

relationships identified above and then comparing the predictions of the models with the actual behavior of isolated tissues. This will now be illustrated.

1.2.1 THE RELATIONSHIP BETWEEN LIGAND CONCENTRATION AND RECEPTOR OCCUPANCY

We begin with the simplest possible representation of the combination of a ligand, A, with its binding site on a receptor, R:

$$A + R \underset{k_{-1}}{\overset{k_{+1}}{\rightleftharpoons}} AR \tag{1.1}$$

Here, binding is regarded as a bimolecular reaction and k_{+1} and k_{-1} are, respectively, the *association rate constant* ($M^{-1} s^{-1}$) and the *dissociation rate constant* (s^{-1}).

The law of mass action states that the rate of a reaction is proportional to the product of the concentrations of the reactants. We will apply it to this simple scheme, making the assumption that equilibrium has been reached so that the rate at which AR is formed from A and R is equal to the rate at which AR dissociates. This gives:

$$k_{+1}[A][R] = k_{-1}[AR]$$

where [R] and [AR] denote the concentrations of receptors in which the binding sites for A are free and occupied, respectively.

It may seem odd to refer to receptor concentrations in this context when receptors can often move only in the plane of the membrane (and even then perhaps to no more than a limited extent, as many kinds of receptors are anchored). However, the model can be formulated equally well in terms of the proportions of a population of binding sites that are either free or occupied by a ligand. If we define p_R as the proportion free,* equal to $[R]/[R]_T$, where $[R]_T$ represents the total concentration of receptors, and p_{AR} as $[AR]/[R]_T$, we have:

$$k_{+1}[A]p_R = k_{-1}p_{AR}$$

Because for now we are concerned only with equilibrium conditions and not with the rate at which equilibrium is reached, we can combine k_{+1} and k_{-1} to form a new constant, $K_A = k_{-1}/k_{+1}$, which has the unit of concentration. K_A is a *dissociation equilibrium constant* (see Appendix 1.2A [Section 1.2.4.1]), though this is often abbreviated to either *equilibrium constant* or *dissociation constant*. Replacing k_{+1} and k_{-1} gives:

$$[A]p_R = K_A p_{AR}$$

Because the binding site is either free or occupied, we can write:

$$p_R + p_{AR} = 1$$

Substituting for p_R:

---

* p_R can be also be defined as N_R/N, where N_R is the number of receptors in which the binding sites are free of A and N is their total number. Similarly, p_{AR} is given by N_{AR}/N, where N_{AR} is the number of receptors in which the binding site is occupied by A. These definitions are used when discussing the action of irreversible antagonists (see Section 1.6.4).

$$\frac{K_A}{[A]} p_{AR} + p_{AR} = 1$$

Hence,*

$$p_{AR} = \frac{[A]}{K_A + [A]} \tag{1.2}$$

This is the important *Hill–Langmuir equation*. A. V. Hill was the first (in 1909) to apply the law of mass action to the relationship between ligand concentration and receptor occupancy at equilibrium and to the rate at which this equilibrium is approached.** The physical chemist I. Langmuir showed a few years later that a similar equation (the *Langmuir adsorption isotherm*) applies to the adsorption of gases at a surface (e.g., of a metal or of charcoal).

In deriving Eq. (1.2), we have assumed that the concentration of A does not change as ligand receptor complexes are formed. In effect, the ligand is considered to be present in such excess that it is scarcely depleted by the combination of a little of it with the receptors, thus [A] can be regarded as constant.

The relationship between p_{AR} and [A] predicted by Eq. (1.2) is illustrated in Figure 1.1. The concentration of A has been plotted using a linear (left) and a logarithmic scale (right). The value of K_A has been taken to be 1 μM. Note from Eq. (1.2) that when [A] = K_A, p_{AR} = 0.5; that is, half of the receptors are occupied.

With the logarithmic scale, the slope of the line initially increases. The curve has the form of an elongated S and is said to be *sigmoidal*. In contrast, with a linear (arithmetic) scale for [A], sigmoidicity is not observed; the slope declines as [A] increases, and the curve forms part of a rectangular hyperbola.

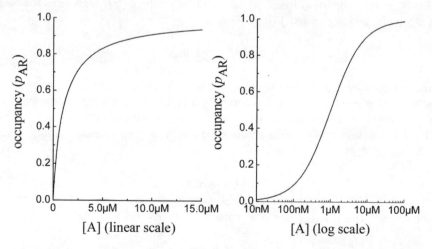

FIGURE 1.1 The relationship between binding-site occupancy and ligand concentration ([A]; linear scale, left; log scale, right), as predicted by the Hill–Langmuir equation. K_A has been taken to be 1 μM for both curves.

---

* If you find this difficult, see Appendix 1.2B at the end of this section.
** Hill had been an undergraduate student in the Department of Physiology at Cambridge where J. N. Langley suggested to him that this would be useful to examine in relation to finding whether the rate at which an agonist acts on an isolated tissue is determined by diffusion of the agonist or by its combination with the receptor.

Equation (1.2) can be rearranged to:

$$\frac{p_{AR}}{1 - p_{AR}} = \frac{[A]}{K_A}$$

Taking logs, we have:

$$\log\left(\frac{p_{AR}}{1 - p_{AR}}\right) = \log[A] - \log K_A$$

Hence, a plot of log ($p_{AR}/(1 - p_{AR})$) against log [A] should give a straight line with a slope of one. Such a graph is described as a *Hill plot*, again after A. V. Hill, who was the first to employ it, and it is often used when p_{AR} is measured directly with a radiolabeled ligand (see Chapter 5). In practice, the slope of the line is not always unity, or even constant, as will be discussed. It is referred to as the *Hill coefficient* (n_H); the term *Hill slope* is also used.

1.2.2 THE RELATIONSHIP BETWEEN RECEPTOR OCCUPANCY AND TISSUE RESPONSE

This is the second of the two questions identified at the start of Section 1.2, where it was noted that the earliest pharmacologists had no choice but to use indirect methods in their attempts to account for the relationship between the concentration of a drug and the tissue response that it elicits. In the absence at that time of any means of obtaining direct evidence on the point, A. V. Hill and A. J. Clark explored the consequences of assuming: (1) that the law of mass action applies, so that Eq. (1.2), derived above, holds; and (2) that the response of the tissue is linearly related to receptor occupancy. Clark went further and made the tentative assumption that the relationship might be one of direct proportionality (though he was well aware that this was almost certainly an oversimplification, as we now know it usually is).

Should there be direct proportionality, and using y to denote the response of a tissue (expressed as a percentage of the maximum response attainable with a large concentration of the agonist), the relationship between occupancy* and response becomes:

$$\frac{y}{100} = p_{AR} \tag{1.3}$$

Combining this with Eq. (1.2) gives an expression that predicts the relationship between the concentration of the agonist and the response that it elicits:

$$\frac{y}{100} = \frac{[A]}{K_A + [A]} \tag{1.4}$$

This is often rearranged to:

$$\frac{y}{100 - y} = \frac{[A]}{K_A} \tag{1.5}$$

---

* Note that no distinction is made here between *occupied* and *activated* receptors; it is tacitly assumed that all the receptors occupied by agonist molecules are in an active state, hence contributing to the initiation of the tissue response that is observed. As we shall see in the following sections, this is a crucial oversimplification.

Taking logs,

$$\log\left(\frac{y}{100-y}\right) = \log[A] - \log K_A$$

The applicability of this expression (and by implication Eq. (1.4)) can be tested by measuring a series of responses (y) to different concentrations of A and then plotting $\log(y/(100-y))$ against $\log[A]$ (the Hill plot). If Equation (1.4) holds, a straight line with a slope of 1 should be obtained. Also, were the underlying assumptions to be correct, the value of the intercept of the line on the abscissa (i.e., when the response is half maximal) would give an estimate of K_A. A. J. Clark was the first to test this using the responses of isolated tissues, and Figure 1.2 illustrates some of his results. Figure 1.2A shows that Eq. (1.4) provides a reasonably good fit to the experimental values. Also, the slopes of the Hill plots in Figure 1.2B are close to unity (0.9 for the frog ventricle, 0.8 for the rectus abdominis). While these findings are in keeping with the simple model that has been outlined, they do not amount to proof that it is correct. Indeed, later studies with a wide range of tissues have shown that many concentration–response relationships cannot be fitted by Eq. (1.4). For example, the Hill coefficient is almost always greater than unity for responses mediated by ligand-gated ion channels (see Appendix 1.2C [Section 1.2.4.3] and Chapter 6). What is more, it is now known that with many tissues the maximal response (for example, contraction of intestinal smooth muscle) can occur when an agonist such as acetylcholine occupies less than a tenth of the available receptors, rather than all of them as postulated in Eq. (1.3). By the same token, when an agonist is applied at the concentration (usually termed the $[A]_{50}$ or EC_{50}) required to produce a half-maximal response, receptor occupancy may be as little as 1% in some tissues,* rather than the 50% expected if the response is directly proportional to occupancy. An additional complication is that many tissues contain enzymes (e.g., cholinesterase) or uptake processes (e.g., for noradrenaline) for which agonists are substrates. Because of this, the agonist concentration in the inner regions of an isolated tissue may be much less than in the external solution.

Pharmacologists have therefore had to abandon (sometimes rather reluctantly and belatedly) not only their attempts to explain the shapes of the dose–response curves of complex tissues in terms of the simple models first explored by Clark and by Hill, but also the hope that the value of the concentration of an agonist that gives a half-maximal response might provide even an approximate estimate of K_A. Nevertheless, as Clark's work showed, the relationship between the concentration of an agonist and the response of a tissue commonly has the same general form shown in Figure 1.1. In keeping with this, concentration–response curves can often be described empirically, and at least to a first approximation, by the simple expression:

$$y = y_{max} \frac{[A]^{n_H}}{[A]_{50}^{n_H} + [A]^{n_H}} \tag{1.6}$$

This is usually described as the *Hill equation* (see also Appendix 1.2C [Section 1.2.4.3]). Here, n_H is again the *Hill coefficient*, and y and y_{max} are, respectively, the observed response and the maximum response to a large concentration of the agonist, A. $[A]_{50}$ is the concentration of A at which y is half maximal. Because it is a constant for a given concentration–response relationship, it is sometimes denoted by K. While this is algebraically neater (and was the symbol used by Hill), it should be remembered that K in this context does not necessarily correspond to an equilibrium constant. Employing $[A]_{50}$ rather than K in Eq. (1.6) helps to remind us that the relationship between

---

* For evidence on this, see Section 1.6 on irreversible antagonists.

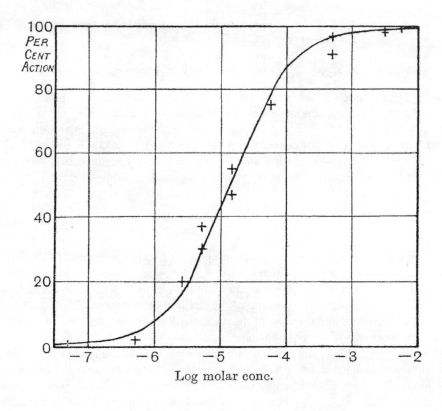

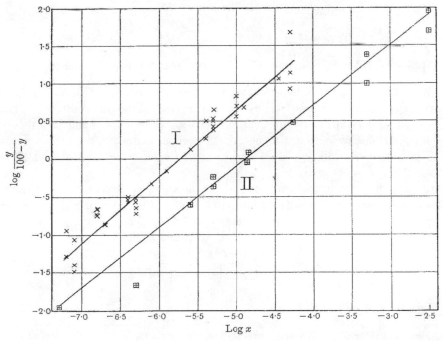

FIGURE 1.2 (Upper) Concentration–response relationship for the action of acetylcholine in causing contraction of the frog rectus abdominis muscle. The curve has been drawn using Eq. (1.4). (Lower) Hill plots for the action of acetylcholine on frog ventricle (curve I) and rectus abdominis (curve II). (From Clark, A. J., *J. Physiol.*, 61, 530–547, 1926.)

[A] and response is here being *described* rather than *explained* in terms of a model of receptor action. This is an important difference.

1.2.3 The Distinction between Agonist Binding and Receptor Activation

Finally, we return to models of receptor action and to a further limitation of the early attempts to account for the shapes of concentration–response curves. As already noted, the simple concepts expressed in Eqs. (1.3) and (1.4) do not distinguish between the occupation and the activation of a receptor by an agonist. This distinction, it is now appreciated, is crucial to the understanding of the action of agonists and partial agonists. Indeed all contemporary accounts of receptor activation take as their starting point a mechanism of the following kind:*

$$\underset{inactive}{\overset{vacant}{A + R}} \overset{K_A}{\rightleftharpoons} \underset{inactive}{\overset{occupied}{AR}} \overset{E}{\rightleftharpoons} \underset{active}{\overset{occupied}{AR*}} \tag{1.7}$$

Here, the occupied receptors can exist in two forms, one of which is inactive (AR) and the other active (AR*) in the sense that its formation leads to a tissue response. AR and AR* can interconvert (often described as isomerization), and at equilibrium the receptors will be distributed among the R, AR, and AR* conditions.** The position of the equilibrium between AR and AR*, and hence the magnitude of the maximum response of the tissue, will depend on the value of the equilibrium constant E.*** Suppose that a very large concentration of the agonist A is applied, so that all the binding sites are occupied (i.e., the receptors are in either the AR or the AR* state). If the position of the equilibrium strongly favors AR, with few active (AR*) receptors, the response will be relatively small. The reverse would apply for a very effective agonist. This will be explained in greater detail in Sections 1.4.3–7, where we will also look into the relationship between agonist concentration and the fraction of receptors in the active state.

1.2.4 Appendices to Section 1.2

1.2.4.1 Appendix 1.2A: Equilibrium, Dissociation, and Affinity Constants

Confusingly, all of these terms are in current use to express the position of the equilibrium between a ligand and its receptors. The choice arises because the ratio of the rate constants k_{-1} and k_{+1} can be expressed either way up. In this chapter, we take K_A to be k_{-1}/k_{+1}, and it is then strictly a *dissociation equilibrium constant*, often abbreviated to either *dissociation constant* or *equilibrium constant*. The inverse ratio, k_{+1}/k_{-1}, gives the *association equilibrium constant*, which is usually referred to as the *affinity constant*.

One way to reduce the risk of confusion is to express ligand concentrations in terms of K_A. This "normalized" concentration is defined as $[A]/K_A$ and will be denoted here by the symbol $\cent_A$. We can therefore write the Hill–Langmuir equation in three different though equivalent ways:

$$p_{AR} = \frac{[A]}{K_A + [A]} = \frac{K_A'[A]}{1 + K_A'[A]} = \frac{\cent_A}{1 + \cent_A}$$

where the terms are as follows:

---

* This will be described as the *del Castillo–Katz scheme*, as it was first applied to receptor action by J. del Castillo and B. Katz (University College London) in 1957 (see also Section 1.4.3).

** The scheme is readily extended to include the possibility that some of the receptors may be active even in the absence of agonist (see Section 1.4.7).

*** This constant is sometimes denoted by L or by K_2. E has been chosen for this introductory account because of the relation to efficacy and also because it is the term used in an important review by Colquhoun (1998) on binding, efficacy, and the effects thereon of receptor mutations.

	Abbreviation	Unit
Dissociation equilibrium constant	K_A	M
Affinity constant	K'_A	M^{-1}
Normalized concentration	ϕ_A	—

1.2.4.2 Appendix 1.2B: Step-by-Step Derivation of the Hill–Langmuir Equation

We start with the two key equations given in Section 1.2.1:

$$[A]p_R = K_A p_{AR} \qquad (A.1)$$

$$p_R + p_{AR} = 1 \qquad (A.2)$$

From Eq. (A.1), $p_R = \dfrac{K_A}{[A]} p_{AR}$ (A.3) Remember, if $ax = by$, then $x = (b/a)y$.

Next, use Eq. (A.3) to replace p_R in Eq. (A.2). This is done because we wish to find p_{AR}:

$$\frac{K_A}{[A]} p_{AR} + p_{AR} = 1$$

$$\boxed{p_{AR}\left(\frac{K_A}{[A]} + 1\right) = 1}$$ Remember, $ax + x = x(a + 1)$.

$$p_{AR}\left(\frac{K_A + [A]}{[A]}\right) = 1$$ Remember, $(s/t) + 1 = (s + t)/t$.

$$\boxed{p_{AR} = \frac{[A]}{K_A + [A]}}$$ Remember, if $x(u/v) = 1$, then $x = (v/u)$.

The Hill–Langmuir equation may be rearranged by cross-multiplying:

$$p_{AR}K_A + p_{AR}[A] = [A]$$

For cross-multiplication, if $(a/b) = (c/d)$, then $(a \times d) = (c \times b)$. Remember, $y = x/(a + x)$ is the same as $(y/1) = x/(a + x)$, which is ready for cross-multiplication.

$$p_{AR}K_A = [A](1 - p_{AR})$$

$$\boxed{\frac{p_{AR}}{1 - p_{AR}} = \frac{[A]}{K_A}}$$

Taking logs,

$$\log\left(\frac{p_{AR}}{1 - p_{AR}}\right) = \log[A] - \log K_A$$ Remember, $\log(a/b) = \log a - \log b$.

1.2.4.3 Appendix 1.2C: The Hill Equation and Hill Plot

In some of his earliest work, published in 1910, A. V. Hill examined how the binding of oxygen to hemoglobin varied with the oxygen partial pressure. He found that the relationship between the two could be fitted by the following equation:

$$y = \frac{K'x^n}{1 + K'x^n}$$

Here, y is the fractional binding, x is the partial pressure of O_2, K' is an affinity constant, and n is a number which in Hill's work varied from 1.5 to 3.2.

This equation can also be written as:

$$y = \frac{x^n}{K_e + x^n} \tag{1.8a}$$

where $K_e = 1/K'$, and as:

$$y = \frac{x^n}{K^n + x^n} \tag{1.8b}$$

This final variant is convenient because K has the same units as x and, moreover, is the value of x for which y is half maximal.

Eq. (1.8b) can be rearranged and expressed logarithmically as:

$$\log\left(\frac{y}{1-y}\right) = n \log x - n \log K$$

Hence, a Hill plot (see earlier discussion) should give a straight line of slope n.

Hill plots are often used in pharmacology, where y may be either the fractional response of a tissue or the amount of a ligand bound to its binding site, expressed as a fraction of the maximum binding, and x is the concentration. It is sometimes found (especially when tissue responses are measured) that the Hill coefficient differs markedly from unity. What might this mean?

One of the earliest explanations to be considered was that n molecules of ligand might bind simultaneously to a single binding site, R:

$$nA + R \rightleftharpoons A_nR$$

This would lead to the following expression for the proportion of binding sites occupied by A:

$$p_{A_nR} = \frac{[A]^n}{K + [A]^n}$$

where K is the dissociation equilibrium constant. Hence, the Hill plot would be a straight line with a slope of n. However, this model is quite unlikely to apply. Extreme conditions aside, few examples exist of chemical reactions in which three or more molecules (e.g., two of A and one of R) must combine simultaneously. Another explanation has to be sought. One possibility arises when the tissue response measured is indirect, in the sense that a sequence of cellular events links receptor activation to the response that is finally observed. The Hill coefficient may not then be unity (or even a constant) because of a nonlinear and variable relation between the proportion of receptors activated and one or more of the events that follow.

Even when it is possible to observe receptor activation directly, the Hill coefficient may still be found not to be unity. This has been studied in detail for ligand-gated ion channels such as the nicotinic receptor for acetylcholine. Here the activity of individual receptors can be followed as it occurs by measuring the tiny flows of electrical current through the ion channel intrinsic to the receptor (see Section 1.4.3 and Chapter 6). On determining the relationship between this response and agonist concentration, the Hill coefficient is observed to be greater than unity (characteristically 1.3–2) and to change with agonist concentration. The explanation is to be found in the structure of this class of receptor. Each receptor macromolecule is composed of several (often five) subunits, of which two carry binding sites for the agonist. Both of these sites must be occupied for the receptor to become activated, at least in its normal mode. The scheme introduced in Section 1.2.3 must then be elaborated:

$$A + R \rightleftharpoons AR + A \rightleftharpoons A_2R \rightleftharpoons A_2R* \tag{1.9}$$

Suppose that the two sites are identical (an oversimplification) and that the binding of the first molecule of agonist does not affect the affinity of the site that remains vacant. The dissociation equilibrium constant for each site is denoted by K_A and the equilibrium constant for the isomerization between A_2R and A_2R* by E, so that $[A_2R*] = E[A_2R]$.

The proportion of receptors in the active state (A_2R*) is then given by:

$$p_{A_2R*} = \frac{E[A]^2}{(K_A + [A])^2 + E[A]^2} \tag{1.10}$$

This predicts a nonlinear Hill plot. Its slope will vary with [A] according to:

$$n_H = \frac{2(K_A + [A])}{K_A + 2[A]}$$

When [A] is small in relation to K_A, n_H approximates to 2. However, as [A] is increased, n_H tends toward unity.

On the same scheme, the amount of A that is bound (expressed as a fraction, p_{bound}, of the maximum binding when [A] is very large, so that all the sites are occupied) is given by:

$$p_{bound} = \frac{[A](K_A + [A]) + E[A]^2}{(K_A + [A])^2 + E[A]^2} \tag{1.11}$$

The Hill plot for binding would be nonlinear with a Hill coefficient given by:

$$n_{\mathrm{H}} = \frac{(K_{\mathrm{A}} + [\mathrm{A}])^2 + E[\mathrm{A}](2K_{\mathrm{A}} + [\mathrm{A}])}{(K_{\mathrm{A}} + [\mathrm{A}])\{K_{\mathrm{A}} + (1+E)[\mathrm{A}]\}} \tag{1.12}$$

This approximates to unity if [A] is either very large or very small. In between, n_{H} may be as much as 2 for very large values of E. It is noteworthy that this should be so even though the affinities for the first and the second binding steps have been assumed to be the same, provided only that some isomerization of the receptor to the active form occurs. This is because isomerization increases the total amount of binding by displacing the equilibria shown in Eq. (1.9) to the right — that is, toward the bound forms of the receptor.

We now consider what would happen if the binding of the first molecule of agonist altered the affinity of the second identical site. The dissociation equilibrium constants for the first and second bindings will be denoted by $K_{\mathrm{A}(1)}$ and $K_{\mathrm{A}(2)}$, respectively, and E is defined as before.

The proportion of receptors in the active state ($\mathrm{A_2R^*}$) is then given by:

$$p_{\mathrm{A_2R^*}} = \frac{E[\mathrm{A}]^2}{K_{\mathrm{A}(1)}K_{\mathrm{A}(2)} + 2K_{\mathrm{A}(2)}[\mathrm{A}] + (1+E)[\mathrm{A}]^2} \tag{1.13}$$

and the Hill coefficient n_{H} would be:

$$n_{\mathrm{H}} = \frac{2(K_{\mathrm{A}(1)} + [\mathrm{A}])}{K_{\mathrm{A}(1)} + 2[\mathrm{A}]}$$

These relationships are discussed further in Chapter 6 (see Eqs. (6.4) and (6.5)).

Using the same scheme, the amount of A that is bound is given by:

$$p_{bound} = \frac{K_{\mathrm{A}(2)}[\mathrm{A}] + (1+E)[\mathrm{A}]^2}{K_{\mathrm{A}(1)}K_{\mathrm{A}(2)} + 2K_{\mathrm{A}(2)}[\mathrm{A}] + (1+E)[\mathrm{A}]^2} \tag{1.14}$$

The Hill plot would again be nonlinear with the Hill coefficient given by:

$$n_{\mathrm{H}} = \frac{K_{\mathrm{A}(1)}K_{\mathrm{A}(2)} + (1+E)[\mathrm{A}](2K_{\mathrm{A}(1)} + [\mathrm{A}])}{(K_{\mathrm{A}(1)} + [\mathrm{A}])\{K_{\mathrm{A}(2)} + (1+E)[\mathrm{A}]\}} \tag{1.15}$$

This approximates to unity if [A] is either very large or very small. In between, n_{H} may be greater (up to 2) or less than 1, depending on the magnitude of E and on the relative values of $K_{\mathrm{A}(1)}$ and $K_{\mathrm{A}(2)}$. If, for simplicity, we set E to 0 and if $K_{\mathrm{A}(2)} < K_{\mathrm{A}(1)}$, then $n_{\mathrm{H}} > 1$, and there is said to be positive cooperativity. Negative cooperativity occurs when $K_{\mathrm{A}(2)} > K_{\mathrm{A}(1)}$ and n_{H} is then < 1. This is discussed further in Chapter 5 where plots of Eqs. (1.14) and (1.15) are shown (Figure 5.3) for widely ranging values of the ratio of $K_{\mathrm{A}(1)}$ to $K_{\mathrm{A}(2)}$, and with E taken to be zero.

1.2.4.4 Appendix 1.2D: Logits, the Logistic Equation, and their Relation to the Hill Plot and Equation

The *logit transformation* of a variable p is defined as:

$$\text{logit}[p] = \log_e\left(\frac{p}{1-p}\right)$$

Hence, the Hill plot can be regarded as a plot of logit (p) against the logarithm of concentration (though it is more usual to employ logs to base 10 than to base e).

It is worth noting the distinction between the *Hill equation* and the *logistic equation*, which was first formulated in the 19th century as a means of describing the time-course of population increase. It is defined by the expression:

$$p = \frac{1}{1 + e^{-(a+bx)}} \tag{1.16}$$

This is easily rearranged to:

$$\frac{p}{1-p} = e^{a+bx}$$

Hence,

$$\text{logit}[p] = \log_e\left(\frac{p}{1-p}\right) = a + bx$$

If we redefine a as $-\log_e K$, and x as $\log_e z$, then

$$p = \frac{z^b}{K + z^b} \tag{1.17}$$

which is a form of the Hill equation (see Eq. (1.8a)). However, note that Eq. (1.17) has been obtained from Eq. (1.16) only by transforming one of the variables. It follows that the terms *logistic equation* (or *curve*) and *Hill equation* (or *curve*) should not be regarded as interchangeable. To illustrate the distinction, if the independent variable in each equation is set to zero, the dependent variable becomes $1/(1 + e^{-a})$ in Eq. (1.16) as compared with zero in Eq. (1.17).

1.3 THE TIME COURSE OF CHANGES IN RECEPTOR OCCUPANCY

1.3.1 INTRODUCTION

At first glance, the simplest approach to determining how quickly a drug combines with its receptors might seem to be to measure the rate at which it acts on an isolated tissue, but two immediate problems arise. The first is that the exact relationship between the effect on a tissue and the proportion of receptors occupied by the drug is often not known and cannot be assumed to be simple, as we have already seen. A half-maximal tissue response only rarely corresponds to half-maximal receptor occupation. We can take as an example the action of the neuromuscular blocking agent tubocurarine on the contractions that result from stimulation of the motor nerve supply to skeletal muscle *in vitro*. The rat phrenic nerve–diaphragm preparation is often used in such experiments. Because neuromuscular transmission normally has a large safety margin, the contractile response to nerve stimulation begins to fall only when tubocurarine has occupied on average more than 80% of the binding sites on the nicotinic acetylcholine receptors located on the superficial muscle fibers. So, when the twitch of the whole muscle has fallen to half its initial amplitude, receptor occupancy by tubocurarine in the surface fibers is much greater than 50%.

The second complication is that the rate at which a ligand acts on an isolated tissue is often determined by the diffusion of ligand molecules through the tissue rather than by their combination with the receptors. Again taking as our example the action of tubocurarine on the isolated diaphragm, the slow development of the block reflects not the rate of binding to the receptors but rather the failure of neuromuscular transmission in an increasing number of individual muscle fibers as tubocurarine slowly diffuses between the closely packed fibers into the interior of the preparation. Moreover, as an individual ligand molecule passes deeper into the tissue, it may bind and unbind several times (and for different periods) to a variety of sites (including receptors). This repeated binding and dissociation can greatly slow diffusion into and out of the tissue.

For these reasons, kinetic measurements are now usually done with isolated cells (e.g., a single neuron or a muscle fiber) or even a patch of cell membrane held on the tip of a suitable microelectrode. Another approach is to work with a cell membrane preparation and examine directly the rate at which a suitable radioligand combines with, or dissociates from, the receptors that the membrane carries. Our next task is to consider what binding kinetics might be expected under such conditions.

1.3.2 INCREASES IN RECEPTOR OCCUPANCY

In the following discussion, we continue with the simple model for the combination of a ligand with its binding sites that was introduced in Section 1.2.1 (Eq. (1.1)). Assuming as before that the law of mass action applies, the rate at which receptor occupancy (p_{AR}) changes with time should be given by the expression:

$$\frac{d(p_{AR})}{dt} = k_{+1}[A]p_R - k_{-1}p_{AR} \tag{1.18}$$

In words, this states that the rate of change of occupancy is simply the difference between the rate at which ligand–receptor complexes are formed and the rate at which they break down.*

At first sight, Eq. (1.18) looks difficult to solve because there are no less than four variables: p_{AR}, t, [A], and p_R. However, we know that $p_R = (1 - p_{AR})$. Also, we will assume, as before, that [A] remains constant; that is, so much A is present in relation to the number of binding sites that the combination of some of it with the sites will not appreciably reduce the overall concentration. Hence, only p_{AR} and t remain as variables, and the equation becomes easier to handle.

Substituting for p_R, we have:

$$\frac{d(p_{AR})}{dt} = k_{+1}[A](1 - p_{AR}) - k_{-1}p_{AR} \tag{1.19}$$

Rearranging terms,

$$\frac{d(p_{AR})}{dt} = k_{+1}[A] - (k_{-1} + k_{+1}[A])p_{AR} \tag{1.20}$$

This still looks rather complicated, so we will drop the subscript from p_{AR} and make the following substitutions for the constants in the equation:

---

* If the reader is new to calculus or not at ease with it, a slim volume (*Calculus Made Easy*) by Silvanus P. Thompson is strongly recommended.

$$a = k_{+1}[A]$$

$$b = k_{-1} + k_{+1}[A]$$

Hence,

$$\frac{dp}{dt} = a - bp$$

This can be rearranged to a standard form that is easily integrated to determine how the occupancy changes with time:

$$\int_{p_1}^{p_2} \frac{dp}{a - bp} = \int_{t_1}^{t_2} dt$$

Integrating,

$$\log_e \left(\frac{a - bp_2}{a - bp_1} \right) = -b(t_2 - t_1)$$

We can now consider how quickly occupancy rises after the ligand is first applied, at time zero ($t_1 = 0$). Receptor occupancy is initially 0, so that p_1 is 0. Thereafter, occupancy increases steadily and will be denoted $p_{AR}(t)$ at time t:

$t_1 = 0$	$p_1 = 0$
$t_2 = t$	$p_2 = p_{AR}(t)$

Hence,

$$\log_e \left\{ \frac{a - bp_{AR}(t)}{a} \right\} = -bt$$

$$\frac{a - bp_{AR}(t)}{a} = e^{-bt}$$

$$p_{AR}(t) = \frac{a}{b}(1 - e^{-bt})$$

Replacing a and b by the original terms, we have:

$$p_{AR}(t) = \frac{k_{+1}[A]}{k_{-1} + k_{+1}[A]} \left\{ 1 - e^{-(k_{-1} + k_{+1}[A])t} \right\} \tag{1.21}$$

Recalling that $k_{-1}/k_{+1} = K_A$, we can write:

$$p_{AR}(t) = \frac{[A]}{K_A + [A]} \left\{ 1 - e^{-(k_{-1} + k_{+1}[A])t} \right\}$$

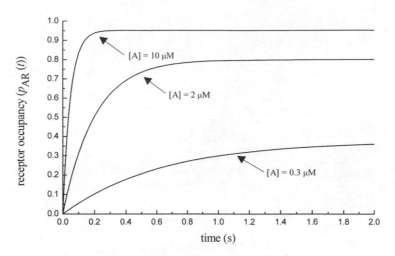

FIGURE 1.3 The predicted time course of the rise in receptor occupancy following the application of a ligand at the three concentrations shown. The curves have been drawn according to Eq. (1.22), using a value of 2×10^6 $M^{-1}sec^{-1}$ for k_{+1} and of 1 sec^{-1} for k_{-1}.

When t is very great, the ligand and its binding sites come into equilibrium. The term in large brackets then becomes unity (because $e^{-\infty} = 0$) so that

$$p_{AR}(\infty) = \frac{[A]}{K_A + [A]}$$

We can then write:

$$p_{AR}(t) = p_{AR}(\infty)\{1 - e^{-(k_{-1}+k_{+1}[A])t}\} \qquad (1.22)$$

This is the expression we need. It has been plotted in Figure 1.3 for three concentrations of A. Note how the rate of approach to equilibrium increases as [A] becomes greater. This is because the time course is determined by $(k_{-1} + k_{+1}[A])$. This quantity is sometimes replaced by a single constant, so that Eq. (1.22) can be rewritten as either:

$$p_{AR}(t) = p_{AR}(\infty)(1 - e^{-\lambda t}) \qquad (1.23)$$

or

$$p_{AR}(t) = p_{AR}(\infty)(1 - e^{-t/\tau}) \qquad (1.24)$$

where

$$\lambda = k_{-1} + k_{+1}[A] = 1/\tau$$

where τ (tau) is the *time constant* and has the unit of *time*; λ (lambda) is the *rate constant*, which is sometimes written as k_{on} (as in Chapter 5) and has the unit of $time^{-1}$.

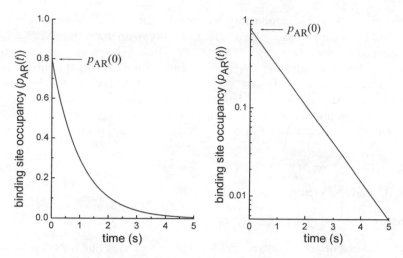

FIGURE 1.4 The predicted time course of the decline in binding-site occupancy. The lines have been plotted using Eq. (1.26), taking k_{-1} to be 1 sec^{-1} and $p_{AR}(0)$ to be 0.8. A linear scale for $p_{AR}(t)$ has been used on the left, and a logarithmic one on the right.

1.3.3 Falls in Receptor Occupancy

Earlier, we had assumed for simplicity that the occupancy was zero when the ligand was first applied. It is straightforward to extend the derivation to predict how the occupancy will change with time even if it is not initially zero. We alter the limits of integration to

$t_1 = 0$	$p_1 = p_{AR}(0)$
$t_2 = t$	$p_2 = p_{AR}(t)$

Here, $p_{AR}(0)$ is the occupancy at time zero, and the other terms are as previously defined.

Exactly the same steps as before then lead to the following expression to replace Eq. (1.22):

$$p_{AR}(t) = p_{AR}(\infty) + \{p_{AR}(0) - p_{AR}(\infty)\}e^{-(k_{-1}+k_{+1}[A])t} \tag{1.25}$$

We can use this to examine what would happen if the ligand is rapidly removed. This is equivalent to setting [A] abruptly to zero, at time zero, and $p(\infty)$ also becomes zero because eventually all the ligand receptor complexes will dissociate. Eq. (1.25) then reduces to:

$$p_{AR}(t) = p_{AR}(0)e^{-k_{-1}t} \tag{1.26}$$

This expression has been plotted in Figure 1.4.

The time constant, τ, for the decline in occupancy is simply the reciprocal of k_{-1}. A related term is the half-time ($t_{1/2}$). This is the time needed for the quantity ($p_{AR}(t)$ in this example) to reach halfway between the initial and the final value and is given by:

$$t_{1/2} = \frac{0.693}{k_{-1}}$$

For the example illustrated in Figure 1.4, $t_{1/2} = 0.693$ sec. Note that τ and $t_{1/2}$ have the unit of *time*, as compared with *time*$^{-1}$ for k_{-1}.

It has been assumed in this introductory account that so many binding sites are present that the average number occupied will rise or fall smoothly with time after a change in ligand concentration; events at single sites have not been considered. When a ligand is abruptly removed, the period for which an individual binding site remains occupied will, of course, vary from site to site, just as do the lifetimes of individual atoms in a sample of an element subject to radioactive decay. It can be shown that the *median* lifetime of the occupancy of individual sites is given by $0.693/k_{-1}$. The *mean* lifetime is $1/k_{-1}$. The introduction of the single-channel recording method has made it possible to obtain direct evidence about the duration of receptor occupancy (see Chapter 6).

1.4 PARTIAL AGONISTS

1.4.1 INTRODUCTION AND EARLY CONCEPTS

The development of new drugs usually requires the synthesis of large numbers of structurally related compounds. If a set of agonists of this kind is tested on a particular tissue, the compounds are often found to fall into two categories. Some can elicit a maximal tissue response and are described as *full agonists* in that experimental situation. Others cannot elicit this maximal response, no matter how high their concentration, and are termed *partial agonists*. Examples include:

Partial Agonist	Full Agonist	Acting at:
Prenalterol	Adrenaline, isoprenaline	β-Adrenoceptors
Pilocarpine	Acetylcholine	Muscarinic receptors
Impromidine	Histamine	Histamine H_2 receptors

Figure 1.5 shows concentration–response curves that compare the action of the β-adrenoceptor partial agonist prenalterol with that of the full agonist isoprenaline on a range of tissues and responses. In every instance, the maximal response to prenalterol is smaller, though the magnitude of the difference varies greatly.

It might be argued that a partial agonist cannot match the response to a full agonist because it fails to combine with all the receptors. This can easily be ruled out by testing the effect of increasing concentrations of a partial agonist on the response of a tissue to a fixed concentration of a full agonist. Figure 1.6 (right, upper curve) illustrates such an experiment for two agonists acting at H_2 receptors. As the concentration of the partial agonist impromidine is raised, the response of the tissue gradually falls from the large value seen with the full agonist alone and eventually reaches the maximal response to the partial agonist acting on its own. The implication is that the partial agonist is perfectly capable of combining with all the receptors, provided that a high enough concentration is applied, but the effect on the tissue is less than what would be seen with a full agonist. The partial agonist is in some way less able to elicit a response.

The experiment of Figure 1.7 points to the same conclusion. When very low concentrations of histamine are applied in the presence of a relatively large fixed concentration of impromidine, the overall response is mainly due to the receptors occupied by impromidine; however, the concentration–response curves cross as the histamine concentration is increased. This is because the presence of impromidine reduces receptor occupancy by histamine (at all concentrations) and vice versa. When the lines intersect, the effect of the reduction in impromidine occupancy by histamine is exactly offset by the contribution from the receptors occupied by histamine. Beyond this point, the presence of impromidine lowers the response to a given concentration of histamine. In effect, it acts as an antagonist. Again, the implication is that the partial agonist can combine with all the receptors but is less able to produce a response.

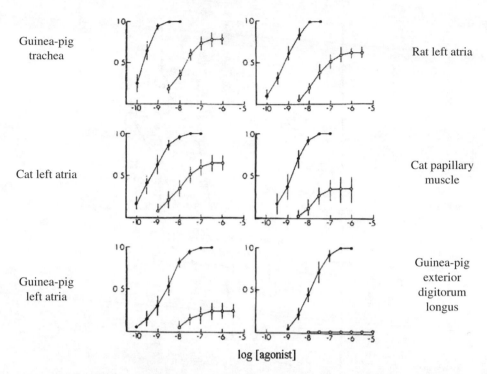

Guinea-pig trachea

Rat left atria

Cat left atria

Cat papillary muscle

Guinea-pig left atria

Guinea-pig exterior digitorum longus

log [agonist]

FIGURE 1.5 Comparison of the log concentration–response relationships for β-adrenoceptor-mediated actions on six tissues of a full and a partial agonist (isoprenaline [closed circles] and prenalterol [open circles], respectively). The ordinate shows the response as a fraction of the maximal response to isoprenaline. (From Kenakin, T, P. and Beek, D., *J. Pharmacol. Exp. Ther.*, 213, 406–413, 1980.)

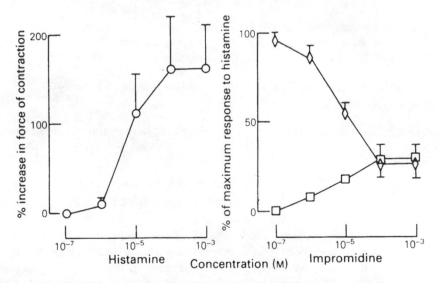

FIGURE 1.6 Interaction between the full agonist histamine and the H_2-receptor partial agonist impromidine on isolated ventricular strips from human myocardium. The concentration–response curve on the left is for histamine alone, and those on the right show the response to impromidine acting either on its own (open squares) or in the presence of a constant concentration (100 μM) of histamine (open diamonds). (From English, T. A. H. et al., *Br. J. Pharmacol.*, 89, 335–340, 1986.)

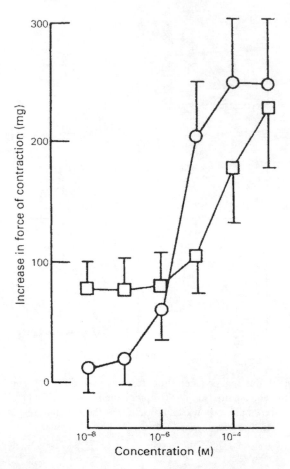

FIGURE 1.7 Log concentration–response curves for histamine applied alone (open circles) or in the presence (open squares) of a constant concentration of the partial agonist impromidine (10 μM). Tissue and experimental conditions as in Figure 1.6. (From English, T. A. H. et al., *Br. J. Pharmacol.*, 89, 335–340, 1986.)

1.4.2 EXPRESSING THE MAXIMAL RESPONSE TO A PARTIAL AGONIST: INTRINSIC ACTIVITY AND EFFICACY

In 1954 the Dutch pharmacologist E. J. Ariëns introduced the term *intrinsic activity*, which is now usually defined as:

$$\text{Intrinsic activity} = \frac{\text{maximum response to test agonist}}{\text{maximum response to a full agonist acting through the same receptors}}$$

For full agonists, the intrinsic activity (often denoted by α) is unity, by definition, as compared with zero for a competitive antagonist. Partial agonists have values between these limits. Note that the definition is entirely descriptive; nothing is assumed about mechanism. Also, *intrinsic* should not be taken to mean that a given agonist has a characteristic activity, regardless of the experimental circumstances. To the contrary, the intrinsic activity of a partial agonist such as prenalterol can vary greatly not only between tissues, as Figure 1.5 illustrates, but also in a given tissue, depending on the experimental conditions (see later discussion). Indeed, the same compound can be a full agonist with one tissue and a partial agonist with another. For this reason, the term *maximal agonist effect* is perhaps preferable to *intrinsic activity*.

Similarly, the finding that a pair of agonists can each elicit the maximal response of a tissue (i.e., they have the same intrinsic activity, unity) should not be taken to imply that they are equally able to activate receptors. Suppose that the tissue has many spare receptors (see Section 1.6.3). One of the agonists might have to occupy 5% of the receptors in order to produce the maximal response, whereas the other might require only 1% occupancy. Evidently, the second agonist is more effective, despite both being full agonists. A more subtle measure of the ability of an agonist to activate receptors is clearly necessary, and one was provided by R. P. Stephenson, who suggested that receptor activation resulted in a "stimulus" or "signal" (S) being communicated to the cells, and that the magnitude of this stimulus was determined by the product of what he termed the *efficacy* (e) of the agonist and the proportion, p, of the receptors that it occupies:*

$$S = ep \tag{1.27}$$

An important difference from Ariëns's concept of intrinsic activity is that efficacy, unlike intrinsic activity, has no upper limit; it is always possible that an agonist with a greater efficacy than any existing compound may be discovered. Also, Stephenson's proposal was not linked to any specific assumption about the relationship between receptor occupancy and the response of the tissue. (Ariëns, like A. J. Clark, had initially supposed direct proportionality, an assumption later to be abandoned.) According to Stephenson,

$$y = f(S_A) = f(e_A p_{AR}) = f\left(e_A \frac{[A]}{K_A + [A]}\right) \tag{1.28}$$

Here, y is the response of the tissue, and e_A is the efficacy of the agonist A. $f(S_A)$ means merely "some function of S_A" (i.e., y depends on S_A in some as yet unspecified way). Note that, in keeping with the thinking at the time, Stephenson used the Hill–Langmuir equation to relate agonist concentration, [A], to receptor occupancy, p_{AR}. This most important assumption is reconsidered in the next section.

In order to be able to compare the efficacies of different agonists acting through the same receptors, Stephenson proposed the convention that the stimulus S is unity for a response that is 50% of the maximum attainable with a full agonist. This is the same as postulating that a partial agonist that must occupy all the receptors to produce a half-maximal response has an efficacy of unity. We can see this from Eq. (1.27); if our hypothetical partial agonist has to occupy all the receptors (i.e., $p = 1$) to produce the half-maximal response, at which point S also is unity (by Stephenson's convention), then e must also be 1.

R. F. Furchgott later suggested a refinement of Stephenson's concept. Recognizing that the response of a tissue to an agonist is influenced by the number of receptors as well as by the ability of the agonist to activate them, he wrote:

$$e = \varepsilon[R]_T$$

Here, $[R]_T$ is the total "concentration" of receptors, and ε (epsilon) is the *intrinsic efficacy* (not to be confused with *intrinsic activity*); ε can be regarded as a measure of the contribution of individual receptors to the overall efficacy.

The efficacy of a particular agonist, as defined by Stephenson, can vary between different tissues in the same way as can the intrinsic activity, and for the same reasons. Moreover, the value of both the intrinsic activity and the efficacy of an agonist in a given tissue will depend on the experimental

---

* No distinction is made here between *occupied* and *activated* receptors. This point is of key importance, as already noted in Section 1.2.3, and is discussed further in the following pages.

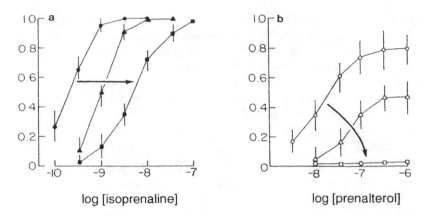

FIGURE 1.8 The effect of carbachol at two concentrations, 1 μM (triangles) and 10 μM (squares), on the relaxations of tracheal smooth muscle caused by a partial agonist, prenalterol, and by a full agonist, isoprenaline. The responses are plotted as a fraction of the maximum to isoprenaline. (From Kenakin, T. P. and Beek, D., *J. Pharmacol. Exp. Ther.*, 213, 406–413, 1980.)

conditions, as illustrated in Figure 1.8. Relaxations of tracheal muscle in response to the β-adrenoceptor agonists isoprenaline and prenalterol were measured first in the absence (circles) and then in the presence (triangles, squares) of a muscarinic agonist, carbachol, which causes contraction and so tends to oppose β-adrenoceptor-mediated relaxation. Hence, greater concentrations of the β-agonists are needed, and the curves shift to the right. With isoprenaline, the maximal response can still be obtained, despite the presence of carbachol at either concentration. The pattern is quite different with prenalterol. Its inability to produce complete relaxation becomes even more evident in the presence of carbachol at 1 μM. Indeed, when administered with 10 μM carbachol, prenalterol causes little or no relaxation; its intrinsic activity and efficacy (in Stephenson's usage) have become negligible.

In the same way, reducing the number of available receptors (for example, by applying an alkylating agent; see Section 1.6.1) will always diminish the maximal response to a partial agonist. In contrast, the log concentration–response curve for a full agonist may first shift to the right, and the maximal response will become smaller only when no spare receptors are available for that agonist (see Section 1.6.3). Conversely, increasing the number of receptors (e.g., by upregulation or by deliberate overexpression of the gene coding for the receptor) will cause the maximal response to a partial agonist to become greater, whereas the log concentration–response curve for a full agonist will move to the left.

1.4.3 INTERPRETATION OF PARTIAL AGONISM IN TERMS OF EVENTS AT INDIVIDUAL RECEPTORS

The concepts of intrinsic activity and efficacy just outlined are purely descriptive, without reference to mechanism. We turn now to how differences in efficacy might be explained in terms of the molecular events that underlie receptor activation, and we begin by considering some of the experimental evidence that has provided remarkably direct evidence of the nature of these events.

Just a year after Stephenson's classical paper of 1956, J. del Castillo and B. Katz published an electrophysiological study of the interactions that occurred when pairs of agonists with related structures were applied simultaneously to the nicotinic receptors at the endplate region of skeletal muscle. Their findings could be best explained in terms of a model for receptor activation that has already been briefly introduced in Section 1.2.3 (see particularly Eq. (1.7)). In this scheme, the occupied receptor can isomerize between an active and an inactive state. This is very different from the classical model of Hill, Clark, and Gaddum in which no clear distinction was made between the *occupation* and *activation* of a receptor by an agonist.

ACh, 100 nм

SubCh, 100 nм

DecCh, 50 nм

CCh, 5 μM

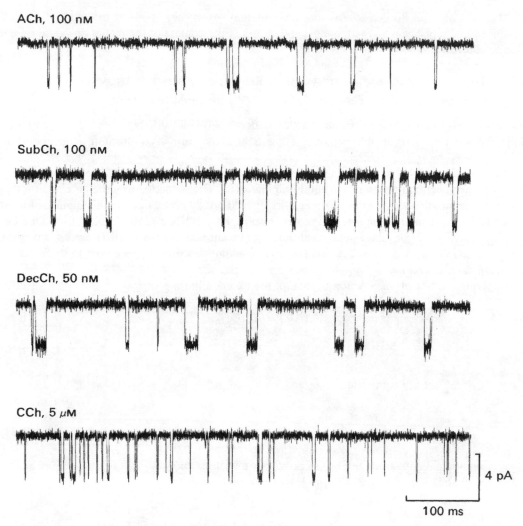

4 pA

100 ms

FIGURE 1.9 Records of the minute electrical currents (downward deflections) that flow through single ligand-gated ion channels in the junctional region of frog skeletal muscle. The currents arise from brief transitions of individual nicotinic receptors to an active (channel open) state in response to the presence of various agonists (ACh = acetylcholine; SubCh = suberyldicholine; DecCh = the dicholine ester of decan-1,10-dicarboxylic acid; CCh = carbamylcholine). (From Colquhoun, D. and Sakmann, B., *J. Physiol.*, 369, 501–557, 1985. With permission.)

Direct evidence for this action was to come from the introduction by E. Neher and B. Sakmann in 1976 of the single-channel recording technique, which allowed the minute electrical currents passing through the ion channel intrinsic to the nicotinic receptor, and other ligand-gated ion channels, to be measured directly and as they occurred. For the first time it became possible to study the activity of individual receptors *in situ* (see also Chapter 6). It was quickly shown that for a wide range of nicotinic agonists, these currents had exactly the same amplitude. This is illustrated for four such agonists in Figure 1.9. What differed among agonists was the fraction of time for which the current flowed (i.e., for which the channels were open). This is just what would be expected from the del Castillo–Katz scheme if the active state (AR*) of the occupied receptor is the same (in terms of the flow of ions through the open channel) for different agonists. However, with a weak partial agonist, the receptor is in the AR* state for only a small fraction of the time, even if all the binding sites are occupied.

The next question to consider is the interpretation of efficacy (both in the particular sense introduced by Stephenson and in more general terms) in the context of the model proposed by del Castillo and Katz.

1.4.4 THE DEL CASTILLO–KATZ MECHANISM: 1. RELATIONSHIP BETWEEN AGONIST CONCENTRATION AND FRACTION OF RECEPTORS IN AN ACTIVE FORM

Our first task is to apply the law of mass action to derive a relationship between the concentration of agonist and the proportion of receptors that are in the active form at equilibrium. This proportion will be denoted by p_{AR*}.

As in all the derivations in this chapter, this one requires only three steps. The first is to apply the law of mass action to each of the equilibria that exist. The second is to write an equation that expresses the fact that the fractions of receptors in each condition that can be distinguished must add up to 1 (the "conservation rule"). The del Castillo–Katz scheme in its simplest form (see Eq. (1.7) in Section 1.2.3) has three such conditions: R (vacant and inactive), AR (inactive, though A is bound), and AR* (bound and active). The corresponding fractions of receptors in these conditions* are p_R, p_{AR}, and p_{AR*}.

Applying the law of mass action to each of the two equilibria gives:

$$[A]p_R = K_A p_{AR} \tag{1.29}$$

$$p_{AR*} = E p_{AR} \tag{1.30}$$

where K_A and E are the equilibrium constants indicated in Eq. (1.7).

Also,

$$p_R + p_{AR} + p_{AR*} = 1 \tag{1.31}$$

We can now take the third and last step. What we wish to know is p_{AR*}, so we use Eqs. (1.29) and (1.30) to substitute for p_R and p_{AR} in Eq. (1.31), obtaining:

$$\frac{K_A}{E[A]} p_{AR*} + \frac{1}{E} p_{AR*} + p_{AR*} = 1$$

$$\therefore p_{AR*} = \frac{E[A]}{K_A + (1+E)[A]} \tag{1.32}$$

This is the expression we require. Although it has the same general form as the Hill–Langmuir equation, two important differences are to be noted:

1. As [A] is increased, p_{AR*} tends not to unity but to

$$\frac{E}{1+E}$$

---

* The term "state" rather than "condition" is often used in this context. However, the latter seems preferable in an introductory account. This is because the del Castillo–Katz mechanism is often described as a "two-state" model of receptor action, meaning here that the occupied receptor exists in *two* distinct (albeit interconvertible) forms, AR and AR*, whereas *three* conditions of the receptor (R, AR, and AR*) have to be identified when applying the law of mass action to the binding of the ligand, A.

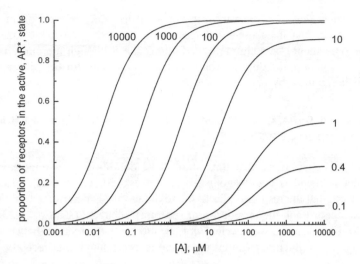

FIGURE 1.10 The relationship between p_{AR*} and [A] predicted by Eq. (1.32) for a range of values of E (given with each line). Note that as E rises above 10, the curves move to the left even though the value of K_A, the dissociation equilibrium constant for the initial combination of A with its binding site, is 200 μM for each curve.

Thus, the value of E will determine the maximal response to A. Only if E is very large in relation to one will almost all the receptors be activated, as illustrated in Figure 1.10, which plots Eq. (1.32) for a range of values of E.

2. Equation (1.32) gives the proportion of *active* receptors (p_{AR*}), rather than *occupied* receptors ($p_{occ} = p_{AR} + p_{AR*}$). To obtain the occupancy, we can use Eq. (1.30) to express p_{AR} in terms of p_{AR*}:

$$p_{occ} = p_{AR} + p_{AR*} = \left(\frac{1+E}{E}\right)p_{AR*} \qquad (1.33)$$

$$= \frac{(1+E)[A]}{K_A + (1+E)[A]}$$

$$= \frac{[A]}{\dfrac{K_A}{1+E} + [A]} \qquad (1.34)$$

This can be rewritten as:

$$p_{occ} = \frac{[A]}{K_{eff} + [A]} \qquad (1.35)$$

where K_{eff}, the *effective dissociation equilibrium constant*, is defined as:

$$K_{eff} = \frac{K_A}{1+E} \qquad (1.36)$$

Because K_{eff} applies to a scheme that involves more that one equilibrium (see Eq. (1.7)), it is referred to as a *macroscopic equilibrium constant*, to distinguish it from the *microscopic equilibrium constants* K_A and E, which describe the individual equilibria.

These results show that if the relationship between the concentration of an agonist and the proportion of receptors that it occupies is measured directly (e.g., using a radioligand binding method), the outcome should be a simple hyperbolic curve. Although the curve is describable by the Hill–Langmuir equation, the dissociation equilibrium constant for the binding will be not K_A but K_{eff}, which is determined by both E and K_A.

1.4.5 THE DEL CASTILLO–KATZ MECHANISM: 2. INTERPRETATION OF EFFICACY FOR LIGAND-GATED ION CHANNELS

In general terms, it is easy to see that the value of the equilibrium constant E in Eq. (1.7) will determine whether a ligand is a full agonist, a partial agonist, or an antagonist. We first recall Stephenson's concept that the response of a tissue to an agonist is determined by the product, S, of the efficacy of the agonist and the proportion of receptors occupied (see Eq. (1.27)). To relate this to the del Castillo–Katz scheme, we rewrite Eq. (1.33) to show the relation between the proportion of active receptors, p_{AR*} (which determines the tissue response) and total receptor occupancy:

$$p_{AR*} = \frac{E}{1+E} \, p_{occ} \tag{1.37}$$

From this we can see that the term $E/(1 + E)$ is equivalent, in a formal sense at least, to Stephenson's efficacy. If an agonist is applied at a very high concentration, so that all the receptors are occupied, the proportion in the active state is $E/(1 + E)$. If this agonist is also very effective (i.e., if E is $\gg 1$), the proportion of active receptors becomes close to unity, the upper limit. Consider next a hypothetical partial agonist that, even when occupying all the receptors ($p_{occ} = 1$), causes only half of them to be in the active form (i.e., $p_{AR} = p_{AR*} = 0.5$). From Eq. (1.37), we can see that E must be unity for this agonist. In Stephenson's scheme, such an agonist would have an efficacy of unity, provided that the response measured is a direct indication of the proportion of activated receptors.

The realization that the ability of an agonist to activate a receptor can be expressed in this way has led to great interest in measuring the rate constants (two each for K_A and E, at the simplest) that determine not only the values of K_A and E but also the kinetics of agonist action. The single-channel recording technique allows this to be achieved for ligand-gated ion channels, as described in Chapter 6. Note, however, the complication that such receptors generally carry two binding sites for the agonist, so the simple scheme just considered, Eq. (1.7), has to be elaborated (see Eq. (1.9) in Appendix 1.2C [Section 1.2.4.3] and also Chapter 6).

A difficulty encountered in such work, and one that has to be considered in any study of the relationship between the concentration of an agonist and its action, is the occurrence of *desensitization*. The response declines despite the continued presence of the agonist. Several factors can contribute. One that has been identified in work with ligand-gated ion channels is that receptors occupied by agonist and in the active state (AR*) may isomerize to an inactive, desensitized, state, AR_D. This can be represented as:

$$A + R \underset{}{\overset{K_A}{\rightleftharpoons}} \underset{(inactive)}{AR} \underset{}{\overset{E}{\rightleftharpoons}} \underset{(active)}{AR*} \underset{}{\overset{K_D}{\rightleftharpoons}} \underset{(inactive)}{AR_D}$$

$\underset{(inactive)}{A + R}$

As explained in Chapter 6, quantitative studies of desensitization at ligand-gated ion channels have shown that even this scheme is an oversimplification, and it is necessary to include the possibility that receptors without ligands can exist in a desensitized state.

Desensitization can occur in other ways. With G-protein-coupled receptors, it can result from phosphorylation of the receptor by one or more protein kinases that become active following the application of agonist.* This activation is sometimes followed by the loss of receptors from the cell surface. An agonist-induced reduction in the number of functional receptors over a relatively long time period is described as *downregulation*. Receptor *upregulation* can also occur, for example, following the prolonged administration of antagonists *in vivo*.

1.4.6　Interpretation of Efficacy for Receptors Acting through G-Proteins

Some of the most revealing studies of partial agonism (including Stephenson's seminal work) have been done with tissues in which G-proteins (see Chapters 2 and 7) provide the link between receptor activation and initiation of the response. In contrast to the situation with "fast" receptors with intrinsic ion channels (see above), it is not yet possible to observe the activity of individual G-protein-coupled receptors (with the potential exception of some that are linked to potassium channels); however, enough is known to show that the mechanisms are complex. The interpretation of differences in efficacy for agonists acting at such receptors is correspondingly less certain.

An early model for the action of such receptors was as follows:

$$A + R \underset{}{\overset{K_A}{\rightleftharpoons}} AR$$

$$AR + G \underset{}{\overset{K_{ARG}}{\rightleftharpoons}} ARG*$$

Here, the agonist–receptor complex (AR) combines with a G-protein (G) to form a ternary complex (ARG*), which can initiate further cellular events, such as the activation of adenylate cyclase. However, this simple scheme (the ternary complex model) was not in keeping with what was already known about the importance of isomerization in receptor activation (see Sections 1.2.3 and 1.4.3), and it also failed to account for findings that were soon to come from studies of mutated receptors. In all current models of G-protein-coupled receptors, receptor activation by isomerization is assumed to occur so that the model becomes:

$$A + R \underset{}{\overset{K_A}{\rightleftharpoons}} AR \underset{}{\overset{E}{\rightleftharpoons}} AR*$$

$$AR* + G \underset{}{\overset{K_{ARG}}{\rightleftharpoons}} AR* G*$$

(1.38)

Here, combination of the activated receptor (AR*) with the G-protein causes the latter to enter an active state (G*) which can initiate a tissue response through, for example, adenylate cyclase, phospholipase C, or the opening or closing of ion channels. In this scheme, what will determine whether a particular agonist can produce a full or only a limited response? Suppose that a high concentration of the agonist is applied, so that all the receptors are occupied. They will then be distributed among the AR, AR*, and AR*G* conditions, of which AR*G* alone leads to a response. The values of both E and K_{ARG} will then influence how much AR*G* is formed, and hence whether the agonist in question is partial or otherwise. In principle, each of these two equilibrium constants

---

* Some of these protein kinases are specific for particular receptors (e.g., β-adrenergic receptor kinase [βARK], now referred to as GRK2).

could vary from agonist to agonist. By analogy with ligand-gated ion channels, it is tempting to suppose that only E is agonist dependent and that the affinity of the active, AR*, state of the receptor for the G-protein is the same for all agonists. However, in the absence of direct evidence, this must remain an open question. Note that, in any case, the magnitude of the response may also depend on the availability of the G-protein. If very little is available, only a correspondingly small amount of AR*G* can be formed, regardless of the concentration of agonist and the number of receptors. Similarly, if few receptors are present in relation to the total quantity of G-protein, that too will limit the formation of AR*G*. Thus, the maximum response to an agonist is influenced by tissue factors as well as by K_A, E, and K_{ARG}. This can be shown more formally by applying the law of mass action to the three equilibria shown in Eq. (1.38). The outcome, with some further discussion, is given in Appendix 1.4B (Section 1.4.9.2).

Complicated though these schemes might seem, they are in fact oversimplifications. Factors that have not been considered include:

1. It is likely that some receptors are coupled to G-proteins even in the absence of agonist.
2. The activated receptor combines with the G-protein in its G_{GDP} form, with the consequence that guanosine triphosphate (GTP) can replace previously bound guanosine diphosphate (GDP). The extent to which this can occur will be influenced by the local concentration of GTP.
3. The structure of the G-protein is heterotrimeric. Following activation by GTP binding, the trimer dissociates into its α and $\beta\gamma$ subunits, each of which may elicit cell responses.
4. G-protein activation has a cyclical nature. The α subunit can hydrolyze the GTP that is bound to it, thereby allowing the heterotrimer to reform. The lifetime of individual α_{GTP} subunits will vary (*cf.* the lifetimes of open ion channels).
5. More than one type of G-protein, each with characteristic cellular actions, may be present in many cells.
6. Some G-protein-coupled receptors have been found to be constitutively active (see the following section).
7. It is possible (although as yet unproven) that the affinity of the active form of the occupied receptor (AR*) for the G-protein may vary from agonist to agonist.
8. Recent evidence suggests that several G-protein-coupled receptors exist as dimers.

In principle, these features can be built into models of receptor activation, although the large number of disposable parameters makes testing difficult. Some of the rate and equilibrium constants must be known beforehand. One experimental tactic is to alter the relative proportions of receptors and G-protein and then determine whether the efficacy of agonists changes in the way expected from the model. The discovery that some receptors are constitutively active has provided another new approach as well as additional information about receptor function, as we shall now see.

1.4.7 CONSTITUTIVELY ACTIVE RECEPTORS AND INVERSE AGONISTS

The del Castillo–Katz scheme (in common, of course, with the simpler model explored by Hill, Clark, and Gaddum) supposes that the receptors are inactive in the absence of agonist. It is now known that this is not always so; several types of receptor are constitutively active. Examples include mutated receptors responsible for several genetically determined diseases. Thus, hyperthyroidism can result from mutations that cause the receptors for thyrotropin (TSH, or thyroid-stimulating hormone) to be active even in the absence of the hormone. Also, receptor variants that are constitutively active have been created in the laboratory by site-directed mutagenesis. Finally, deliberate overexpression of receptors by receptor-gene transfection of cell lines and even laboratory animals has revealed that many "wild-type" receptors also show some activity in the absence of agonist. What might the mechanism be? The most likely possibility, and one which is in keeping

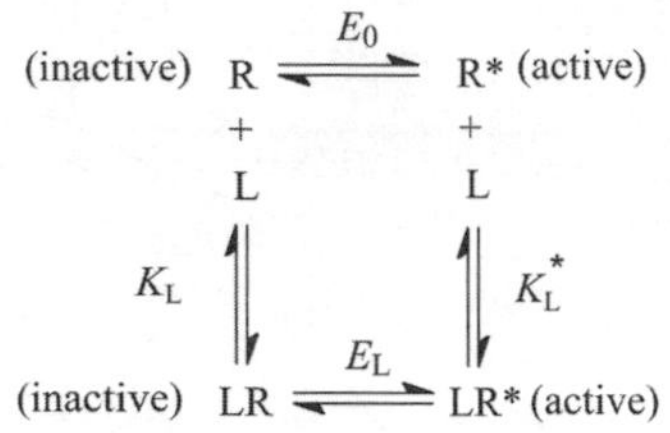

$$(\text{inactive}) \quad R \; \underset{}{\overset{E_0}{\rightleftharpoons}} \; R^* \; (\text{active})$$

$$+ \qquad\qquad +$$

$$L \qquad\qquad L$$

$$K_L \Big\Updownarrow \qquad\qquad \Big\Updownarrow K_L^*$$

$$(\text{inactive}) \quad LR \; \underset{}{\overset{E_L}{\rightleftharpoons}} \; LR^* \; (\text{active})$$

FIGURE 1.11 A model to show the influence of a ligand, L, on the equilibrium between the active and inactive forms of a constitutively active receptor, R. Note that if L, R, and LR are in equilibrium, and likewise L, R* and LR*, then the same must hold for LR and LR* (see Appendix 1.6B (Section 1.6.7.2) for further explanation).

with what has been learned about how ion channels work, is that such receptors can isomerize spontaneously to and from an active form:

$$\underset{(\text{inactive})}{R} \; \rightleftharpoons \; \underset{(\text{active})}{R^*}$$

In principle, both forms could combine with agonist, or indeed with any ligand, L, with affinity, as illustrated in Figure 1.11.

Suppose that L combines only with the inactive, R, form. Then the presence of L, by promoting the formation of LR at the expense of the other species, will reduce the proportion of receptors in the active, R*, state. L is said to be an *inverse agonist* or *negative antagonist* and to possess *negative efficacy*. If, in contrast, L combines with the R* form alone, it will act as a *conventional* or *positive* agonist of very high intrinsic efficacy.

Exploring the scheme further, a partial agonist will bind to both R and R* but with some preferential affinity for one or the other of the two states. If the preference is for R, the ligand will be a *partial inverse agonist*, as its presence will reduce the number of receptors in the active state, though not to zero.

As shown in Section 1.10 (see the solution to Problem 1.4), application of the law of mass action to the scheme of Figure 1.11 provides the following expression for the fraction of receptors in the active state (i.e., $p_{R*} + p_{LR*}$) at equilibrium:

$$p_{\text{active}} = \frac{E_0}{E_0 + \left(\dfrac{1 + \dfrac{[L]}{K_L}}{1 + \dfrac{[L]}{K_L^*}} \right)} \tag{1.39}$$

Here, the equilibrium constant E_0 is defined by p_{R*}/p_R, K_L by $[L]p_R/p_{LR}$, and K_L^* by $[L]p_{R*}/p_{LR*}$. Figure 1.12 plots this relationship for three hypothetical ligands that differ in their relative affinities for the active and the inactive states of the receptor. The term α has been used to express the ratio of K_L to K_L^*. When $\alpha = 0.1$, the ligand is an inverse agonist; whereas when $\alpha = 100$, it is a conventional agonist. In the third example, with a ligand that shows no selectivity between the active and inactive forms of the receptor ($\alpha = 1$), the proportion of active receptors remains unchanged as [L] (and therefore receptor occupancy) is increased.

Such a ligand, however, will reduce the action of either a conventional or an inverse agonist, and so in effect is an antagonist. More precisely, it is a neutral competitive antagonist. If large

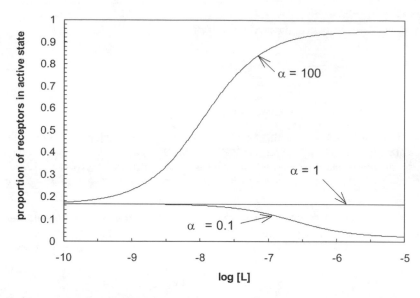

FIGURE 1.12 The relationship between the total fraction of receptors in the active state ($p_{R*} + p_{AR*}$) and ligand concentration ([L]) for a constitutively active receptor. The curve has been drawn according to Eq. (1.39), using the following values: $E_0 = 0.2$, $K_L = 200$ nM, $\alpha = K_L/K_L^* = 0.1$, 1, and 100, as shown. Note that on this model some of the receptors (a fraction given by $E_0/(1 + E_0) = 0.167$) are active in the absence of ligand.

numbers of competitive antagonists of the same pharmacological class (e.g., β-adrenoceptor block-ers) are carefully tested on a tissue or cell line showing constitutive activity, some will be found to cause a small increase in basal activity. They are, in effect, weak conventional partial agonists. Others will reduce the basal activity and so may be inverse agonists with what could be a substantial degree of negative efficacy.* Few of the set can be expected to have exactly the same affinity for the active and inactive forms of the receptor and so be neutral antagonists. However, some com-pounds of this kind have been identified, and Figure 1.13 illustrates the effect of one on the response to both a conventional and an inverse agonist acting on 5HT$_{1A}$ receptors expressed in a cell line.

As with the experiments of Figure 1.13, constitutive activity is often investigated in cultured cell lines that do not normally express the receptor to be examined but have been made to do so by transfection with the gene coding for either the native receptor or a mutated variant of it. The number of receptors per cell (receptor density) may be much greater in these circumstances than in cells that express the receptors naturally. While overexpression of this kind has the great advantage that small degrees of constitutive activity can be detected and studied, it is worth noting that constitutive activity is often much less striking *in situ* than in transfected cells. Hence, the partial agonist action (conventional or inverse) of an antagonist may be much less marked, or even negligible, when studied in an intact tissue so that simple competitive antagonism is observed, as described in Section 1.5.

Nevertheless, the evidence that some receptors have sufficient constitutive activity to influence cell function *in vivo* even in the absence of agonist makes it necessary to extend the simple models already considered for the activation of G-protein-coupled receptors. In principle, the receptor can now exist in no less than eight different conditions (R, R*, LR, LR*, RG, R*G, LRG, LR*G), which is best represented graphically as a cube with one of the conditions at each vertex (see Figure 1.14). The calculation of the proportions of activated and occupied receptors is straightforward, if lengthy (see the answer to Problem 1.5 in Section 1.10). Finding the proportion in the active form is more difficult if the supply of G-protein is limited but can be done using numerical methods.

---

* The possibility that the depression in basal activity may have some other explanation (e.g., an inhibitory action on one or more of the events that follow receptor activation) should not be overlooked.

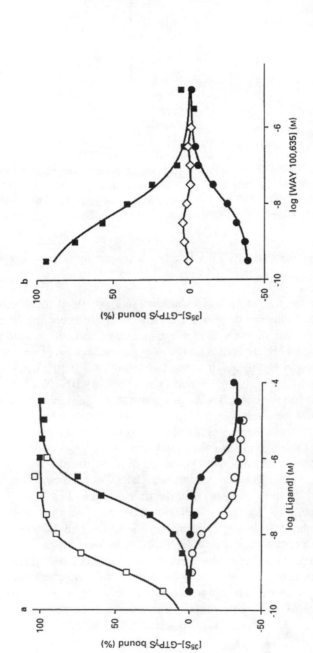

FIGURE 1.13 The effects of a conventional agonist, an inverse agonist, and a neutral antagonist on the activity of a constitutively active G-protein-coupled 5HT$_{1A}$ receptor. The panel on the left shows the log concentration–response curves for the conventional agonist (open squares) and the inverse agonist (open circles). The closed symbols show how the curves change when the antagonist (WAY 100,635 at 10 nM) is included in the incubation fluid. Note the parallel, and similar, shift in the lines. The panel on the right illustrates the effects of a wide range of concentrations of the same antagonist applied on its own (open diamonds) or in the presence of a high concentration of either the conventional agonist (closed squares) or the inverse agonist (closed circles). Note that the antagonist by itself causes little change, showing that it has no preference for the active or inactive forms of the receptor. In keeping with this, high concentrations of the antagonist abolish the response to both types of agonist (the curves converge). (From Newman-Tancredi, A. et al., *Br. J. Pharmacol.*, 120, 737–739, 1997.)

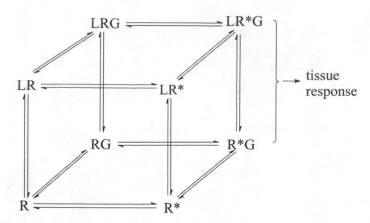

FIGURE 1.14 An elaboration of the model shown in Figure 1.11, which is reproduced as the front face of the cube. Each of its four elements (R, R*, LR, and LR*) can combine with a G-protein to form RG, R*G, LRG, and LR*G, respectively. Of these, only R*G and LR*G lead to a tissue response. The top face of the cube shows ligand-bound states of the receptor. Further details can be found in Section 1.10 (see solution to Problem 1.5).

1.4.8 ATTEMPTING TO ESTIMATE THE EFFICACY OF A PARTIAL AGONIST FROM THE END RESPONSE OF A COMPLEX TISSUE

Though observations of receptor function at the molecular level (e.g., single-channel recording or changes in receptor fluorescence following the binding of a ligand) are becoming increasingly practicable, it still often happens that the only available measure of receptor activation is the response of an intact tissue. This could be the contraction or relaxation of a piece of smooth muscle, secretion by a gland, or a change in heartbeat. How can the action of a partial agonist best be characterized in such a situation? Clearly, the maximum agonist activity (the so-called *intrinsic activity*; see previous discussion) and the concentration of agonist that produces half the maximal response that the agonist can elicit are invaluable descriptive measures. As we have already seen, R. P. Stephenson took matters further by supposing that the response to an agonist is determined by the product of the efficacy of the agonist and the proportion of receptors occupied (see Eq. (1.27)). He also described experimental methods that promised to allow the efficacies of agonists acting on intact tissues to be compared. These procedures were later extended by others and quite widely applied. An example is given in the section on irreversible antagonists.

However, as already discussed, it has now become clear that the occupancy and activation of a receptor by an agonist are not equivalent; hence, Stephenson's use of the Hill–Langmuir equation to relate agonist concentration to receptor occupancy in Eq. (1.27) is an oversimplification. Our final task in this account of partial agonism is to reexamine Stephenson's formulation of efficacy, and the results of experiments based on it, in the light of the new knowledge about how receptors function.

A first step is to recast Stephensons's equations in terms of total receptor occupancy (p_{occ}, occupied but inactive plus occupied and active). Taking this course, and assuming that the del Castillo–Katz mechanism applies in its simplest form (Eq. (1.7)), we can write:

$$S = e_A^* p_{occ(A)} = e_A^* \frac{[A]}{K_{eff} + [A]} \tag{1.40}$$

where K_{eff} is defined as in Eq. (1.36) in Section 1.4.4. Before going further, it has to be made clear that this modification of Stephenson's scheme departs fundamentally from his original concept that efficacy and affinity can be regarded as separable and potentially independent quantities. To emphasize the point, the symbol e^* rather than e is used. We have already seen in the last section

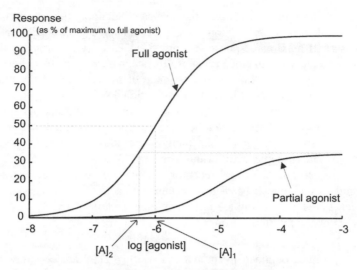

FIGURE 1.15 Estimating the efficacy of a partial agonist by comparing its concentration–response curve with that for a full agonist (see text for further details).

that the macroscopic dissociation equilibrium constant K_{eff} is determined not only by the value of K_A but also by E, which is directly related to efficacy. In the same vein, both the efficacy and the macroscopic affinity of an agonist acting through a G-protein-coupled receptor depend on tissue factors such as the relative and absolute quantities of G-protein and receptors, as well as on the microscopic equilibrium constants.

With these reservations in mind, we will next consider three approaches that have been used in the past to measure the efficacy of a partial agonist acting on an intact tissue. Each will be analyzed in two ways with the details given in Appendix 1.4C (Section 1.4.9.3). The first is of historical interest only and is based on Stephenson's original formulation, as expressed in Eq. (1.27) (Section 1.4.2) and with receptor occupancy given by the Hill–Langmuir equation in its simplest form, which we have already seen to be inadequate for agonists. The second analysis defines receptor occupancy as all the receptors that are occupied, active plus inactive.

The first two of the three methods presuppose that the measurements are made with a tissue that has a large receptor reserve. It is also assumed that a full agonist is available that can evoke a maximal response when occupying only a small fraction of the receptors.

Method 1. Concentration–response curves are constructed for the full agonist (A) and for the partial agonist [P], the efficacy of which is to be determined (Figure 1.15). Two concentrations are read off the curve for the full agonist. The first, $[A]_1$, causes a half-maximal response. The second, $[A]_2$, elicits the same response as the maximum seen with the partial agonist. The efficacy of the partial agonist is given by the ratio of $[A]_2$ to $[A]_1$ (see Appendix 1.4C, part A).

Method 2. Exactly the same measurements and assumptions are made as before (see again Figure 1.15). From the concentration–response curves for the full and partial agonists, the values of [A] and [P] that elicit the same response are read off for several levels of response. A plot of $1/[A]$ against $1/[P]$ is constructed and should yield a straight line from which the efficacy of the partial agonist could be obtained if the underlying assumptions are correct (see Appendix 1.4C, part B).

Method 3. This method is more general than the other two in the sense that it is also applicable to full agonists, at least in principle. Suppose that we had some reliable means of determining the dissociation equilibrium constant for the combination of the agonist with its receptors. One procedure that has been used in the past is Furchgott's irreversible antagonist method, as described in Section 1.6.4. We can then apply the appropriate occupancy relationship to calculate the proportion of receptors occupied at the concentration of agonist that produces a half-maximal response. Because S is then unity, according to the convention introduced by Stephenson, the reciprocal of this occupancy gives the value of e (from Eq. (1.27)). This is the basis of Furchgott's estimate of the efficacy of histamine acting on isolated guinea-pig ileum (see Figure 1.24 in Section 1.6.3.). Clearly, this method stands or falls by the validity of the procedures used to measure the dissociation equilibrium constant and to relate agonist concentration to occupancy. We shall see in Section 1.6.4 that Furchgott's irreversible antagonist method provides an estimate, not, as was first thought, of the microscopic equilibrium constant, K_A, but rather of the macroscopic equilibrium constant, K_{eff}. Hence, receptor occupancies calculated from it using the Hill–Langmuir equation will be of total occupancy, active plus inactive. It follows that efficacies calculated in this way are to be regarded as defined by Eq. (1.40) and not Eq. (1.28), as formulated by Stephenson.

Are the efficacy values obtained in these ways useful? They are certainly no substitute for measurements, if these can be made, of the microscopic equilibrium constants that govern the proportion of receptors in the occupied and active forms. Also, because e^* is influenced by tissue factors (e.g., $[G]_T$ and $[R]_T$, as well as E and K_{ARG} for G-protein-coupled receptors), a particular value can result from several combinations of these variables; E, the isomerization equilibrium constant for the formation of active receptors, is not the only determinant. Hence, the value of e^* (or of e) cannot be used as a reliable measure of E. Comparison of e^* values for different agonists acting on a particular tissue is more informative because tissue-dependent factors such as $[G]_T$ and $[R]_T$ are the same. The ratio of e^* for two agonists should then give an estimate of the inverse ratio of the total receptor occupancies required to elicit a certain response. However, the key question of how these occupied receptors are distributed between the active and inactive states remains unanswered in the absence of other kinds of evidence. Despite the great importance of Stephenson's concept of efficacy, we have to conclude that numerical estimates of efficacy, as originally defined, and based on measuring the responses of intact tissues, are of little more than descriptive value.

1.4.9 Appendices to Section 1.4

1.4.9.1 Appendix 1.4A: Definition of a Partial Agonist

The term *partial agonist* has come to be used in two slightly different senses. The first, as in this account, is to refer to an agonist that in a particular tissue or organism, under specified conditions, cannot elicit as great an effect (even when applied in large amounts) as can a full agonist acting through the same receptors. The second, more restricted, usage adds the condition that the response is submaximal because not enough of the receptors occupied by the partial agonist convert to the active form.

The distinction can be illustrated by considering the action of decamethonium on the nicotinic receptors of skeletal muscle. Like acetylcholine, decamethonium causes the ion channels intrinsic to these receptors to open, so that the electrical conductance of the endplate region of the muscle fibers rises. However, even at very high concentrations, decamethonium cannot match the conductance increase caused by acetylcholine. This is not because decamethonium is much less able to cause the receptors to isomerize to the active form; rather, the smaller maximal response is largely a consequence of the greater tendency of decamethonium to block the nicotinic receptor ion channel. Hence, decamethonium would not be regarded as a partial agonist in the second sense defined above. However, if compared with acetylcholine for its ability to contract a piece of skeletal muscle, then it would be found to produce a smaller maximum response and so would be described as a partial agonist in the first, more general, sense.

1.4.9.2 Appendix 1.4B: Expressions for the Fraction of G-Protein-Coupled Receptors in the Active Form

Application of the law of mass action to each of the three equilibria shown in Eq. (1.38) and the use of the conservation rule (see earlier) lead to the following expression* for p_{AR*G*}:

$$p_{AR*G*} = \frac{E[G]_T[A]}{K_A K_{ARG} + \{E[G]_T + K_{ARG}(1+E)\}[A]} \quad (1.41)$$

Though this looks complicated, it still predicts a simple hyperbolic relationship (as with the Hill–Langmuir equation; see Figure 1.1 and the accompanying text) between agonist concentration and the proportion of receptors in the state (AR*G*) that leads to a response. If a very large concentration of A is applied, so that all the receptors are occupied, the value of p_{AR*G*} asymptotes to:

$$\frac{E[G]_T}{E[G]_T + K_{ARG}(1+E)}$$

Thus, the intrinsic efficacy** of an agonist is influenced by both K_{ARG} and $[G]_T$ as well as, of course, by E.

In deriving Eq. (1.41), it has been assumed that the concentration of G does not fall as a consequence of the formation of AR*G*. This would be so if the total concentration of G, $[G]_T$, greatly exceeds the concentration of receptors ($[R]_T$), so that the concentration of G could be regarded as a constant, approximately equal to $[G]_T$. But, can we really regard [G] as constant? Suppose, instead, that $[R]_T \gg [G]_T$, rather than the reverse. Then, Eq. (1.41) must be replaced by:

$$p_{AR*G*} = \frac{E[G]_T[A]}{K_A K_{ARG} + \{E[R]_T + K_{ARG}(1+E)\}[A]} \quad (1.42)$$

The maximum response would now be:

$$\frac{E[G]_T}{E[R]_T + K_{ARG}(1+E)}$$

so the intrinsic efficacy of the agonist would be influenced by $[R]_T$ as well as by K_{ARG} and $[G]_T$.

Clearly, it would be best to avoid the need to have to make any assumptions about either the constancy of [G] or the relative magnitudes of $[R]_T$ and $[G]_T$. This can be done for the scheme of Eq. (1.38), and the outcome is a somewhat more complex expression for the concentration of AR*G*, which is obtainable from the roots of a quadratic equation:

---

* This expression is derived in Section 1.10; see the solution to Problem 1.3.

** This term has increasingly come to be employed (as here) in a rather different sense from that introduced by R. F. Furchgott (Section 1.4.2). With this newer usage, *intrinsic efficacy* indicates the maximum receptor activation (often expressed as the fraction of receptors in the active state) that can be achieved by an agonist acting through a mechanism that can be formulated and studied at the molecular level, as in the present example. The intention of this redefinition is to focus on the receptor itself and its immediate transduction mechanism (e.g., G-protein activation), rather than on the cellular events that follow.

$$[AR^*G^*]^2 - (Q + [G]_T + [R]_T)[AR^*G^*] + [R]_T[G]_T = 0 \qquad (1.43)$$

where

$$Q = K_{ARG}\left\{1 + \frac{1}{E}\left(1 + \frac{K_A}{[A]}\right)\right\}$$

This predicts a nonhyperbolic relationship between $[AR^*G^*]$ and $[A]$, as well as between binding and $[A]$. In general, the intrinsic efficacy is determined by E and K_{ARG} as well as by $[R]_T$ and $[G]_T$.

1.4.9.3 Appendix 1.4C: Analysis of Methods 1 and 2 in Section 1.4.8

A. Analysis of Method 1 (Section 1.4.8) proposed for the determination of the efficacy of a partial agonist acting on an intact tissue:

Analysis following Stephenson's formulation of efficacy, and using his assumptions and terms.

For a half-maximal response, $S = 1$ (by Stephenson's convention) and $p_{AR} \approx [A]_1/K_A$. This approximation holds because if A occupies few receptors (i.e., $[A] \ll K_A$), then

$$\frac{[A]}{K_A + [A]} \approx \frac{[A]}{K_A}$$

Hence, recalling that $S_A = e_A p_{AR}$, we have:

$$1 = e_A \frac{[A]_1}{K_A} \qquad (1.44)$$

When the partial agonist P occupies all the binding sites in order to produce its maximal response, $p_{PR} = 1$. Hence, the stimulus (S_P) attributable to P is simply e_P. Assuming that the same tissue response, whether elicited by A or by P, corresponds to the same value of S, we can write:

$$S_P = S_A$$
$$\therefore e_P = e_A \frac{[A]_2}{K_A} \qquad (1.45)$$

Dividing Eq. (1.45) by (1.44), we obtain:

$$e_P = \frac{[A]_2}{[A]_1}$$

Analysis based on redefining the stimulus as the product of efficacy (e^*) and the total receptor occupancy by the agonist (i.e., p_{occ}).

For a half-maximal response, $S = 1$ (by Stephenson's convention) and $p_{occ(A)} \approx [A]_1/K_{eff(A)}$. This approximation holds because if A occupies few receptors, then

$$\frac{[A]}{K_{eff(A)} + [A]} \approx \frac{[A]}{K_{eff(A)}}$$

Hence, recalling the redefinition of S_A as $e^*_A p_{occ(A)}$, we have:

$$1 = e^*_A \frac{[A]_1}{K_{eff(A)}} \qquad (1.46)$$

When the partial agonist occupies all the receptors in order to produce its maximal response, $p_{occ(P)} = 1$. Hence, the stimulus (S_P) attributable to P is e^*_P. Assuming that the same tissue response corresponds to the same value of S, we can write:

$$S_P = S_A$$
$$\therefore e^*_P = e^*_A \frac{[A]_2}{K_{eff(A)}} \qquad (1.47)$$

Dividing Eq. (1.47) by (1.46), we obtain:

$$e^*_P = \frac{[A]_2}{[A]_1}$$

B. Analysis of Method 2 (Section 1.4.8) proposed for the determination of the efficacy of a partial agonist acting on an intact tissue:

Analysis following Stephenson's formulation of efficacy.
Just as before, we assume that $S_A = S_P$ for the same magnitude of response. Therefore,

$$e_A \frac{[A]}{K_A + [A]} = e_P \frac{[P]}{K_P + [P]}$$

If A occupies few receptors (so that $[A] \ll K_A$; see Method 1), we can write:

$$e_A \frac{[A]}{K_A} \approx e_P \frac{[P]}{K_P + [P]}$$

$$\Rightarrow \frac{1}{[A]} = \frac{e_A K_P}{e_P K_A} \frac{1}{[P]} + \frac{e_A}{e_P K_A}$$

Hence, a plot of 1/[A] against 1/[P] should provide a straight line of slope $e_A K_P / e_P K_A$ and intercept $e_A / e_P K_A$. The ratio of the slope to the intercept should give an estimate of K_P. If the partial agonist can produce a response equal to or greater than 50% of that to the full agonist, the value of e_P can then be calculated by using K_P to work out the proportion of receptors occupied by the partial agonist when it elicits the half-maximal response; the reciprocal of this occupancy gives e_P (because S is then unity, by definition). If, however, the partial agonist can produce only a small response, then Method 1 can be applied to estimate e_P.

Analysis based on redefining the stimulus as the product of efficacy (e*) and the total receptor occupancy by the agonist, as before.
We again assume that $S_A = S_P$, for the same magnitude of response. Therefore,

$$e_A^* \frac{[A]}{K_{eff(A)} + [A]} = e_P^* \frac{[P]}{K_{eff(P)} + [P]}$$

If A occupies few receptors (so that $[A] \ll K_{eff(A)}$; see Method 1), we can write:

$$e_A^* \frac{[A]}{K_{eff(A)}} \approx e_P^* \frac{[P]}{K_{eff(P)} + [P]}$$

$$\Rightarrow \frac{1}{e_A^*} \frac{K_{eff(A)}}{[A]} = \frac{1}{e_P^*} \frac{K_{eff(P)}}{[P]} + \frac{1}{e_P^*}$$

$$\Rightarrow \frac{1}{[A]} = \frac{e_A^* K_{eff(P)}}{e_P^* K_{eff(A)}} \frac{1}{[P]} + \frac{e_A^*}{e_P^* K_{eff(A)}}$$

Hence, a plot of 1/[A] against 1/[P] should provide a straight line of slope $e^*_A K_{eff(P)} / e^*_P K_{eff(A)}$ and intercept $e^*_A / e^*_P K_{eff(A)}$. The ratio of the slope to the intercept should give an estimate of $K_{eff(P)}$. The value of e^*_P can then be calculated as described on the left for e_P.

1.5 INHIBITORY ACTIONS AT RECEPTORS: I. SURMOUNTABLE ANTAGONISM

1.5.1 OVERVIEW OF DRUG ANTAGONISM

Many of the most useful drugs are antagonists: substances that reduce the action of another agent, which is often an endogenous agonist (e.g., a hormone or neurotransmitter). Though the most common mechanism is simple competition, antagonism can occur in a variety of ways.

1.5.1.1 Mechanisms Not Involving the Agonist Receptor Macromolecule

1. *Chemical antagonism.* The antagonist combines directly with the substance being antagonized; receptors are not involved. For example, the chelating agent EDTA is used to treat lead poisoning (a less toxic chelate is formed and excreted).
2. *Functional or physiological antagonism.* The "antagonist" is actually an agonist that produces a biological effect opposite to the substance being antagonized. Each substance

acts through its own receptors. See also *indirect antagonism* (below). For example, adrenaline relaxes bronchial smooth muscle, thus reducing the bronchoconstriction caused by histamine and the leukotrienes.

3. *Pharmacokinetic antagonism.* Here, the "antagonist" effectively reduces the concentration of the active drug at its site of action. For example, repeated administration of phenobarbitone induces an increase in the activity of hepatic enzymes that inactivate the anticoagulant drug warfarin. Hence, if phenobarbitone and warfarin are given together, the plasma concentration of warfarin is reduced, so it becomes less active.

4. *Indirect antagonism.* The antagonist acts at a second, downstream receptor that links the action of the agonist to the final response observed. For example, β-adrenoceptor blockers such as propranolol reduce the rise in heart rate caused by indirectly acting sympathomimetic amines such as tyramine. This is because tyramine acts by releasing noradrenaline from noradrenergic nerve endings, and the released noradrenaline acts on β-adrenoceptors to increase heart rate:

tyramine → release of noradrenaline → β-receptor activation → response

Another possibility is that the antagonist interferes with other post-receptor events that contribute to the tissue response. For example, calcium channel blockers such as verapamil block the influx of calcium necessary for maintained smooth muscle contraction; hence, they reduce the contractile response to acetylcholine. Some pharmacologists prefer to describe this as a variant of functional antagonism (see above).

1.5.1.2 Mechanisms Involving the Agonist Receptor Macromolecule

1. *The binding of agonist and antagonist is mutually exclusive.* This may be because the agonist and antagonist compete for the same binding site or combine with adjacent sites that overlap. A third possibility is that different sites are involved but they interact in such a way that agonist and antagonist molecules cannot be bound to the receptor macromolecule at the same time. This type of antagonism has two main variants:

    a. The agonist and antagonist form only short-lasting combinations with the receptor, so that equilibrium between agonist, antagonist, and receptors can be reached during the presence of the agonist. The interaction between the antagonist and the binding site is freely reversible. Hence, the blocking action can always be surmounted by increasing the concentration of agonist, which will then occupy a higher proportion of the binding sites. This is described as *reversible competitive antagonism* (see later). For example, atropine competitively blocks the action of acetylcholine on muscarinic receptors.

    b. The antagonist combines irreversibly (or effectively so within the time scale of the agonist application) with the binding site for the agonist. When enough receptors have been irreversibly blocked in this way, the antagonism is *insurmountable* (i.e., no amount of agonist can produce a full response because too few unblocked receptors are left). Note that most pharmacologists now describe this as *irreversible competitive antagonism*, which is the term used in this account; others have regarded it as *noncompetitive*. For example, phenoxybenzamine forms a covalent bond at or near the agonist binding sites on the α-adrenoceptor, resulting in insurmountable antagonism.

2. *Noncompetitive antagonism occurs when the agonist and the antagonist can be bound, at the same time, to different regions of the receptor macromolecule.* It is sometimes also referred to as *allotopic* or *allosteric* antagonism (*allotopic* means "different place" in contrast to *syntopic*, meaning "same place"; for a note on *allosteric*, see Appendix 1.6A [Section 1.6.7.1]). In principle, noncompetitive antagonists can be either reversible or

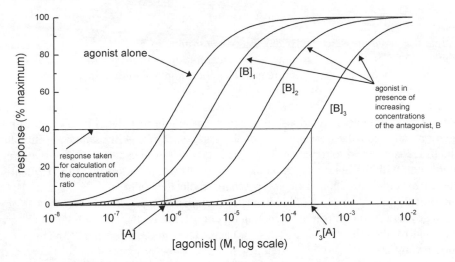

FIGURE 1.16 The predicted effect of three concentrations of a reversible competitive antagonist, B, on the log concentration–response relationship for an agonist. The calculation of the concentration ratio (r_3) for the highest concentration of antagonist, $[B]_3$, is illustrated.

irreversible. An example of the former is that hexamethonium reversibly reduces the action of acetylcholine at the nicotinic receptor of sympathetic ganglion cells by blocking the ion channel that is intrinsic to the nicotinic receptor. Note that the term *noncompetitive* is sometimes extended to include forms of antagonism that do not involve the agonist receptor macromolecule (see, for example, *indirect antagonism* in the preceding section).

1.5.2 REVERSIBLE COMPETITIVE ANTAGONISM

We start by examining how a reversible competitive antagonist (for example, atropine) alters the concentration–response relationship for the action of an agonist (for example, acetylcholine). It is found experimentally that the presence of such an antagonist causes the log concentration–response curve for the agonist to be shifted to the right, often without a change in slope or maximal response. The antagonism is *surmountable*, commonly over a wide range of antagonist concentrations, as illustrated in Figure 1.16.

The extent of the shift is best expressed as a *concentration ratio*,* which is defined as the factor by which the agonist concentration must be increased to restore a given response in the presence of the antagonist. The calculation of the concentration ratio is done as follows. First, a certain magnitude of response is selected. This is often 50% of the maximum attainable, but in principle any value would do;** 40% has been taken in the illustration. In the absence of antagonist, this response is elicited by a concentration of agonist, [A]. When the antagonist is present, the agonist concentration has to be increased by a factor r (i.e., to $r[A]$). Thus, for antagonist concentration $[B]_3$ in Figure 1.16, the concentration ratio is r_3 (= $r_3[A]/[A]$).

The negative logarithm of the concentration of antagonist that causes a concentration ratio of x is commonly denoted by pA_x. This term was introduced by H. O. Schild as an empirical measure of the activity of an antagonist. The value most often quoted is pA_2, where

---

* Or *dose ratio* — both terms are used.

** Clearly it is sensible to avoid the extreme ends of the range. The concentration ratio can also be estimated using a least-squares minimization procedure to fit the Hill equation (see Sections 1.2.2 and 1.2.4.3), or some other suitable function, to each of the concentration–response curves. This also allows the parallelism of the curves to be assessed. A further possibility is to fit all the curves (i.e., with and without antagonist) simultaneously by assuming that the Gaddum equation holds (see next page) and by making use of the Hill equation, or another function, to relate receptor activation to the measured tissue response.

$$pA_2 = -\log[B]_{r=2}$$

To illustrate this notation we consider the ability of atropine to block the muscarinic receptors for acetylcholine. The presence of atropine at a concentration of only 1 nM makes it necessary to double the acetylcholine concentration required to elicit a given submaximal response of a tissue. Hence, $pA_2 = 9$ for this action of atropine ($-\log(10^{-9}) = 9$).

We next look at why a parallel shift in the curves occurs, and at the same time we will derive a simple but most important relationship between the amount of the shift, as expressed by the concentration ratio, and the concentration of the antagonist. We will assume for simplicity that when the tissue is exposed to the agonist and the antagonist at the same time, the two drugs come into equilibrium with the binding sites on the receptor. At a given moment, an individual site may be occupied by either an agonist or an antagonist molecule, or it may be vacant. The relative proportions of the total population of binding sites occupied by agonist and antagonist are governed, just as Langley had surmised (see Introduction (Section 1.1)), by the concentrations of agonist and antagonist and by the affinities of the sites for each. Because the agonist and the antagonist bind reversibly, raising the agonist concentration will increase the proportion of sites occupied by the agonist, at the expense of antagonist occupancy. Hence, the response will become greater.

The law of mass action was first applied to competitive antagonism by Clark, Gaddum, and Schild at a time before the importance of receptor activation by isomerization was established. It was assumed, therefore, that the equilibrium among agonist, antagonist, and their common binding site could be represented quite simply by the reactions:

$$A + R \rightleftharpoons AR$$

$$B + R \rightleftharpoons BR$$

As shown in Section 1.5.5, application of the law of mass action to these simultaneous equilibria leads to the following expression for the proportion of the binding sites occupied by agonist:

$$p_{AR} = \frac{[A]}{K_A\left(1 + \dfrac{[B]}{K_B}\right) + [A]} \tag{1.48}$$

Here, K_A and K_B are the dissociation equilibrium constants for the binding of agonist and antagonist, respectively. This is the *Gaddum equation*, named after J. H. Gaddum, who was the first to derive it in the context of competitive antagonism. Note that if [B] is set to zero, we have the Hill–Langmuir equation (Section 1.2.1).

If, instead, we take as our starting point the del Castillo–Katz mechanism for receptor activation (see Eq. (1.7)), three equilibria should be considered:

$$A + R \underset{}{\overset{K_A}{\rightleftharpoons}} AR \underset{}{\overset{E}{\rightleftharpoons}} AR^*$$

$$B + R \underset{}{\overset{K_B}{\rightleftharpoons}} BR$$

Applying the law of mass action (see Section 1.5.5), we obtain the following expression for the proportion of receptors in the active state:

$$p_{AR^*} = \frac{E[A]}{K_A\left(1 + \dfrac{[B]}{K_B}\right) + (1 + E)[A]} \tag{1.49}$$

Here, K_A and E are as defined in Section 1.2.3, and K_B, as before, is the dissociation equilibrium constant for the combination of the antagonist with the binding site. If [B] is set to zero, we have Eq. (1.32).

Equations (1.48) and (1.49) embody the law that Langley had concluded must relate the amounts of the "compounds" he postulated to the concentrations of the agonist and antagonist (see Section 1.1). However, in order to apply this law to the practical problem of understanding how a competitive antagonist will affect the response to the agonist, we need to make some assumption about the relationship between the response and the proportion of active receptors. Gaddum and Schild recognized that the best way to proceed was to assume that the same response (say, 30% of the maximum attainable) corresponded to the same receptor activation by agonist whether the agonist was acting alone or at a higher concentration in the presence of the competitive antagonist. This assumption makes it unnecessary to know the exact form of the relationship between receptor activation and response. This was a most important advance, however obvious it might seem on looking back.

We can now consider an experiment in which a certain response (e.g., 30% of the maximum) is elicited first by a concentration of agonist, [A], acting alone and then by a greater concentration (r[A]), when A is applied in the presence of the antagonist. Here, r is the concentration ratio, as already defined. Because p_{AR*} is assumed to be the same in the two situations, we can then write, from Eq. (1.49):*

$$\frac{E[A]}{K_A + (1+E)[A]} = \frac{Er[A]}{K_A\left(1 + \dfrac{[B]}{K_B}\right) + (1+E)r[A]}$$

Here, the left-hand side gives the fraction of receptors in the active state when A is applied on its own. This fraction is assumed to be the same when an identical response is elicited by applying the agonist at an increased concentration (r[A]) in the presence of the antagonist at concentration [B] (right-hand side of the equation).

Dividing each term on the right-hand side by r, we have:

$$\frac{E[A]}{K_A + (1+E)[A]} = \frac{E[A]}{K_A\left(\dfrac{1 + \dfrac{[B]}{K_B}}{r}\right) + (1+E)[A]}$$

If the expressions on the left and right are to take the same value, the following equality must hold:

$$\frac{1 + \dfrac{[B]}{K_B}}{r} = 1$$

Hence,

$$r - 1 = \frac{[B]}{K_B} \tag{1.50}$$

This is the *Schild equation*, which was first stated and applied to the study of competitive antagonism by H. O. Schild in 1949. It is probably the most important single quantitative relationship in

---

* We assume here that the del Castillo–Katz model applies. Using the Gaddum equation, based on the simpler scheme explored by Hill and by Clark, leads to exactly the same conclusion, as the reader can easily show by following the same steps but starting with Eq. (1.48).

pharmacology and has been shown to apply to the action of many competitive antagonists over a wide range of concentrations. Though originally derived on the basis of the simple scheme for receptor activation described in Sections 1.2.1 and 1.2.2, it holds equally for the del Castillo–Katz scheme, as we have just shown, as well as for more complex models in which the receptor is constitutively active.

One of the predictions of the Schild equation is that a reversible competitive antagonist should cause a parallel shift in the log agonist concentration–response curve (as illustrated in Figure 1.16; see also Figure 1.18). This is because if the equation holds, the concentration ratio, r, is determined only by the values of [B] and of K_B, regardless of the concentration and even the identity of the agonist (provided that it acts through the same receptors as the antagonist). With a logarithmic scale, a constant value of r corresponds to a constant separation of the concentration–response curves, i.e., parallelism, because $\log(r[A]) - \log[A] = \log r + \log[A] - \log[A] = \log r$, whatever the value of [A].

Probably the most important application of the Schild equation is that it provides a way of estimating the dissociation equilibrium constant for the combination of an antagonist with its binding site. A series of agonist concentration–response curves is established, first without and then with increasing concentrations of antagonist present, and is tested for parallelism. If this condition is met, the value of $(r - 1)$ is plotted against the antagonist concentration, [B]. This should give a straight line of slope equal to the reciprocal of K_B.

More usually, both $(r - 1)$ and [B] are plotted on logarithmic scales (the *Schild plot*). The outcome should be a straight line with a slope of unity, and the intercept on the x-axis provides an estimate of $\log K_B$. The basis for these statements can be seen by expressing the Schild equation in logarithmic form:

$$\log(r - 1) = \log[B] - \log K_B \tag{1.51}$$

A Schild plot (based on the results of a student class experiment on the effect of atropine on the contractile response of guinea-pig ileum to acetylcholine) is shown in Figure 1.17. Note that the line is straight, and its slope is close to unity, as Eq. (1.51) predicts.

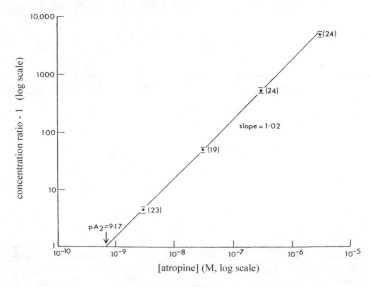

FIGURE 1.17 Schild plot for the action of atropine in antagonizing the action of acetylcholine on guinea-pig ileum. Each point gives the mean ± the standard error of the mean of the number of observations shown.

How might the value of pA_2 be interpreted in these terms? If the Schild equation is obeyed, pA_2 then gives an estimate of $-\log K_B$, because, from Eq. (1.51):

$$\log(2-1) = \log(1) = 0 = \log[B]_{r=2} - \log K_B$$

$$\therefore -\log[B]_{r=2} = pA_2 = -\log K_B$$

The term pK_B is often used to denote $-\log K_B$.*

To summarize to this point, reversible competitive antagonism has the following characteristics:

1. The action of the antagonist can be overcome by a sufficient increase in the concentration of agonist (i.e., the antagonism is surmountable).
2. In the presence of the antagonist, the curve relating the log of the agonist concentration to the size of the response is shifted to the right in a parallel fashion.
3. The relationship between the magnitude of the shift (as expressed by the concentration ratio) and the antagonist concentration obeys the Schild equation.

1.5.3 PRACTICAL APPLICATIONS OF THE STUDY OF REVERSIBLE COMPETITIVE ANTAGONISM

The quantitative study of competitive antagonism by the methods just described has important uses:

1. *The identification and characterization of receptors.* Measuring the value of K_B for the action of a well-characterized competitive antagonist can allow the identification of a particular type of receptor in a tissue or cell preparation. For example, if a tissue is found to respond to acetylcholine, and if the response is antagonized by atropine with a pK_B value of about 9, then the receptor involved is likely to be muscarinic. Preferably, more than one antagonist should be used, which can allow receptor subtypes to be identified. For example, if the response just mentioned is blocked by the muscarinic antagonist pirenzepine with a pK_B of 7.9–8.5, and the corresponding value for the antagonist himbacine is found to be 7–7.2, then the receptor is very probably of the M_1 subtype.
2. *The assessment of new competitive antagonists.* The procedures developed by Gaddum and Schild have been invaluable for the development of new competitive antagonists. Examples include the H_2-receptor antagonists such as cimetidine which reduce gastric acid secretion (see below), and the $5HT_3$-receptor antagonists such as ondansetron, which can control the nausea and vomiting caused by cytotoxic drugs. These competitive antagonists, and others, were discovered by careful examination of the relationship between chemical structure and biological activity, as assessed by the methods of Gaddum and Schild. Having a reliable measure of the change in affinity that results from modifying the chemical structure of a potential drug provides the medicinal chemist with a powerful tool with which to discover compounds with greater activity and selectivity.
3. *The classification of agonists.* At first sight, this may seem a surprising application of a method developed primarily for the study of antagonists. However, recall that only the

---

* The distinction between pK_B and pA_2 is subtle but can be important. pA_2, as Schild defined it, is an *empirical* measure of the action of an antagonist, without reference to theory. It can be measured whether or not the predictions of the Schild equation have been met. Thus, the intercept of a Schild plot on the abscissa gives an estimate of pA_2 even if the slope of the line is not unity. If, however, the line is adequately defined experimentally and is straight (but has a slope that is not unity, though not differing significantly from it), then it is common, and appropriate, to constrain the slope to unity. The intercept on the abscissa then provides an estimate not of pA_2 but of pK_B, as defined above. pK_B and pA_2 coincide only if the slope is exactly unity and no complicating factors are present. If the slope of the Schild plot differs significantly from unity, so that the Schild equation does not hold, K_B cannot be estimated.

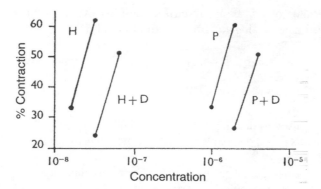

FIGURE 1.18 Responses of guinea-pig ileum to histamine (H) and pyridylethylamine (P) in the absence and presence of diphenhydramine (D, at 3.3 ng/ml). The equal shift in the lines (from H to H+D and from P to P+D) suggests that the two agonists act on the same receptor. (From Arunlakshana, O. and Schild, H. O., *Br. J. Pharmacol.*, 14, 48–58, 1959.)

ratio of agonist concentrations appears in the Schild equation, not the actual values of the concentrations. It follows that for a given competitive antagonist acting at a fixed concentration, the concentration ratio should be the same for all agonists acting through the receptors at which the antagonist acts. So it is possible to test if a new agonist acts at a given receptor by examining whether the concentration ratio is the same for the novel agonist as it is for a well-characterized agonist known to act at that receptor. Figure 1.18, from the work of Arunlakshana and Schild, illustrates the approach. It can be seen that the competitive antagonist diphenhydramine, which acts at H_1-receptors, caused exactly the same shift (i.e., the same concentration ratio) of the log concentration–response curve for pyridylethylamine as for histamine. This strongly suggested that pyridylethylamine was acting through the same receptors as histamine, even though it is almost 100 times less active as an agonist.

The application of these principles is well illustrated by the classical work of J. W. Black and colleagues, which led to the discovery of the first competitive antagonists acting at the H_2-receptors for histamine. Although the overall aim of the study was to develop compounds that would reduce gastric acid secretion in disease, much of the work was done not with secretory tissue but with two isolated tissue preparations: guinea-pig atria and rat uterus. These could be used because they were shown to possess histamine receptors of the same kind (H_2) as in gastric acid secretion. Also, their responses to histamine (increased rate of contraction of the atria and relaxation of the rat uterus) were more easily measured than was gastric secretion. This allowed large numbers of compounds to be tested.

The successful outcome included the synthesis of burimamide, the first H_2-receptor antagonist to be tested in humans. Table 1.1 compares its ability to antagonize the actions of three agonists on guinea-pig atria: histamine, 4-methylhistamine, and 2-methylhistamine. The K_B values are almost the same, despite the varying potencies of the agonists, suggesting that all three agonists were acting through the same receptors (see item 3 in the list above).

Table 1.2 shows that the value of K_B for the blockade by burimamide of the action of histamine on the rat uterus is almost the same as for the guinea-pig atria, as would be expected if the receptors in the two tissues are the same (see item 1 in list above). In contrast, when burimamide was tested for its inhibitory action against the H_1-mediated contractile action of histamine on guinea-pig ileum, it was found to be approximately 40-fold less active (as judged by the apparent K_B value). Moreover, the characteristics of the inhibition no longer conformed to the predictions of competitive antagonism. Thus, the slope of the Schild plot, at 1.32, was significantly greater than unity. Further, when burimamide was tested against carbachol (carbamoyl choline), which also contracts the guinea-pig ileum

TABLE 1.1

Comparison of the Antagonism by Burimamide of the Actions of Histamine and Two Related Agonists on Guinea-Pig Atria

Agonist	EC_{50} on Guinea-Pig Atria (μM)	Dissociation Equilibrium Constant (K_B) for the Blocking Action of Burimamide (μM)
Histamine	1.1	7.8
4-Methylhistamine	3.1	7.2
2-Methylhistamine	19.8	6.9

Source: From Black, J. W. et al., *Nature*, 236, 385–390, 1972.

TABLE 1.2

Comparison of the Ability of Burimamide to Block the Actions of Histamine on Guinea-Pig (G.-P.) Ileum and Atrium and on Rat Uterus

Tissue	Agonist	n_s (Slope of Schild Plot)	Apparent Dissociation Equilibrium Constant (K_B) for the Blocking Action of Burimamide (μM)
G.-P. atrium (H_2)	Histamine	0.98	7.8
Rat uterus (H_2)	Histamine	0.96	6.6
G.-P. ileum (H_1)	Histamine	1.32	288
G.-P. ileum	Carbachol	1.44	174

Source: From Black, J. W. et al., *Nature*, 236, 385–390, 1972.

(although through muscarinic rather than H_1 receptors), the slope was similarly divergent, and the apparent K_B value was of the same order. This suggested that the inhibition by burimamide of the response of the ileum to the two agonists was more likely to have resulted from a nonspecific depression of the tissue rather than from weak competitive antagonism at both H_1 and muscarinic receptors.

1.5.4 COMPLICATIONS IN THE STUDY OF REVERSIBLE COMPETITIVE ANTAGONISM

Though the predictions of competitive antagonism are often fulfilled over a wide range of agonist and antagonist concentrations, divergences sometimes occur and much can be learned from them. Two examples follow.

Example 1

Figure 1.19 shows two Schild plots, one of which (open circles) is far from the expected straight line of unit slope. Both sets of experiments were done with a smooth muscle preparation, the isolated nictitating membrane of the cat's eye. This tissue receives a dense noradrenergic innervation and contracts in response to noradrenaline, which was the agonist used. The adrenoceptors concerned are of the α-subtype and can be blocked by the reversible competitive antagonist phentolamine. To account for the nonlinear Schild plot, the key observation was that, when the experiments were repeated but with a nictitating membrane that had previously been denervated (i.e., the adrenergic nerve supply had been cut and allowed to degenerate), the concentration ratios became larger, and the Schild plot became linear, with a slope near to unity.

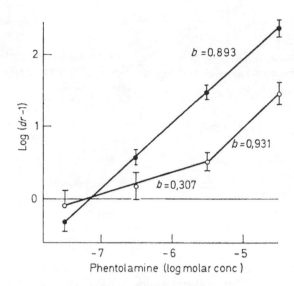

FIGURE 1.19 Schild plots for the antagonism of noradrenaline by phentolamine, studied in the isolated nictitating membrane of the cat. The values plotted are the means (± S.E.) for four to five experiments. Closed circles, denervated nictitating membrane; open circles, normal membrane; b indicates the slope. The slope values for normal membrane were calculated for the three lowest concentrations and the two highest concentrations of phentolamine. (From Furchgott, R. F., *Handbook of Experimental Pharmacology*, Vol. 23, 1972, pp. 283–335; based on the results of Langer, S. Z. and Trendelenburg, U., *J. Pharmacol. Exp. Ther.*, 167, 117–142, 1969.)

This finding suggested an explanation in terms of the presence in the normal but not the denervated muscle of the neuronal uptake mechanism (uptake$_1$) for noradrenaline. This uptake process can be so effective that, when noradrenaline is added to the bathing fluid, the concentration attained in the interior of the preparation (especially if it is relatively thick) may be much less than that applied. As noradrenaline diffuses in, some of it is taken up by the adrenergic nerves, so that a large concentration gradient is maintained. In keeping with this, blockade of uptake$_1$ (for example, by cocaine) can greatly potentiate the action of noradrenaline, as illustrated schematically in Figure 1.20. The left-most full line shows the control concentration–response curve for an adrenergically innervated tissue. The dotted line (extreme left) represents the consequence of blocking the uptake process; much lower concentrations of noradrenaline are now sufficient to elicit a given response.* The full line on the right shows the displacement of the control curve caused by the application of phentolamine, and the dotted line just to its left depicts the effect of blocking uptake when phentolamine is present. Note that this dotted line is closer to the full line than is seen with the pair of curves on the left. This is because the influence of uptake (which is a saturable process) on the local concentration of noradrenaline will be proportionately smaller when a large noradrenaline concentration is applied, as is required to restore the response in the presence of phentolamine. Hence, the concentration ratio will be greater if uptake$_1$ is lacking, as it is in the chronically denervated tissue.

Example 2

Figure 1.21, like Figure 1.19, shows two Schild plots, one of which (open circles) departs greatly from the expected behavior. The deviation occurs when noradrenaline is the agonist and again it can be accounted for in terms of the reduction in local concentration caused by the uptake$_1$ process

---

* The curves in Figure 1.20 are stylized; the leftward displacement due to the blockade of noradrenaline uptake would not be expected to be exactly parallel.

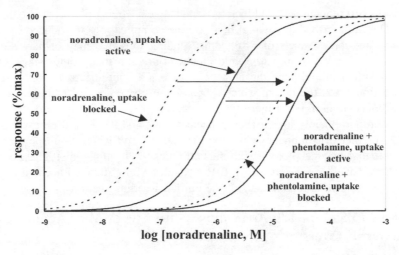

FIGURE 1.20 Hypothetical concentration–response curves to illustrate how the uptake$_1$ process can influence the study of the antagonism of noradrenaline by phentolamine. The two full lines show the response to noradrenaline, first in the absence and then in the presence of phentolamine. If the experiment is repeated, but with the uptake process blocked, the dotted lines would be obtained. Noradrenaline has become more active, and phentolamine now causes a greater shift (compare the lengths of the two horizontal arrows), as explained in the text.

(the tissue used, the atrium of the guinea pig, has a dense adrenergic innervation). Isoprenaline is not subject to uptake$_1$. Accordingly, the Schild plot with this agonist is linear with a slope close to unity. In keeping with this explanation (and with the prediction that the concentration ratio should be the same for different agonists, provided that they act through the same receptors; see Section 1.5.3), blockade of uptake$_1$ by the inclusion of cocaine in the bathing fluid causes the concentration ratio for noradrenaline to increase to the same value as seen with isoprenaline as agonist.

Deviations from the expected behavior will also be seen when the antagonist has additional actions at the concentrations examined. An example is provided by the ability of the reversible

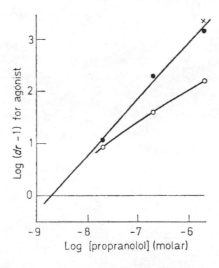

FIGURE 1.21 Schild plots for the antagonism by propranolol of the actions of noradrenaline (open circles) and isoprenaline (closed circles) on the contractile force of the isolated atrium of the guinea pig. The × shows the value obtained with noradrenaline as agonist but in the presence of cocaine (20 μM). (From Furchgott, R. F., *Handbook of Experimental Pharmacology,* Vol. 23, 1972, pp. 283–335; based on the results of Blinks, J. R., *Ann. N.Y. Acad. Sci.,* 139, 673–685, 1967.)

competitive antagonist tubocurarine to block the ion channels which open when nicotinic receptors are activated. This is described in Chapter 6, as are the complications introduced by the presence on such ligand-gated ion channels of two agonist binding sites that may or may not have equal affinities for the antagonist. Nonlinear Schild plots can arise in many other ways. One cause is failure to allow sufficient time for the antagonist to reach equilibrium with the receptors. As discussed in Section 1.3.2, the rate at which a ligand equilibrates with its binding sites becomes slower at lower concentrations (see Figure 1.3). Hence, if the exposure is too short, the concentration ratio will be disproportionately low at such concentrations, and the Schild plot will be steeper in this region than predicted. Nonlinear Schild plots can also result when the response of a tissue is mediated by more than one receptor with different affinities for the antagonist. These complications, and several others, have been described by T. P. Kenakin, whose detailed account of the analysis of competitive antagonism is recommended (see Further Reading section).

1.5.5 Appendix to Section 1.5: Application of the Law of Mass Action to Reversible Competitive Antagonism

Classical analysis of competitive antagonism, following Gaddum and Schild

We begin by assuming that both the agonist (A) and the antagonist (B) combine with their binding site according to the law of mass action and in a way that can be represented by the two reactions:

$$A + R \rightleftharpoons AR$$

$$B + R \rightleftharpoons BR$$

Our task is to work out how the proportion of receptors occupied by the agonist varies with the concentrations of the agonist and the antagonist. Equilibrium is assumed. Applying the law of mass action gives:

$$[A][R] = K_A[AR]$$

$$[B][R] = K_B[BR]$$

As in Section 1.2.1, these equations can be rewritten in terms of the proportions of binding sites that are free (p_R) or occupied by either A (p_{AR}) or B (p_{BR}):

$$[A]p_R = K_A p_{AR} \qquad (1.52)$$

$$[B]p_R = K_B p_{BR} \qquad (1.53)$$

An individual receptor is either vacant or occupied by an agonist or an antagonist molecule. Hence,

$$p_R + p_{AR} + p_{BR} = 1 \qquad (1.54)$$

Competitive antagonism on the del Castillo–Katz scheme for receptor activation (see Section 1.2.3, Eq. (1.7)).

Receptor isomerization to the active form occurs when the binding site is occupied by A but not by the antagonist B:

$$A + R \overset{K_A}{\rightleftharpoons} AR \overset{E}{\rightleftharpoons} AR*$$

$$B + R \overset{K_B}{\rightleftharpoons} BR$$

Applying the law of mass action to each of the three equilibria, we have:

$$[A][R] = K_A[AR]$$

$$[AR*] = E[AR]$$

$$[B][R] = K_B[BR]$$

where K_B is the dissociation equilibrium constant for the combination of B with the binding site, and K_A and E are as previously defined. These equations can be rewritten in terms of the fractions of receptors in different conditions:

$$[A]p_R = K_A p_{AR}$$

$$p_{AR*} = E p_{AR}$$

$$[B]p_R = K_B p_{BR}$$

Adding up the fractions of receptors, we have:

$$p_R + p_{AR} + p_{AR*} + p_{BR} = 1$$

We need to know p_{AR}, so we use Eqs. (1.52) and (1.53) to substitute for p_R and p_{BR} in Eq. (1.54):

$$\frac{K_A}{[A]} \cdot p_{AR} + p_{AR} + \frac{[B]}{K_B} \cdot \frac{K_A}{[A]} \cdot p_{AR} = 1$$

$$\Rightarrow p_{AR} = \frac{[A]}{K_A \left(1 + \frac{[B]}{K_B}\right) + [A]}$$

Substituting to obtain p_{AR*} gives:

$$\frac{K_A}{E[A]} p_{AR*} + \frac{p_{AR*}}{E} + p_{AR*} + \frac{[B]}{K_B} \frac{K_A}{E[A]} p_{AR*} = 1$$

Hence,

$$p_{AR*} = \frac{E[A]}{K_A \left(1 + \frac{[B]}{K_B}\right) + (1 + E)[A]}$$

1.6 INHIBITORY ACTIONS AT RECEPTORS: II. INSURMOUNTABLE ANTAGONISM

1.6.1 IRREVERSIBLE COMPETITIVE ANTAGONISM

In this form of drug antagonism, the antagonist forms a long-lasting or even irreversible combination with either the agonist binding site or a region related to it in such a way that agonist and antagonist molecules cannot be bound at the same time. Irreversible in this context means that the dissociation of the antagonist from its binding site is very slow *in relation to the duration of the agonist application*. This is an important qualification because the rate of dissociation can vary greatly from antagonist to antagonist. For some, hours or even days may be necessary so that there is no appreciable fall in occupancy during the 60 sec or so for which the agonist might be applied. Others may dissociate more quickly and the surmountability of the block will then depend on how long the agonist is present and also on how well the response to the agonist is maintained in the particular tissue.

Under physiological conditions, a naturally occurring agonist (e.g., a neurotransmitter) may be present for a very brief time indeed — only a millisecond or less for acetylcholine released from the motor nerve endings on skeletal muscle. This is unlikely to be long enough to allow an appreciable fall in receptor occupancy by a competitive antagonist such as tubocurarine, which would therefore be effectively irreversible *on this time scale*. If, however, the interaction between acetylcholine and tubocurarine is studied in the classical pharmacological manner, in which both agents are applied for enough time for equilibrium to be reached, the blocking action then shows all the characteristics of reversible competitive antagonism (albeit with the additional feature that tubocurarine also blocks open ion channels).

An example of an irreversible antagonist with a very long action (usually many hours) is phenoxybenzamine, which blocks α-adrenoceptors and, less potently, H_1-histamine and muscarinic receptors. Its structure is shown below. Also illustrated is benzilylcholine mustard, a highly active and selective irreversible blocker of muscarinic receptors.

phenoxybenzamine   benzilylcholine mustard

Both compounds are β-haloalkylamines; that is, they contain the grouping:

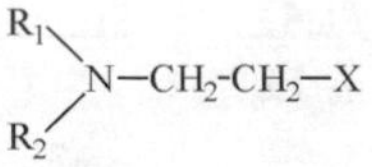

$$R_1 \diagdown$$
$$N-CH_2-CH_2-X$$
$$R_2 \diagup$$

where X is a halogen atom. Once in aqueous solution, such agents cyclize to form an unstable ethyleneiminium ion (Figure 1.22).* This ion is likely to have a greater affinity than the parent molecule for the binding site on the receptor, because an ionic bond can now be formed. When the ethyleneiminium ion docks with the binding site, two outcomes are possible. One is that after a short interval, the ion dissociates from the site. The other is that the ethyleneiminium ring opens to create a reactive intermediate, with the consequence that a covalent bond between the drug molecule and the binding site can be formed. In effect, the receptor becomes alkylated, as illustrated in Figure 1.22.**

Groups that can be alkylated in this way include $-SH$, $-OH$, $=NH$, and $-COOH$; however, not all irreversible antagonists act by forming a covalent bond. Some may "fit" the binding site so well that the combined strength of the other kinds of intermolecular interaction (ionic, hydrophobic, van der Waals, hydrogen bonds) that come into play approaches that of a covalent link.

1.6.2 SOME APPLICATIONS OF IRREVERSIBLE ANTAGONISTS

1.6.2.1 Labeling Receptors

Alkylation of the kind illustrated in Figure 1.22, but using a radiolabeled ligand, provides a means of labeling the binding site(s) of receptor macromolecules.*** The tissue is exposed to the labeled antagonist for long enough to allow combination with most of the receptors. It is then washed with ligand-free solution so that unbound or loosely bound antagonist can diffuse away, leaving (ideally) only the receptors covalently labeled. A related approach is to use a photo-affinity label. This is a compound that has not only affinity for the receptor but also the property of breaking down to form a reactive intermediate following absorption of light energy of the appropriate wavelength. Light sensitivity of this kind can often be achieved by attaching an azido group $(-N_3)$ to a drug molecule. The resulting photo-affinity label is allowed to equilibrate with a tissue or membrane preparation, which is then exposed to intense light. The outcome (for an azide) is the formation of a highly reactive nitrene that combines with immediately adjacent structures (including, it is hoped, the

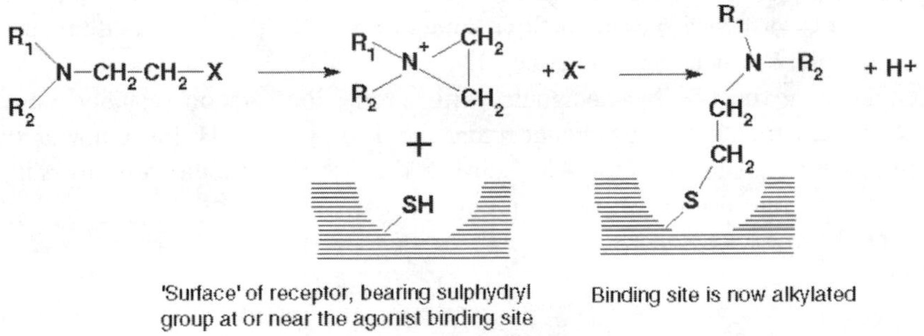

'Surface' of receptor, bearing sulphydryl   Binding site is now alkylated
group at or near the agonist binding site

FIGURE 1.22 Alkylation of a receptor by a β-haloalkylamine.

---

* The terms *ethyleneimmonium* or *aziridinium ion* are also used.
** This process might occur via the formation of a reactive carbonium ion: $R_1R_2NCH_2CH_2^+$.
*** As well as β-haloalkylamines, substances with haloalkyl groups attached to carbons bonded to oxygen can be used. An interesting example is bromoacetylcholine, which acts as a "tethered agonist" acting on nicotinic receptors.

binding regions of the receptor), to form covalent bonds, thus "tagging" the binding site(s).* This can provide a first step toward receptor isolation.

1.6.2.2 Counting Receptors

If the antagonist can be radiolabeled, the same general procedure may be used to estimate the number of receptors in an intact tissue, provided that the specific activity (i.e., the radioactivity expressed in terms of the quantity of material) of the ligand is known. An early example was the application of ^{125}I- or ^{131}I-labeled α-bungarotoxin to determine the number of nicotinic receptors at the endplate region of skeletal muscle. This revealed that the muscular weakness that characterizes myasthenia gravis, a disease affecting the transmission of impulses from motor nerves to skeletal muscle, results from a reduction in the number of nicotinic receptors. A variant of the technique, using α-bungarotoxin labeled with a fluorescent group, allows these receptors to be visualized by light microscopy.

1.6.2.3 Receptor Protection Experiments

The rate at which an irreversible antagonist inactivates receptors will be reduced by the simultaneous presence of a reversible agonist or competitive antagonist that acts at the same binding site. The reversible agent, by occupying sites, lowers the number irreversibly blocked within a given period; the receptors are said to be "protected." This can be a useful tool for the characterization of drugs as well as of receptors. For example, R. F. Furchgott (who introduced the method) tested the ability of three agonists (noradrenaline, adrenaline, and isoprenaline) to protect against the alkylating agent dibenamine (a phenoxybenzamine-like compound) applied to rabbit aortic strips. Each agonist protected the response to the other two. Thus, after the tissue had been exposed to dibenamine in the presence of a large concentration of noradrenaline, followed by a drug-free washing period, adrenaline and isoprenaline as well as noradrenaline were still able to cause contraction. The same exposure to dibenamine on its own abolished the response to the subsequent application of each of the same agonists. This provided evidence that all three agonists caused contraction by acting at a common receptor (now well established to be the α-adrenoceptor subtype), which was uncertain at the time.

Another example of receptor protection, but using a competitive antagonist rather than an agonist, is provided by the ability of tubocurarine to slow the onset of the blocking action of α-bungarotoxin at the neuromuscular junction. Note that the degree of receptor protection will depend not only on the relative concentrations and affinities of the reversible and irreversible antagonists, but also on the period allowed for their interaction with the receptors, as described in Chapter 5. Given enough time, a completely irreversible antagonist will eventually occupy all the binding sites, even in the presence of a high concentration of a reversible ligand.

1.6.3 Effect of an Irreversible Competitive Antagonist on the Response to an Agonist

An adequate exposure of a tissue to an irreversible antagonist results in insurmountable antagonism — the response cannot be fully restored by increasing the concentration of agonist, applied for the usual period. This is because an individual binding site, once firmly occupied by antagonist, is "out of play," in contrast to the dynamic equilibrium between agonist and antagonist that is characteristic of reversible competitive antagonism. Hence, it is usual in work with irreversible antagonists that form covalent bonds to apply the compound for just long enough for it to occupy the required fraction of the binding sites, and then to wash the tissue with drug-free solution so that unbound

---

* Some drugs are intrinsically photolabile; examples include tubocurarine and chlorpromazine, each of which has been used to label the binding regions of receptors.

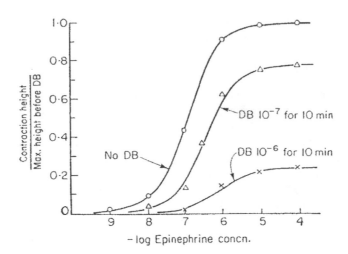

- log Epinephrine concn.

FIGURE 1.23 Effect of a 10-min exposure to two concentrations of a phenoxybenzamine-like compound, dibenamine (DB), on the contractile response of a strip of rabbit aorta to adrenaline (epinephrine). (From Furchgott, R. F., *Adv. Drug Res.*, 3, 21–55, 1966.)

antagonist can diffuse away. The change in the response to the agonist can now be studied. The results of experiments of this kind are illustrated in Figures 1.23 and 1.24.

The family of concentration–response curves in Figure 1.23 shows the effect of an alkylating agent on the contractile response of rabbit aorta to adrenaline. Note the reduction in the maximal response, the departure from parallelism, and the fact that the exposure times as well as the concentrations of the antagonist have been given for each curve.

Figure 1.24 illustrates the influence of the same irreversible antagonist on the contractile response of the guinea-pig ileum to histamine. The full line is the control concentration–response curve, and the dotted lines show the consequences of five successive exposures to 1 μM dibenamine, with testing of histamine after each exposure. A striking feature is that the first application of the antagonist caused an almost parallel shift of the curve. Only after further applications of dibenamine did the maximal response become smaller in the expected way (compare Figure 1.23). The most likely explanation is as follows. Although the first application of dibenamine blocked many receptors, enough remained to allow histamine (albeit at a higher concentration) to produce a full response. Only when the number of receptors had been reduced even further by the subsequent applications of dibenamine was there an appreciable fall in the maximal response attainable. The implication is that in this tissue, not all the receptors have to be occupied by histamine in order to elicit a maximal response. In effect, spare receptors are available, and the tissue is said to have a receptor reserve for this agonist. This does not, of course, mean that we have two kinds of receptors, spare and used; the receptors do not differ. However, only a few must be activated to cause a large or even maximal response. This can occur when the response of the tissue is limited not by the number of active receptors but by one or more of the events that follow receptor activation. For example, the maximal shortening of a piece of smooth muscle may occur in response to a rise in cytosolic calcium that is much less than can be elicited by activating all the receptors.

The situation is different with a partial agonist (see Section 1.4.1). Inactivation of any of the receptors by, for example, dibenamine or phenoxybenzamine will now reduce the maximal response to the partial agonist, without the initial parallel shift in the log concentration–response curve that would be seen (e.g., Figure 1.24) with a full agonist if the tissue has a substantial receptor reserve.

The existence of a receptor reserve in many tissues has the implication that the value of the EC_{50} for a full agonist cannot give even an approximate estimate of the dissociation equilibrium constant for the combination of the agonist with its binding sites; as already mentioned, when the response is half maximal, only a small fraction of the receptors may be occupied rather than the

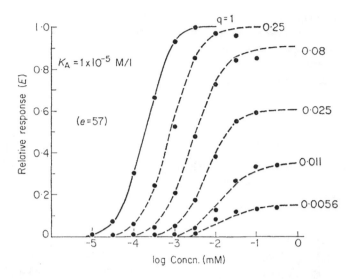

FIGURE 1.24 The effect of progressive receptor blockade by dibenamine on the response of guinea-pig ileum to histamine. Five successive exposures to 1 µM dibenamine, each for 10 min, were used, and the response to histamine was tested after each exposure. The results were analyzed as described in Section 1.6.4, and the value of q listed for each curve gives an estimate of the fraction of receptors remaining unblocked. The dashed curves were constructed from the original, pre-dibenamine curve by inserting these estimates of q, and also the value of K_A shown, into the equations set out in Section 1.6.4 (which see, together with the related discussion). (From Furchgott, R. F., *Adv. Drug Res.*, 3, 21–55, 1966; based on data obtained by Ariëns, E. J. et al., *Arch. Int. Pharmacodynamie*, 127, 459–478, 1960.)

50% envisaged in Clark's tentative assumption of direct proportionality between occupancy and response. So, pharmacologists have had to look for other approaches to determine the affinities of receptors for full agonists. One possibility was suggested by the availability of irreversible competitive antagonists, and this is the next topic to be considered.

1.6.4 CAN AN IRREVERSIBLE COMPETITIVE ANTAGONIST BE USED TO FIND THE DISSOCIATION EQUILIBRIUM CONSTANT FOR AN AGONIST?

The characteristic changes (see Figure 1.24) in the shape and position of an agonist concentration–response relationship caused by a limited exposure of a tissue to an irreversible antagonist suggested a possible way of estimating the dissociation equilibrium constant for an agonist. It was first described by R.F. Furchgott. The experimental procedure is to compare the concentrations of agonist required to produce a selected response (say, 40% of the maximum) before and after the tissue has been exposed to the irreversible antagonist. In the fresh tissue, this response is elicited by a concentration that we represent by [A]; after the antagonist has acted, this has to be increased to [A]′. The fraction of receptors left free after the application of antagonist is denoted by q. (If only 10% of the receptors remained unblocked, q would be 0.1.) We now ask what relationship would be expected to hold between [A], [A]′, and q. This question will be approached in two ways. First we follow Furchgott in taking as our starting point the simplest possible model for agonist action, that of Hill and Clark (see Sections 1.2.1 and 1.2.2). Although we have already seen that this scheme is deficient in its failure to distinguish between the occupation and activation of receptors, it is included for historical interest. The second approach is based on a more realistic, if still basic, representation of receptor activation. This is the del Castillo–Katz model (see Sections 1.2.3 and 1.4.4–1.4.6). The application of Furchgott's method to G-protein-coupled receptors is considered briefly in Section 1.10 (see the answer to Problem 1.3).

Classical approach, following Furchgott, and based on the early view that all the receptors occupied by an agonist are activated: First, we recall one of our two earlier definitions of p_{AR}, the proportion of binding sites occupied by A:

$$p_{AR} = \frac{N_{AR}}{N}$$

Here, N_{AR} is the number of receptors in which A occupies its binding site, and N refers to the total number. Hence,

$$N_{AR} = N \frac{[A]}{K_A + [A]}$$

from the Hill–Langmuir equation. After the irreversible antagonist has acted, N is reduced to qN, and a greater concentration of agonist, $[A]'$, must now be applied in order to achieve the same value of N_{AR} as before:

$$N_{AR} = qN \frac{[A]'}{K_A + [A]'}$$

Furchgott then went on to assume that the same (submaximal) response of the tissue before and after the application of antagonist corresponds to the same receptor occupancy by the agonist. Hence, he equated:

$$N \frac{[A]}{K_A + [A]} = qN \frac{[A]'}{K_A + [A]'}$$

Canceling N and inverting give:

$$\frac{K_A}{[A]} + 1 = \frac{1}{q} \frac{K_A}{[A]'} + \frac{1}{q}$$

$$\frac{1}{[A]} = \frac{1}{q} \frac{1}{[A]'} + \frac{1}{K_A} \left(\frac{1}{q} - 1 \right)$$

Hence, a plot of $1/[A]$ against $1/[A]'$ should give a straight line with a slope of $1/q$ and an intercept of $(1 - q)/q.K_A$. The value of q is obtained from the reciprocal of the slope, and that of K_A from (slope − 1)/intercept.

Analysis based on the del Castillo–Katz model of receptor activation (see Sections 1.2.3 and 1.4.4): The fraction of receptors in the active state is defined by:

$$p_{AR*} = \frac{N_{AR*}}{N}$$

Here, N_{AR*} is the number of receptors in the active (AR*) form of a total N. Hence,

$$N_{AR*} = N \frac{E[A]}{K_A + (1 + E)[A]}$$

from Eq. (1.32). After the irreversible antagonist has acted, N is reduced to qN, and a greater concentration of agonist, $[A]'$, is necessary to achieve the same value of N_{AR*} as before:

$$N_{AR*} = qN \frac{E[A]'}{K_A + (1 + E)[A]'}$$

We next assume that the same (submaximal) response of the tissue before and after the antagonist corresponds to the same number, N_{AR*}, of activated receptors. So we equate:

$$N \frac{E[A]}{K_A + (1 + E)[A]} = qN \frac{E[A]'}{K_A + (1 + E)[A]'}$$

Canceling N and inverting give:

$$\frac{K_A}{E[A]} + \frac{1 + E}{E} = \frac{K_A}{qE[A]'} + \frac{1 + E}{Eq}$$

$$\frac{1}{[A]} = \frac{1}{q} \frac{1}{[A]'} + \left(\frac{1 + E}{K_A} \right) \left(\frac{1}{q} - 1 \right)$$

Hence, a plot of $1/[A]$ against $1/[A]'$ should give a straight line with a slope of $1/q$ and an intercept of:

$$\left(\frac{1 + E}{K_A} \right) \left(\frac{1}{q} - 1 \right)$$

The value of q is obtained from the reciprocal of the slope, and that of $K_A/(1 + E)$ from (slope − 1)/intercept.

Applying the analysis in the left-hand column to the results of Figure 1.24, Furchgott estimated K_A to be 10 μM for the combination of histamine with its receptors. He used this figure, and the values of q obtained as just described, to construct the dashed curves in the illustration. These lie close to the experimental points, which is certainly in keeping with the predictions of the approach taken. Just as certainly, this does not provide decisive proof that either the experimental or the theoretical suppositions that underlie it are correct. An important assumption, and one that is difficult to test, is that the irreversible antagonist has had no action other than to inactivate the receptors under study. Were it, for example, to have interfered with one or more of the steps that link receptor activation to the observed response, the approach would be invalid. Furchgott later showed that this was not a complication under the conditions he used.

Continuing with Furchgott's analysis of the experiment of Figure 1.24, we note that, in the fresh tissue, the concentration of histamine necessary to produce a half maximal contraction was about 180 nM. The value of K_A was estimated to be 10 μM, as we have seen. Furchgott substituted these figures in the Hill–Langmuir equation to obtain a value for the receptor occupancy needed to elicit half the maximal response. This came to only 0.0177, indicating a large receptor reserve. Furchgott's final step was to use this value to obtain an estimate of the efficacy of histamine, in the sense used by Stephenson. Because the response is half-maximal, the "stimulus" as defined by Stephenson is unity, so that, from Eq. (1.27), the efficacy is 1/0.0177 = 57, the value given in Figure 1.24 (see also Method 3 in Section 1.4.8).

The validity of these estimates and of their interpretation, however, depends crucially on the appropriateness of the model for receptor activation on which the analysis is based. It is important to appreciate that the satisfactory fit of the "theoretical" (dotted) lines in Figure 1.24 does not allow one to distinguish between the two models of receptor action (Hill and Clark vs. del Castillo–Katz) that have been used to analyze these results. Both models make exactly the same predictions about the form of the relationship between [A], [A]′, and q. Also, the interpretation of the value of q is the same for each model. What differs, and this is the key issue, is that acceptance of the concept that the receptor must isomerize to an active form carries the implication that Furchgott's irreversible antagonist method yields an estimate of the macroscopic dissociation equilibrium constant ($K_{eff} = K_A/(1 + E)$; see Section 1.4.4) rather than of the microscopic equilibrium constant, K_A, for the initial binding step. Only if E is very small in relation to unity (i.e., A is a very weak partial agonist) does K_{eff} approximate to K_A. Note, too, that a direct radioligand binding measurement (in the absence of desensitization and any other complications) would also yield an estimate of K_{eff} and not K_A. Finding K_A requires other kinds of measurements and so far has been achieved only for ligand-gated ion channels where the single-channel recording method allows the binding and activation steps to be distinguished, as explained in Chapter 6.

The realization that Furchgott's irreversible antagonist method estimates K_{eff}* rather than K_A has profound implications for the calculation of efficacy as defined by Stephenson. As we have just seen, the experiment of Figure 1.24, as analyzed by Furchgott, had suggested that when histamine caused a half-maximal contraction of guinea-pig ileum, only 1.77% of the receptors were occupied. In light of the foregoing discussion, it is likely that this figure refers to the total receptor occupancy by agonist — that is, "occupied but inactive" plus "occupied and active." Hence, the value of 57 (the reciprocal of 0.0177) for the efficacy of histamine shown in Figure 1.24 has to be regarded as based on Eq. (1.40) rather than Eq. (1.27), as Furchgott had originally envisaged. The limited usefulness of this modified definition of efficacy, e*, has already been discussed in Section 1.4.8.

1.6.5 REVERSIBLE NONCOMPETITIVE ANTAGONISM

In this variant of insurmountable antagonism, the antagonist acts by combining with a separate inhibitory site on the receptor macromolecule. Agonist and antagonist molecules can be bound at

---

* See Eq. (1.36) and also the worked answer in Section 1.10 to Problem 1.3 (Section 1.8).

the same time, though the receptor becomes active only when the agonist site alone is occupied (Figure 1.25). This is sometimes referred to as *allosteric* or *allotopic* antagonism (see Appendix 1.6A [Section 1.6.7.1] for further comments on these terms).

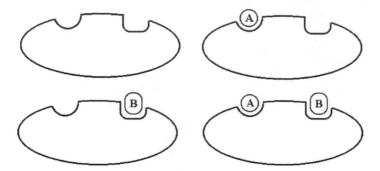

FIGURE 1.25 Noncompetitive antagonism. A stylized receptor carries two sites, one of which can combine with agonist (A) and the other with antagonist (B). Four conditions are possible, only one of which (agonist site occupied, antagonist site empty; see upper right) is active.

In the presence of a large enough concentration of such an antagonist, the inhibition will become insurmountable; too few receptors remain free of antagonist to give a full response, even if all the agonist sites are occupied. The point at which this occurs in a particular tissue will depend on the numbers of spare receptors, just as with an irreversible competitive antagonist (see Section 1.6.3.). If a full agonist is used and the tissue has a large receptor reserve, the initial effect of a reversible noncompetitive antagonist will be to shift the log concentration–response curve to the right. Eventually, when no spare receptors remain, the maximum will be reduced. In contrast, without a receptor reserve, the antagonist will depress the maximum from the outset.

If we apply the law of mass action to this form of antagonism, the proportion of inhibitory sites occupied by the antagonist will be given by the Hill–Langmuir equation:

$$p_{BR} = \frac{[B]}{K_B + [B]}$$

Hence, the proportion free of antagonist will be:

$$1 - p_{BR} = \frac{K_B}{K_B + [B]}$$

We now make the following additional assumptions: (1) Each receptor macromolecule carries one agonist and one antagonist (inhibitory) site. (2) Occupation of the inhibitory site by the antagonist does not alter either the affinity of the other site for the agonist or the equilibrium between the active and the inactive states of the receptor according to the del Castillo–Katz scheme; however, if the antagonist is bound, no response ensues even if the receptor has isomerized to the active form. (3) The affinity for the antagonist is not affected by the binding of the agonist.

Based on these rather extensive and not entirely realistic assumptions,* the fraction of the receptors in the AR* state is given by Eq. (1.32); however, only some of these agonist-combined, isomerized, receptor macromolecules are free of antagonist and thus able to initiate a response. To

---

* A more plausible model follows (see Section 1.6.6).

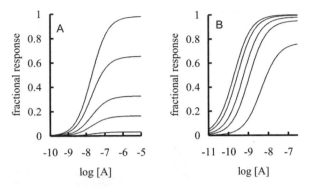

FIGURE 1.26 The effect of a reversible noncompetitive antagonist on the response to an agonist, A. Each set of curves has been constructed using Eq. (1.55) and shows the effect of four concentrations of the antagonist (5, 20, 50, and 300 μM). K_A, K_B, and E have been taken to be 1, 10, and 50 μM, respectively. For (A), the response has been assumed to be directly proportional to the fraction of receptors in the active state. (B) has been constructed using the same values, but now assuming the presence of a large receptor reserve. This condition has been modeled by supposing that the relationship between the response, y, and the proportion of active receptors is given by $y = 1.01 \times p_{active}/(0.01 + p_{active})$, so that a half-maximal response occurs when just under 1% of the receptors are activated.

obtain the proportion (p_{active}) in this condition, we simply multiply the fraction in the AR* state by the fraction free of antagonist:

$$p_{active} = \left(\frac{E[A]}{K_A + (1+E)[A]} \right) \left(\frac{K_B}{K_B + [B]} \right)$$
(1.55)

Figure 1.26 shows log concentration–response curves drawn according to this expression. In A, the response has been assumed to be directly proportional to p_{active}; there are no spare receptors. In B, spare receptors have been assumed to be present, and accordingly the presence of a relatively low concentration of the antagonist causes an almost parallel shift before the maximum is reduced.

The initial near-parallel displacement of the curves in Figure 1.26B raises the question of whether the Schild equation would be obeyed under these conditions. If we consider the two concentrations of agonist that give equal responses before and during the action of the antagonist ([A] and r[A], respectively, where r is the concentration ratio) and repeat the derivation set out in Section 1.5.2 (but using Eq. (1.55) rather than (1.49)), we find that the expression equivalent to the Schild equation is:

$$r - 1 = \frac{[B]}{K_B} \left(1 + \frac{r[A]}{K_{eff}} \right)$$

Here, K_{eff} is as defined in Section 1.4.4. If $r[A]/K_{eff} \ll 1$ (i.e., if the proportion of receptors occupied by the agonist remains small even when the agonist concentration has been increased to overcome the effect of the reversible noncompetitive antagonist), this expression approximates to:

$$r - 1 = \frac{[B]}{K_B}$$

Hence, the Schild equation would apply, albeit over a limited range of concentrations that is determined by the receptor reserve. Moreover, the value of K_B obtained under such conditions will

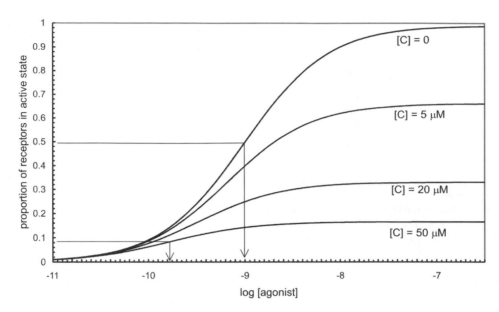

FIGURE 1.27 Curves drawn using Eq. (1.57) to illustrate the effect of three concentrations of an open channel blocker, C, on the response to an agonist acting on a ligand-gated ion channel. Values of 100 nM and 100 and 10 μM were taken for K_A, E, and K_C, respectively. The vertical arrows show the concentrations of agonist causing a half-maximal response in the absence and presence of C at 50 μM.

provide an estimate of the dissociation equilibrium constant for the combination of the antagonist with its binding sites.

A corollary is that a demonstration of the Schild equation holding over a small range of concentrations should not be taken as proof that the action of an antagonist is competitive. Clearly, as wide as practicable a range of antagonist concentrations should be tested, especially if there is evidence for the presence of spare receptors.

Open Channel Block

Studies of the action of ligand-gated ion channels have brought to light an interesting and important variant of reversible noncompetitive antagonism. It has been found that some antagonists block only those channels that are open by entering and occluding the channel itself. In effect, the antagonist combines only with activated receptors. Examples include the block of neuronal nicotinic receptors by hexamethonium, and of N-methyl-D-aspartate (NMDA) receptors by dizocilpine (MK801).

Such antagonists cause a characteristic change in the log concentration–response curve for an agonist. In contrast to what is observed with the other kinds of antagonism so far considered, the value of $[A]_{50}$ will become smaller rather than larger in the presence of the antagonist. This is illustrated in Figure 1.27 and is best understood in terms of the del Castillo–Katz mechanism. Incorporating the possibility that an antagonist, C, is present which combines specifically with active receptors, we have:

$$\underset{\text{(inactive)}}{A + R} \rightleftharpoons \underset{\text{(inactive)}}{AR} \rightleftharpoons \underset{\text{(active)}}{AR^*} + C \rightleftharpoons \underset{\text{(inactive)}}{AR^*C} \tag{1.56}$$

Hence, the receptor has four conditions: R, AR, AR*, and AR*C, of which only one, AR*, is active. This scheme predicts that at equilibrium the proportion of active receptors is given by:

$$p_{AR*} = \frac{E[A]}{K_A + \left\{1 + E\left(1 + \dfrac{[C]}{K_C}\right)\right\}[A]}$$ (1.57)

where K_c is the dissociation equilibrium constant for the combination of C with the activated receptor, AR*. This equation has been used to draw the curves shown in Figure 1.27. Note how $[A]_{50}$ decreases as the antagonist concentration is increased. In effect, the combination of the antagonist with AR* causes a rightward shift in the positions of the other equilibria expressed in Eq. (1.56).

Note, too, the convergence at low agonist concentrations of the curves plotted in Figure 1.27. The antagonist becomes less active when the response is small, because there are fewer receptors in the AR* form available to combine with C. Again, in contrast to the other kinds of antagonism that have been described, there is no initial parallel displacement of the curves (even if many spare receptors are present), and the Schild equation is never obeyed.

Some antagonists combine the ability to block open ion channels with a competitive action at or near the agonist binding site. A well-characterized example is the nicotinic blocker tubocurarine (see Chapter 6). Agonists may also be open channel blockers, thus limiting the maximal response that they can elicit. Such agents (e.g., decamethonium) may therefore behave as partial agonists when tested on an intact tissue.*

The scheme illustrated in Figure 1.25 assumes that the accessory site is inhibitory. It is now known that some agonists (e.g., glutamate) may only be effective in the presence of another ligand (e.g., glycine in the case of the NMDA receptors for glutamate) which binds to its own site on the receptor macromolecule. Glutamate is then referred to as the primary agonist, and glycine as a co-agonist. In principle, an antagonist could act by competing with either the primary agonist or the co-agonist.

1.6.6 A MORE GENERAL MODEL FOR THE ACTION OF AGONISTS, CO-AGONISTS, AND ANTAGONISTS

The realization that many receptors show some degree of constitutive activity (that is, they can isomerize to the active state even in the absence of agonist) suggests a more general and at the same time more physically realistic model for the action of noncompetitive antagonists. It is illustrated in Figure 1.28 and can be regarded as a straightforward extension of the scheme for constitutive activity introduced in Section 1.4.7 (see Figure 1.11). Two ligands, A and B, can bind to different sites on the receptor so that in principle both can be present at the same time, as shown in Figure 1.25, which was the starting point for our discussion of noncompetitive antagonism. The scheme in Figure 1.28 covers a wider range of possibilities and also has the merit that it suggests a molecular mechanism not only for noncompetitive antagonism but also, as we shall see, for several other patterns of drug action. The underlying concept is that any substance that combines with an accessory (allotopic, allosteric) site can be expected to alter the equilibrium between the active and inactive states of the receptor and so affect agonist action.

Four limiting cases of the general scheme will be considered. Each supposes that A is a conventional, "positive" agonist; that is, its presence increases the proportion of active receptors because of its preferential affinity for the active form.

1. The ligand B has a much greater affinity for the inactive (R, AR) than the active (R*, AR*) states of the receptor. Little BR* or ABR* is formed. In the presence of large

---

* As noted in Appendix 1.4A, the characterization of a substance as a partial agonist need not presuppose a particular mechanism for its failure to elicit a maximal effect.

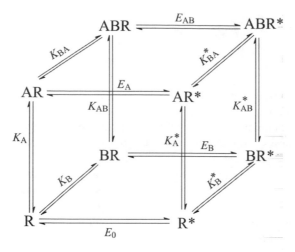

FIGURE 1.28 An extension to two ligands, A and B, of the scheme for the constitutive activity shown in Figure 1.11, which is reproduced as the front face of the cube. We suppose that A and B combine with separate sites on the receptor macromolecule, R, so that both can be present at the same time (top edge of the rear face of the cube). Active and inactive states of the receptor are represented by the right- and left-hand side faces respectively.

concentrations of both A and B, most of the receptors will be in the inactive, ABR condition (top, left, rear vertex of the cube). B then acts as a noncompetitive antagonist (see Figure 1.29A).

2. The dissociation equilibrium constants that determine the formation of ABR and ABR* are so large (i.e., the corresponding affinities are so small) that the quantities of these doubly liganded forms are negligible. In effect, the binding of A and B is mutually exclusive. If, in addition, the affinity of B for the active form of the receptor is very low, B will then act as a competitive antagonist (see Figure 1.29B).*

3. B binds mainly to the active states of the receptor (R* and AR*) and in such a way that the resulting complexes (BR* and ABR*) are inactive. The predicted curves are shown in Figure 1.29C. Open channel block (see Section 1.6.5) provides an example (compare Figure 1.27).

4. Though A binds to R and to R*, the position of the equilibrium between A, R, and R* is now assumed to be such that little AR* is formed in the absence of B. However, if B is also present, many of the receptors enter the active ABR* configuration. Under these circumstances, B acts as a co-agonist for A; full activation requires the simultaneous presence of A and B (see Figure 1.29D).

1.6.7 APPENDICES TO SECTION 1.6

1.6.7.1 Appendix 1.6A: A Note on the Term *Allosteric*

Allosteric has come to be used in receptor pharmacology in at least three different senses, making the concept difficult for the beginner at least. The main usages are:

1. To denote either a binding site other than that for the agonist or a ligand that acts by combining with this other site. For example, the "allosteric antagonist" gallamine influences activation of the muscarinic receptor by binding to a distinct region (an "allosteric

---

* Here, *competitive* is defined as in Section 1.5.1.2 to include the possibility that A and B may combine with different binding sites that interact in such a way that if A is present, B cannot be, and vice versa.

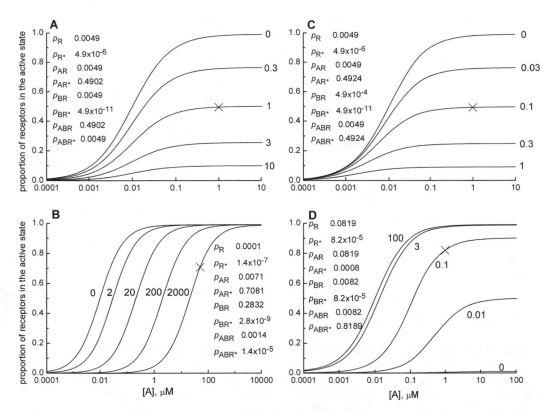

FIGURE 1.29 The effect of a second ligand on the relationship between agonist concentration ([A]) and the proportion of active receptors, as predicted by the scheme shown in Figure 1.28. Each panel illustrates the effect of the additional ligand, B, at the four concentrations (μM) indicated by the number given with each line. For panels A, B, and C, but not D, the agonist has been assumed to have a high intrinsic efficacy so that almost all of the receptors can be activated by it. An additional assumption throughout is that the constitutive activity of the receptor is low, so that in the absence of ligands, few of the receptors are active.

A. Here, the second ligand, B, has been assumed to have a high preferential affinity for the inactive forms of the receptor. The outcome closely mimics 'classical,' noncompetitive antagonism.

B. The two ligands A and B have been assumed to combine with the receptor in an almost mutually exclusive manner. In effect, A and B are in competition, and the model then predicts that increasing concentrations of B cause a near-parallel shift in the curves.

C. Here, B is assumed to combine mainly with the active forms of the receptor to form complexes (BR*, ABR*) that are inactive. An example is the action of an open channel blocker. Note the convergence of the curves at low agonist concentrations (contrast with the pattern expected for noncompetitive antagonism, as in panel A and as shown in Figure 1.26).

D. For this simulation the equilibrium constant for isomerization between AR and the AR* has been set so that few of the receptors are in the active state even in the presence of a large concentration of A on its own. However, with B also present at increasing concentrations, the equilibria shown in Figure 1.28 are shifted toward the active forms so that the maximum response to A rises to a point at which almost all of the receptors can be activated. In effect, B is acting as a co-agonist. Note that it causes little receptor activation when [A] is small.

The columns of numbers given with each panel show the fraction of receptors in each condition at the particular concentration of A indicated by × on one of the curves. The values of the equilibrium constants used in the simulations are listed in Table 1.4.

site") of the receptor macromolecule. Some authors have extended this by describing the agonist site as "orthosteric." Allosteric antagonism can be regarded as a form of non-competitive antagonism as defined and discussed in this chapter.

2. To describe the all-or-none transition between distinct conformational states of enzymes or receptors — an "allosteric transition." In keeping with this usage, the constant that describes the position of the equilibrium between the states (e.g., E_0 in the schemes of Figures 1.11 and 1.28) is sometimes described as the *allosteric constant*.

3. To denote the mechanism whereby the position of the equilibrium between two distinct forms of the receptor changes in the presence of a ligand (agonist or antagonist) for which the affinity of the forms is different.

Though each of these usages is self-consistent and can be justified, it is easy to see that *allosteric*, if unqualified, can mean different things to different people. For example, activation of the nicotinic and muscarinic receptors by acetylcholine can be regarded as an example of an allosteric mechanism as defined in usage 3 above. But, acetylcholine does not act through an allosteric site, as defined in usage 1. Clearly, the term must be qualified in the context in which it is employed. For further discussion, see the account by Colquhoun (1998), who describes the origin of the term and the evolution of the way it is used.

In an attempt to reduce the potential for confusion, the terms *allotopic* and *syntopic* have been suggested as designations for different site and same site, respectively, though it is probably too late to hope to rationalize usage in this context.

1.6.7.2 Appendix 1.6B: Applying the Law of Mass Action to the Scheme of Figure 1.28

A first assumption is that the twelve reversible reactions represented in Figure 1.28 have reached equilibrium. Of the twelve equilibrium constants that specify how many receptors are in each condition, only seven need to be known; the remaining five are determined by the others. This can best be understood by returning to the simpler scheme shown in Figure 1.11. Applying the law of mass action to three of the four equilibria in that scheme, we have:

$$p_{R^*} = E_0 p_R$$

$$[L]p_R = K_L p_{LR}$$

$$[L]p_{R^*} = K_L^* p_{LR^*}$$

Hence, for the remaining equilibrium,

$$E_L = \frac{p_{LR^*}}{p_{LR}} = \frac{p_{R^*}}{p_R} \frac{K_L}{K_L^*} = E_0 \frac{K_L}{K_L^*}$$

We see from this that the value of the fourth equilibrium constant (for isomerization between the active and inactive forms of the occupied receptor) is determined by the other three, E_0, K_L, and K_L^*.

Returning to the scheme of Figure 1.28 and thinking about the choice of the seven constants that must be specified, it is advantageous to separate the seven into three "primary" and four "secondary" constants. The primary ones are taken to be E_0, K_A, and K_B, and the others are expressed as multiples of them. The four multipliers required for this are designated a, b, d, and g, for consistency with previous accounts of this scheme for receptor activation (see, e.g., Colquhoun [1998] and references therein).

Table 1.3 sets out the relationships between the three primary and the nine other equilibrium constants that appear in Figure 1.28. Table 1.4 lists the particular values used to calculate the sets

TABLE 1.3
Equilibrium Constants that Determine the Position of the Equilibria in Figure 1.28

Equilibrium Constant in Figure 1.28	Equilibrium Constants Expressed in Terms of E_0, K_A, or K_B	Notes
E_0, K_A, K_B	—	1. The three primary constants
K_A^*	K_A/a	2. a is the factor by which the affinity of the active form (R*) for A exceeds that of R. It also expresses the increase in the tendency for the receptor to isomerize to the active form when the binding site for A alone is occupied.
K_B^*	K_B/b	3. As above, but for B.
K_{AB}	K_A/g	4. g expresses the ratio of (a) the affinities of BR and R for A, and (b) the affinities of AR and R for B. If g is very small, few bi-liganded receptors (ABR, ABR*) will be present.
K_{BA}	K_B/g	See 4.
K_{AB}^*	K_A/adg	5. d, with a and g, determines the ratio of the affinities of BR* and R for A.
K_{BA}^*	K_B/bdg	6. d, with b and g, determines the ratio of the affinities of AR* and R for B.
E_A	aE_0	See 2.
E_B	bE_0	See 3.
E_{AB}	$abdE_0$	7. The product of a, b, and d relates the isomerization of ABR to ABR* to that of R to R*.

TABLE 1.4
The Values Used In the Simulations Illustrated in Figure 1.29, A–D

Equilibrium Constant*	Value of Multiplier**	Panel A	Panel B	Panel C	Panel D
	a	100000	100000	100000	10
	b	0.00001	0.00001	0.0001	10
	d	10	10	10000	1000
	g	100	0.0001	10	1
E_0		0.001	0.001	0.001	0.001
K_A		1	1	1	1
K_B		1	1	1	1
K_A^*		0.00001	0.00001	0.00001	0.1
K_B^*		100000	10000	10000	0.1
K_{AB}		0.01	10000	0.1	1
K_{BA}		0.01	10000	0.1	1
K_{AB}^*		0.00000001	0.01	1E-10	0.0001
K_{BA}^*		100	10000000	0.1	0.0001
E_A		100	100	100	0.01
E_B		0.00000001	0.00000001	0.0000001	0.01
E_{AB}		0.01	0.01	100	100

* The units of all the dissociation equilibrium constants listed are μM.
** These multipliers are used to calculate the secondary constants (e.g., K_A^*, E_A) from the primary ones (E_0, K_A, K_B), as listed in Table 1.3. For example, if $E_0 = 0.001$ and $a = 100000$, then $E_A = a E_0 = 100$. Similary, $K_A^* = K_A/a = 1/100000 = 0.00001$ μM.

of curves shown in Figure 1.29. Such calculations can be done in several ways, some being better for exposition and others making for easier evaluation with a spreadsheet. The approach that follows is more flexible, though less concise, than an alternative given in the answer in Section 1.10 to Problem 1.5 (Section 1.8).

We start by using the law of mass action to enable us to relate the fraction of receptors in each of the various conditions (R*, AR*, BR*, ABR*, AR, etc.) to the fraction (p_R) in the inactive state (R) with both binding sites vacant:

$$p_{R^*} = E_0 p_R$$

$$p_{AR^*} = \frac{[A]}{K_A^*} p_{R^*} = E_0 \frac{[A]}{K_A^*} p_R$$

$$p_{BR^*} = \frac{[B]}{K_B^*} p_{R^*} = E_0 \frac{[B]}{K_B^*} p_R$$

$$p_{ABR^*} = \frac{[B]}{K_{BA}^*} p_{AR^*} = E_0 \frac{[B]}{K_{BA}^*} \frac{[A]}{K_A^*} p_R$$

$$p_{AR} = \frac{[A]}{K_A} p_R$$

$$p_{BR} = \frac{[B]}{K_B} p_R$$

$$p_{ABR} = \frac{[B]}{K_{BA}} p_{AR} = \frac{[B]}{K_{BA}} \frac{[A]}{K_A} p_R$$

Also,

$$p_{R^*} + p_{AR^*} + p_{BR^*} + p_{ABR^*} + p_R + p_{AR} + p_{BR} + p_{ABR} = 1$$

Substituting for p_{R^*}, p_{AR^*}, etc., in this expression, we have:

$$p_R \left(E_0 + E_0 \frac{[A]}{K_A^*} + E_0 \frac{[B]}{K_B^*} + E_0 \frac{[B]}{K_{BA}^*} \frac{[A]}{K_A^*} + 1 + \frac{[A]}{K_A} + \frac{[B]}{K_B} + \frac{[B]}{K_{BA}} \frac{[A]}{K_A} \right) = 1$$

Hence,

$$p_R = \frac{1}{E_0 \left(1 + \frac{[A]}{K_A^*} + \frac{[B]}{K_B^*} + \frac{[B]}{K_{BA}^*} \frac{[A]}{K_A^*} \right) + 1 + \frac{[A]}{K_A} + \frac{[B]}{K_B} + \frac{[B]}{K_{BA}} \frac{[A]}{K_A}} \tag{1.58}$$

This expression, together with the mass law equilibrium equations just listed, can now be used to calculate the proportions of receptors in any condition or combination of conditions. For example, the fraction in the active state is given by:

$$p_{active} = p_{R^*} + p_{AR^*} + p_{BR^*} + p_{ABR^*}$$

$$= E_0 \left(1 + \frac{[A]}{K_A^*} + \frac{[B]}{K_B^*} + \frac{[B]}{K_{BA}^*} \frac{[A]}{K_A^*} \right) p_R$$

Substituting for p_R using Eq. (1.58) provides the final expression relating the fraction of receptors in the active form to the concentrations of A and B:

$$p_{\text{active}} = \cfrac{E_0}{E_0 + \left(\cfrac{1 + \cfrac{[A]}{K_A} + \cfrac{[B]}{K_B} + \cfrac{[B]}{K_{BA}} \cfrac{[A]}{K_A}}{1 + \cfrac{[A]}{K_A^*} + \cfrac{[B]}{K_B^*} + \cfrac{[B]}{K_{BA}^*} \cfrac{[A]}{K_A^*}} \right)} \tag{1.59}$$

This has been used to construct the sets of curves in Figure 1.29.*

In the same way, the proportion of receptors in which A occupies its binding site is given by:

$$p_{occupied(A)} = p_{AR} + p_{AR*} + p_{ABR} + p_{ABR*}$$

$$= \left(\frac{[A]}{K_A} + E_0 \frac{[A]}{K_A^*} + \frac{[B]}{K_{BA}} \frac{[A]}{K_A} + E_0 \frac{[B]}{K_{BA}^*} \frac{[A]}{K_A^*} \right) p_R$$

Using Eq. (1.58) to substitute for p_R, we have:

$$p_{occupied(A)} = \cfrac{\cfrac{[A]}{K_A} + E_0 \cfrac{[A]}{K_A^*} + \cfrac{[B]}{K_{BA}} \cfrac{[A]}{K_A} + E_0 \cfrac{[B]}{K_{BA}^*} \cfrac{[A]}{K_A^*}}{\cfrac{[A]}{K_A} + E_0 \cfrac{[A]}{K_A^*} + \cfrac{[B]}{K_{BA}} \cfrac{[A]}{K_A} + E_0 \cfrac{[B]}{K_{BA}^*} \cfrac{[A]}{K_A^*} + 1 + E_0 \left(1 + \cfrac{[B]}{K_B^*}\right) + \cfrac{[B]}{K_B}}$$

$$= \cfrac{1}{1 + \left\{ \cfrac{1 + E_0 \left(1 + \cfrac{[B]}{K_B^*}\right) + \cfrac{[B]}{K_B}}{\cfrac{[A]}{K_A} + E_0 \cfrac{[A]}{K_A^*} + \cfrac{[B]}{K_{BA}} \cfrac{[A]}{K_A} + E_0 \cfrac{[B]}{K_{BA}^*} \cfrac{[A]}{K_A^*}} \right\}}$$

Using the relationship $E_0 = \dfrac{K_A^*}{K_A} E_A$,

$$= \cfrac{[A]}{K_A \left\{ \cfrac{1 + E_0 \left(1 + \cfrac{[B]}{K_B^*}\right) + \cfrac{[B]}{K_B}}{1 + E_A \left(1 + \cfrac{[B]}{K_{BA}^*}\right) + \cfrac{[B]}{K_{BA}}} \right\} + [A]}$$

From this we see that the relation between the concentration of A and the amount of it that is bound should follow the Hill–Langmuir equation. K_{eff}, the macroscopic dissociation equilibrium constant, is given by:

---

* For panel C, however, p_{active} is taken to be $p_{R*} + p_{AR*}$, in keeping with the hypothesis that in this instance BR* and ABR* do not contribute to the response.

$$K_{\text{eff}} = \left\{ \frac{1 + E_0 \left(1 + \dfrac{[B]}{K_B^*}\right) + \dfrac{[B]}{K_B}}{1 + E_A \left(1 + \dfrac{[B]}{K_{BA}^*}\right) + \dfrac{[B]}{K_{BA}}} \right\} K_A$$

$$= \left\{ \frac{1 + E_0 + (1 + E_B)\dfrac{[B]}{K_B}}{1 + E_A + (1 + E_{AB})\dfrac{[B]}{K_{BA}}} \right\} K_A$$

Note that the term in the large brackets can be greater or less than unity, depending on the values of the six constants. Hence, the presence of B can either increase or reduce the binding of A.

1.7 CONCLUDING REMARKS

Modeling the action of receptors in the ways outlined in this chapter is likely to continue to be of value. In particular, it allows the actions of drugs to be better described, quantified and analyzed. It should not be forgotten, however, that each of the key advances in the understanding of receptor action has come not from modeling and equation writing but rather from new experimental techniques such as the radioligand binding method, single-channel recording, and, most recently, the procedures of molecular biology that allow the structure of receptors to be not only determined but also modified in precise ways. These and other advances are dealt with in the chapters that follow.

1.8 PROBLEMS

Problem 1.1

A competitive antagonist (B) is applied to a tissue and produces a concentration ratio r_B. A second competitive antagonist (C) acting at the same receptors produces a concentration ratio r_C under identical conditions. The tissue is next exposed to both antagonists together, at the same concentrations as in the separate applications. The concentration ratio is now observed to be r_{B+C}. What relationship might be expected to hold between r_B, r_C, and r_{B+C}? (Assume that the del Castillo–Katz mechanism of receptor activation holds in its simplest form (Eq. (1.7).)

Problem 1.2

When studying competitive antagonism, it is sometimes necessary to include an uptake inhibitor or a ganglion blocker in all the bathing solutions used. If this compound has in addition some competitive blocking action at the receptor being studied, what effect will this have on estimation of the dissociation equilibrium constant for a competitive antagonist?

Problem 1.3

What quantity would Furchgott's irreversible antagonist method (Section 1.6.4) estimate if the occupied receptor, AR, must first isomerize to a second form, AR*, which then attaches to another entity, such as a G-protein, in order to elicit a response (as in Eq. (1.38))? Assume that the G-protein is present in great excess in relation to the receptors.

Problem 1.4

Derive Eq. (1.39) in Section 1.4.7, which expresses how the proportion of active receptors varies with the concentration of a ligand that combines with a receptor with constitutive activity.

Problem 1.5

Apply the law of mass action to work out the proportion of receptors in the active form (p_{active}) for the mechanism for receptor activation shown in Figure 1.14. What will be the value of EC_{50} under these circumstances? (Assume that the response measured is directly proportional to p_{active} and that the concentration of the G protein can be regarded as constant.)

1.9 FURTHER READING

General

More detailed accounts of some of the material in this chapter can be found in four excellent books:

Kenakin, T. P., *Pharmacologic Analysis of Drug–Receptor Interaction*, 3rd ed., Raven Press, New York, 1997.

Kenakin, T. and Angus, J. A., The pharmacology of functional, biochemical and recombinant receptor systems, in *Handbook of Experimental Pharmacology*, Vol. 148, 2000.

Limbird, L. E., *Cell Surface Receptors: A Short Course on Theory and Methods*, 2nd ed., Nijhoff, Boston, 1996.

Pratt, W. B. and Taylor, P., *Principles of Drug Action*, Churchill Livingstone, New York, 1990 (see, in particular, Chapters 1 and 2).

Early Work (Now Mainly of Historical Interest)

Hill–Langmuir equation and the application of the law of mass action to the kinetics of drug–receptor interaction:

Hill, A. V., The mode of action of nicotine and curari, determined by the form of the contraction curve and the method of temperature coefficients, *J. Physiol.*, 39, 361–373, 1909.

The Hill equation:

Hill, A. V., The possible effects of the aggregation of the molecules of haemoglobin on its dissociation curve, *J. Physiol.*, 40, iv–vii, 1910.

Clark's modeling of the concentration–response relationship:

Clark, A. J., The reaction between acetylcholine and muscle cells, *J. Physiol.*, 61, 530–547, 1926.

The Gaddum equation:

Gaddum, J. H., The quantitative effect of antagonistic drugs, *J. Physiol.*, 89, 7–9P, 1937.

Gaddum, J. H., The antagonism of drugs, *Trans. Faraday Soc.*, 39, 323–332, 1943.

The pA scale:

Schild, H. O., pA: a new scale for the measurement of drug antagonism, *Br. J. Pharmacol.*, 2, 189–206, 1947.

The Schild equation:

Schild, H. O., pA_x and competitive drug antagonism, *Br. J. Pharmacol.*, 4, 277–280, 1949.

Schild, H. O., Drug antagonism and pA_x, *Pharmacol. Rev.*, 9, 242–246, 1957.

Efficacy

Colquhoun, D., Affinity, efficacy and receptor classification: is the classical theory still useful?, in *Perspectives on Receptor Classification*, Black, J. W., Jenkinson, D. H., and Gerskowitch, V.P., Eds., Liss, New York, 1987, chap. 11.

Colquhoun, D., Binding, gating, affinity and efficacy. The interpretation of structure–activity relationships and of the effects of mutating receptors, *Br. J. Pharmacol.*, 125, 924–947, 1998.

Samama, P., Cotecchia, S., Costa, T., and Lefkowitz, R. J., A mutation-induced activated state of the β_2-adrenergic receptor: extending the ternary complex model, *J. Biol. Chem.*, 268, 4625–4636, 1993.

Stephenson, R. P., A modification of receptor theory, *Br. J. Pharmacol.*, 11, 379–393, 1956.

Examples of the practical application of Schild's approach to the study of antagonism

Arunlakshana, O. and Schild, H. O., Some quantitative uses of drug antagonists, *Br. J. Pharmacol.*, 14, 48–58, 1959.

Black, J. W., Duncan, W. A. M., Durant, C. J., Ganellin, C. R., and Parsons, E. M., Definition and antagonism of histamine H_2-receptors, *Nature*, 236, 385–390, 1972.

Additional example of analysis of deviations from the Schild equation

Black, J. W., Leff, P., and Shankley, N. P., Further analysis of anomalous pK_B values for histamine H_2-receptor antagonists on the mouse isolated stomach assay, *Br. J. Pharmacol.*, 86, 581–587, 1985.

Application of irreversible antagonists (receptor protection experiments, attempted determination of K_A for agonists)

Eglen, R. M. and Harris, G. C., Selective inactivation of muscarinic M_2 and M_3 receptors in guinea-pig ileum and atria *in vitro*, *Br. J. Pharmacol.*, 109, 946–952, 1993.

Furchgott, R. F., The use of β-haloalkylamines in the differentiation of receptors and in the determination of dissociation constants of receptor-agonist complexes, *Adv. Drug Res.*, 3, 21–55, 1966.

Morey, T. E., Belardinell, L., and Dennis, D. M., Validation of Furchgott's method to determine agonist-dependent A_1-adenosine receptor reserve in guinea-pig atrium, *Br. J. Pharmacol.*, 123, 1425–1433, 1998.

1.10 SOLUTIONS TO PROBLEMS

Problem 1.1

We have three experimental situations to consider:

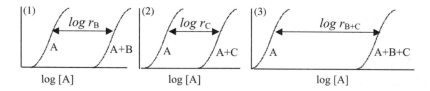

(1) and (2) are straightforward (see Section 1.5.2), whereas (3) breaks new ground.

When B and C are applied together, as in (3) above, and the agonist A is also present, we have four simultaneous equilibria (at least in principle):

$$A + R \underset{K_A}{\rightleftharpoons} AR \underset{E}{\rightleftharpoons} AR^*$$

$$B + R \underset{K_B}{\rightleftharpoons} BR$$

$$C + R \underset{K_C}{\rightleftharpoons} CR$$

Applying the law of mass action:

$$[A]p_R = K_A p_{AR}$$

$$p_{AR^*} = E p_{AR}$$

$$[B]p_R = K_B p_{BR}$$

$$[C]p_R = K_C p_{CR}$$

Also (see Section 1.5.2),

$$p_R + p_{AR} + p_{AR*} + p_{BR} + p_{CR} = 1$$

From these equations,

$$p_{AR*} = \frac{E[A]}{K_A\left(1 + \frac{[B]}{K_B} + \frac{[C]}{K_C}\right) + (1 + E)[A]}$$

Hence, equating equal receptor activations by the agonist (at which it is assumed that the responses would also be equal), first in the absence of any antagonist and then in the simultaneous presence of B and C:

$$\frac{E[A]}{K_A + (1 + E)[A]} = \frac{Er_{B+C}[A]}{K_A\left(1 + \frac{[B]}{K_B} + \frac{[C]}{K_C}\right) + (1 + E)r_{B+C}[A]}$$

$$\frac{E[A]}{K_A + (1 + E)[A]} = \frac{E[A]}{K_A\left(\dfrac{1 + \dfrac{[B]}{K_B} + \dfrac{[C]}{K_C}}{r_{B+C}}\right) + (1 + E)[A]}$$

$$\therefore \frac{1 + \dfrac{[B]}{K_B} + \dfrac{[C]}{K_C}}{r_{B+C}} = 1$$

$$r_{B+C} - 1 = \frac{[B]}{K_B} + \frac{[C]}{K_C}$$

$$r_{B+C} - 1 = (r_B - 1) + (r_C - 1)$$

$$\therefore r_{B+C} = r_B + r_C - 1$$

This relationship has often been used to obtain evidence that two antagonists act at the same site. It can also be derived by taking the Gaddum equation as the starting point rather than expressions based on the del Castillo–Katz mechanism.

Problem 1.2

We will use B to denote the competitive antagonist being investigated and C to represent the substance with some competitive blocking action that is present in all the bathing solutions used in the experiment. When the control curve is determined, the tissue is exposed to both the agonist A and the substance C at concentrations [A] and [C], respectively. Assuming equilibrium, the proportion of receptors in the active state is then:

$$p_{AR*} = \frac{E[A]}{K_A\left(1 + \frac{[C]}{K_C}\right) + (1 + E)[A]}$$

(See Eq. (1.49).)

When the competitive antagonist B is also applied, the concentration of A has to be increased by a factor r, the concentration ratio, to restore the same response. The proportion of receptors in the active state is then:

$$p_{AR*} = \frac{Er[A]}{K_A\left(1 + \dfrac{[B]}{K_B} + \dfrac{[C]}{K_C}\right) + (1 + E)r[A]}$$

(See the answer to Problem 1.1.)

Assuming that equal responses correspond to equal receptor activations in the two situations (i.e., with and without B present), we can write:

$$1 + \frac{[C]}{K_C} = \frac{1 + \dfrac{[B]}{K_B} + \dfrac{[C]}{K_C}}{r}$$

so that

$$r - 1 = \frac{[B]}{K_B\left(1 + \dfrac{[C]}{K_C}\right)}$$

Hence, a Schild plot based on the results of such an experiment will give an estimate not of K_B but of $K_B(1 + [C]/K_C)$.

PROBLEM 1.3

Here the scheme for receptor activation is as shown in Eq. (1.38) in Section 1.4.6. Applying the law of mass action to each of the three equilibria gives:

$$[A]p_R = K_A p_{AR}$$

$$p_{AR*} = E p_{AR}$$

$$[G]p_{AR*} = K_{ARG} p_{AR*G*}$$

Also,

$$p_R + p_{AR} + p_{AR*} + p_{AR*G*} = 1$$

Using the mass law equilibrium equations to substitute for p_R, p_{AR}, and p_{AR*} in this expression, we obtain:

$$p_{AR*G*} = \frac{E[G]_T[A]}{K_A K_{ARG} + \{E[G]_T + K_{ARG}(1 + E)\}[A]}$$

It has been assumed here that G is present in such excess that its total concentration $[G]_T$ does not fall appreciably when AR*G* is formed. [G] in the mass law equation can then be replaced by $[G]_T$.

If we now consider Furchgott's analysis of the effect of an irreversible antagonist on the response to an agonist and make the same assumptions as in Section 1.6.4, we can write:

$$\frac{E[R]_T[G]_T[A]}{K_A K_{ARG} + \{E[G]_T + K_{ARG}(1+E)\}[A]} = \frac{qE[R]_T[G]_T[A]'}{K_A K_{ARG} + \{E[G]_T + K_{ARG}(1+E)\}[A]'}$$

Here, just as before, [A] and [A]' are the concentrations of the agonist A that produce the same response (assumed to correspond to the same concentrations of receptors in the active, AR*G*, form) before and after reducing the total "concentration" of receptors from $[R]_T$ to $q[R]_T$.

Canceling E, $[G]_T$, and $[R]_T$ in the numerators, and inverting, we obtain:

$$\frac{1}{[A]} = \frac{1}{q}\frac{1}{[A]'} + \left(\frac{E[G]_T + K_{ARG}(1+E)}{K_A K_{ARG}}\right)\left(\frac{1}{q}-1\right)$$

Hence, a plot of 1/[A] against 1/[A]' should again give a straight line of slope 1/q, and the quantity estimated by (slope − 1)/intercept would be:

$$\frac{K_A K_{ARG}}{E[G]_T + K_{ARG}(1+E)}$$

This is just what would be estimated by a direct ligand-binding experiment were this scheme for receptor occupation and activation to apply.

Problem 1.4

The model is:

$$\begin{array}{ccc}
\text{(inactive)} \quad R & \underset{}{\overset{E_0}{\rightleftharpoons}} & R^* \text{ (active)} \\
+ & & + \\
L & & L \\
K_L \updownarrow & & \updownarrow K_L^* \\
\text{(inactive)} \quad LR & \underset{E_L}{\overset{}{\rightleftharpoons}} & LR^* \text{ (active)}
\end{array}$$

from which we see that three equilibria must be considered (the fourth is determined by the position of the other three; see Appendix 1.6B). Applying the law of mass action to three of the equilibria, we have:

$$p_{R^*} = E_0 p_R$$

$$[L]p_R = K_L p_{LR}$$

$$[L]p_{R^*} = K_L^* p_{LR^*}$$

where the equilibrium constants E_0, K_L, and K_L^* are as defined in Section 1.4.7.

Also,

$$p_R + p_{R*} + p_{LR} + p_{LR*} = 1$$

By using the mass law equilibrium expressions to substitute for p_R, p_{R*}, and p_{LR} in the last equation, we obtain:

$$p_{LR*} = \frac{E_0[L]}{E_0([L] + K_L^*) + K_L^*\left(1 + \dfrac{[L]}{K_L}\right)}$$

From this, and using the third of the equilibrium expressions, we also have:

$$p_{R*} = \frac{E_0 K_L^*}{E_0([L] + K_L^*) + K_L^*\left(1 + \dfrac{[L]}{K_L}\right)}$$

We wish to know the total fraction of receptors in the active state:

$$p_{active} = p_{R*} + p_{LR*}$$

$$= \frac{E_0([L] + K_L^*)}{E_0([L] + K_L^*) + K_L^*\left(1 + \dfrac{[L]}{K_L}\right)}$$

$$= \frac{E_0}{E_0 + \left(\dfrac{1 + \dfrac{[L]}{K_L}}{1 + \dfrac{[L]}{K_L^*}}\right)}$$

This derivation has followed the same general procedure applied throughout this chapter. Another route, however, is instructive:

$$p_{active} = p_{R*} + p_{LR*}$$

$$= \frac{[R*] + [LR*]}{[R*] + [LR*] + [R] + [LR]}$$

$$= \frac{1}{1 + \left(\dfrac{[R] + [LR]}{[R*] + [LR*]}\right)}$$

Considering just the term in brackets and making use of the three equilibrium equations, we have:

$$\frac{[R] + [LR]}{[R*] + [LR*]} = \frac{[R]}{[R*]}\left(\frac{1 + \dfrac{[LR]}{[R]}}{1 + \dfrac{[LR*]}{[R*]}}\right) = \frac{1}{E_0}\left(\frac{1 + \dfrac{[L]}{K_L}}{1 + \dfrac{[L]}{K_L^*}}\right)$$

Hence, Eq. (1.39) has been derived.

Problem 1.5

Here, the model is formally similar to the one discussed in Appendix 1.6B, which describes the application of the law of mass action to a scheme (Figure 1.28) in which each receptor macromolecule carries a separate binding site for each of two ligands. However, in the mechanism for the action of a G-protein-coupled receptor illustrated in Figure 1.14, only two (R*G and LR*G) of the eight possible conditions of the receptor are active. The diagram below reproduces Figure 1.14 with the addition of the 12 equilibrium constants:

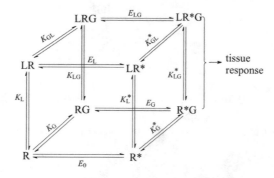

Using the second approach introduced in the solution to the last problem, we can write the fraction of active receptors as:

$$p_{active} = \frac{[R^*G]+[LR^*G]}{[R]+[R^*]+[LR]+[LR^*]+[RG]+[R^*G]+[LRG]+[LR^*G]}$$

$$= \frac{1}{1+\left(\dfrac{[R]+[R^*]+[LR]+[LR^*]+[RG]+[LRG]}{[R^*G]+[LR^*G]}\right)}$$

$$= \frac{1}{1+\dfrac{[R]}{[R^*]}\left(\dfrac{1+\dfrac{[R^*]}{[R]}+\dfrac{[LR]}{[R]}+\dfrac{[LR^*]}{[R]}+\dfrac{[RG]}{[R]}+\dfrac{[LRG]}{[R]}}{\dfrac{[R^*G]}{[R^*]}+\dfrac{[LR^*G]}{R^*]}}\right)}$$

By using the relationships obtained from applying the law of mass action to the individual equilibria in the scheme (see Appendix 1.6B), this can be rewritten as:

$$p_{active} = \frac{E_0}{E_0+\left\{\dfrac{1+E_0+\dfrac{[L]}{K_L}+E_0\dfrac{[L]}{K_L^*}+\dfrac{[G]}{K_G}+\dfrac{[G]}{K_{GL}}\dfrac{[L]}{K_L}}{\dfrac{[G]}{K_G^*}+\dfrac{[G]}{K_{GL}^*}\dfrac{[L]}{K_L^*}}\right\}}$$

Rearrangement and making use of the relationships between the equilibrium constants set out in Table 1.3 (see Appendix 1.6B for more detail) provide the expression we require:

$$p_{active} = \frac{E_G \dfrac{[G]}{K_G}\left(1 + \dfrac{[L]}{K_{LG}^*}\right)}{1 + E_0 + (1 + E_G)\dfrac{[G]}{K_G} + \left\{1 + E_L + (1 + E_{LG})\dfrac{[G]}{K_{GL}}\right\}\dfrac{[L]}{K_L}} \tag{1.60}$$

In the absence of the ligand L, Eq. (1.60) reduces to:

$$p_{active(min)} = \frac{E_G \dfrac{[G]}{K_G}}{1 + E_0 + (1 + E_G)\dfrac{[G]}{K_G}}$$

This predicts the constitutive activity of the G-protein-coupled receptor. Note the dependence on the effective concentration of the G-protein.

If the concentration of L is made very large, the proportion of the receptors in the active state rises to:

$$p_{active(max)} = \frac{E_{LG} \dfrac{[G]}{K_{GL}}}{1 + E_L + (1 + E_{LG})\dfrac{[G]}{K_{GL}}}$$

Assuming, finally, that we are fortunate enough to be dealing with a simple response that is directly proportional to the fraction of receptors in the active condition, we can go on to predict the EC_{50}. This is the concentration of L that causes the response to rise from its value y_{min} in the absence of L to y_{min} plus 50% of the maximum increase $(y_{max} - y_{min})$ that L can induce. More formally, and assuming direct proportionality between y and p_{active}, we can write:

$$p_{actuve(EC_{50})} = p_{active(min)} + \tfrac{1}{2}\left(p_{active(max)} - p_{active(min)}\right)$$

$$= \tfrac{1}{2}\left(p_{active(max)} + p_{active(min)}\right)$$

Using Eq. (1.60) and the expressions for $p_{active(min)}$ and $p_{active(max)}$ just derived, we find that the value of EC_{50} is given by:

$$\left\{\frac{1 + E_0 + (1 + E_G)\dfrac{[G]}{K_G}}{1 + E_L + (1 + E_{LG})\dfrac{[G]}{K_{GL}}}\right\}K_L$$

In Appendix 1.6B we obtained an expression for the macroscopic dissociation equilibrium constant, K_{eff}, for the binding of a ligand on the same scheme as in Figure 1.14. Allowing for the difference in terms, K_{eff} and EC_{50} are seen to be identical.

Section II

Molecular Structure of Receptors

2 Molecular Structure and Function of 7TM G-Protein-Coupled Receptors

Thue W. Schwartz and Birgitte Holst

CONTENTS

0-8493-1029-6/03/$0.00+$1.50

2.1 G-PROTEIN-COUPLED RECEPTORS CONSTITUTE A UNIFYING SIGNAL-TRANSDUCTION MECHANISM

2.1.1 GTP BINDING PROTEINS ACT AS TRANSDUCERS BETWEEN RECEPTORS AND EFFECTOR SYSTEMS

Already in 1969 it was suggested by Martin Rodbell and co-workers that a series of hormones, all of which stimulated adenylate cyclase, acted by binding to specific receptors (*discriminators*), which were linked to intracellular adenylate cyclase (the *amplifier*) through a so-called *transducer* system. The common transducer for all of these hormones was subsequently characterized as being one of several heterotrimeric guanine nucleotide binding proteins, G-proteins. In the signal-transduction mechanism, receptor activation leads to an exchange of guanosine diphosphate (GDP) with guanosine triphosphate (GTP) in the G-protein, which then becomes active and can stimulate various intracellular effector systems until its GTPase activity leads to GTP hydrolysis to GDP, which turns the system off again (see Chapter 7). Besides adenylate cyclase, a number of amplifiers or effector systems, such as phospholipases and phosphodiesterases, as well as ion channels, are regulated by the G-protein subunits in a sophisticated signal-processing system. The number of hormone receptors and receptors for other chemical messengers acting through G-proteins is now known to be very large. It is clear that G-protein-coupled receptors constitute one of the major signal-transduction systems in eukaryotic cells.

2.1.2 G-Protein-Coupled Receptors Comprise a Very Large Superfamily of Proteins with Seven Transmembrane Segments

In 1983, rhodopsin, the light-sensing molecule that binds the chromophore retinal, was the first G-protein-coupled molecule to be cloned. The most conspicuous structural feature of this photoreceptor was the seven hydrophobic segments believed to constitute seven transmembrane (7TM) helices, by analogy with the seven transmembrane helices of the proton pump, bacteriorhodopsin. When the β-adrenergic receptor, as the first neurotransmitter/hormone receptor, was cloned, this protein turned out to be surprisingly homologous to rhodopsin and to have a similar overall structure, with seven transmembrane segments. The subsequent cloning of a multitude of different receptors and characterization of the human genome have demonstrated that 7TM receptors constitute the largest superfamily of proteins in our organism. Although most of the receptors have turned out to be homologous to rhodopsin, several distantly related families of G-protein-coupled receptors were discovered, with the only apparent, common structural feature being the seven hydrophobic segments. Importantly, it has become increasingly clear that 7TM receptors may signal through G-protein-independent pathways, and it is therefore more appropriate to use the name *7TM receptors* than *G-protein-coupled receptors*.

2.1.3 A Multitude of Very Different Chemical Messengers Act through 7TM Receptors

The spectrum of hormones, neurotransmitters, paracrine mediators, etc., that act through G-protein-coupled receptors includes all kinds of chemical messengers: *ions* (calcium ions acting on the parathyroid and kidney chemosensor), *amino acids* (glutamate and γ-aminobutyric acid, or GABA), *monoamines* (catecholamines, acetylcholine, serotonin, etc.), *lipid messengers* (prostaglandins, thromboxane, anandamide, endogenous cannabinoid, platelet-activating factor, etc.), *purines* (adenosine and adenosine triphosphate [ATP]), *neuropeptides* (tachykinins, neuropeptide Y, endogenous opioids, cholecystokinin, vasoactive intestinal polypeptide [VIP], etc.), *peptide hormones* (angiotensin, bradykinin, glucagon, calcitonin, parathyroid hormone, etc.), chemokines (interleukin-8 [IL-8], RANTES, macrophage inflammatory peptide 1α [MIP-1α], etc.), *glycoprotein hormones* (thyroid-stimulating hormone [TSH], follicle-stimulating hormone [FSH], luteinizing hormone [LH]/chorionic gonadotropin, etc.), as well as proteases (thrombin). In our sensory systems, G-protein-coupled receptors are involved both as the light-sensing molecules in the eye (rhodopsin and the color pigment proteins) and as several hundreds of distinct odorant receptors in the olfactory system, in addition to a large number of taste receptors.

2.2 G-PROTEIN-COUPLED RECEPTORS ARE SEVEN-HELICAL BUNDLE PROTEINS EMBEDDED IN THE CELL MEMBRANE

The problem of characterizing the three-dimensional structure of G-protein-coupled receptors by x-ray crystallography or nuclear magnetic resonance (NMR) has been particularly difficult to solve. The receptors are complicated membrane proteins that are difficult to produce in sufficiently large quantities. When they have been available, it has been difficult to make them form useful crystals. However, based especially on cryoelectron microscopic analysis (electron crystallography) of two-dimensional crystals and on systematic electron paramagnetic resonance (EPR) studies of spin-labeled rhodopsin, a number of molecular models of 7TM receptors were developed during the 1990s that added to the vast amount of mutational and other types of biochemical data available.

2.2.1 THE X-RAY STRUCTURE OF RHODOPSIN

In 2000, the first x-ray structure based on three-dimensional crystals of a 7TM receptor was published, showing bovine rhodopsin in the inactive, dark state and having a seven-helical bundle closely corresponding to that described in most of the molecular models. Importantly, 11-*cis*-retinal, the chromophore or ligand, was located almost exactly as expected, clearly being attached to LysVII:10 in TM-VII through the Schiff base linkage and from here passing between TM-III and TM-VI, running rather parallel along TM-III, allowing the β-ionone ring to interact mainly with residues over in TM-V and TM-VI (Figures 2.1 and 2.2). Surprisingly, the ligand was closely covered from the extracellular side, not only by side-chains from the transmembrane helices but also by a well-ordered "plug" consisting of β-sheets formed by extracellular loop-2 (connecting TM-IV and TM-V), which, as expected, was held down to the top of TM-III by a disulfide bond. On the intracellular side, more or less well-ordered loops were observed, but instead of a loop between the end of TM-VII and the palmitoylation site (see later), a well-ordered amphipathic alpha helix (helix VIII) was found running parallel to the membrane below TM-VII, TM-I, and TM-II.

This structure was the first picture of a 7TM receptor, but unfortunately only in its inactive state. It should be noted that even though more structures, including active conformations and hormone/transmitter receptors, will become available in the coming years, these will only give us static pictures. In the future, the dynamic interchange between different conformations of these proteins must be understood. This question is starting to be addressed through various biophysical means — for example, experiments using spin-labels or fluorescent probes.

2.3 G-PROTEIN-COUPLED RECEPTORS ARE COMPOSED OF SEVERAL FAMILIES

Most of the G-protein-coupled receptors are homologous with rhodopsin; however, other quantitatively minor families as well as some individual receptors do not share any of the structural features common to the rhodopsin family (Figure 2.3). The most dominant of these are the glucagon/VIP/calcitonin receptor family, or "family B" (which has approximately 65 members), and the metabotropic glutamate receptor family, or "family C" (which has approximately 15 members), as well as the frizzled/smoothened family of receptors. Thus, the only structural feature that all G-protein-coupled receptors have in common is the seven-transmembrane helical bundle. Nevertheless, most non-rhodopsin-like receptors do have certain minor structural features in common with the rhodopsin-like receptors — for example, a disulfide bridge between the top of TM-III and the middle of extracellular loop-3, and a cluster of basic residues located just below TM-VI.

2.3.1 MANY 7TM RECEPTORS ARE STILL ORPHAN RECEPTORS

Total consensus regarding the total number of 7TM receptors has not been reached. However, it is clear that among members of the two large families, close to half of the receptors are still orphans; that is, the endogenous ligand has not yet been identified. Although the de-orphanization process is becoming more and more efficient, it is expected that still some years will pass before these hundreds of orphan receptors have been characterized, including determining which ligand they may bind, if any. After that, the physiological role and the pharmacological potential of these many

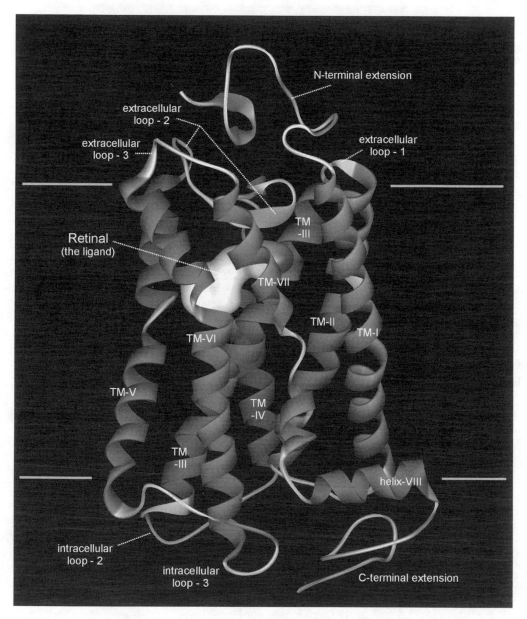

FIGURE 2.1 A side view of the structure of the prototype G-protein-coupled, 7TM receptor rhodopsin. The x-ray structure of bovine rhodopsin is shown with horizontal gray lines, indicating the limits of the cellular lipid membrane. The retinal ligand is shown in a space-filling model as the cloud in the middle of the structure. The seven transmembrane (7TM) helices are shown in solid ribbon form. Note that TM-III is rather tilted (see TM-III at the extracellular and intracellular end of the helix) and that kinks are present in several of the other helices, such as TM-V (to the left), TM-VI (in front of the retinal), and TM-VII. In all of these cases, these kinks are due to the presence of a well-conserved proline residue, which creates a weak point in the helical structure. These kinks are believed to be of functional importance in the activation mechanism for 7TM receptors in general. Also note the amphipathic helix-VIII which is located parallel to the membrane at the membrane interface.

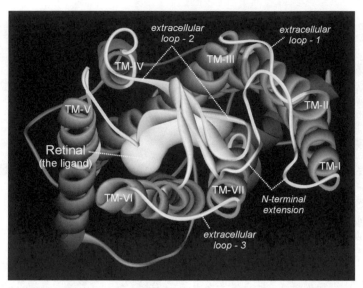

FIGURE 2.2 A top view of the structure of the prototype G-protein-coupled 7TM receptor rhodopsin. The x-ray structure of bovine rhodopsin is shown as viewed from the extracellular space. The extracellular ends of each of the transmembrane helices are indicated. Note how the retinal ligand is totally covered by a "plug" consisting of a β-sheet structure formed by the N-terminal extracellular extension and extracellular loop-2. A solid gray line from the extracellular end of TM-III to the first β-strand in extracellular loop-2 indicates the location of the structurally highly important disulfide bridge, which is conserved not only among family A, rhodopsin-like receptors but also among all 7TM receptors (see text for the few exceptions).

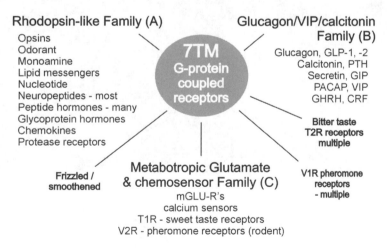

FIGURE 2.3 The three main families of mammalian G-protein-coupled 7TM receptors in mammals. No obvious sequence identity is found between the rhodopsin-like family A, the glucagon/VIP/calcitonin family B, and the metabotropic glutamate/chemosensor family C of G-protein-coupled 7TM receptors, with the exception of the disulfide bridge between the top of TM-III and the middle of extracellular loop-2 (see Figure 2.2). Similarly, no apparent sequence identity exists among members of these three families and, for example the 7TM bitter taste receptors, the V1R pheromone receptors, and the 7TM frizzled proteins, which all are either known or believed to be G-protein-coupled receptors. Bacteriorhodopsins, which are not G-protein-coupled proteins but proton pumps, are totally different in respect to amino-acid sequence but have a seven-helical bundle arranged rather similarly to that for the G-protein-coupled receptors.

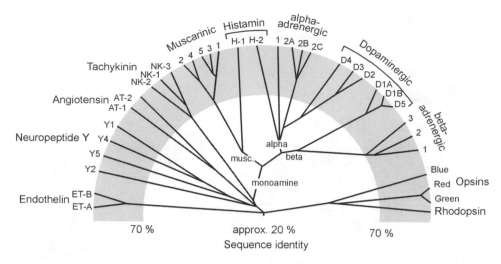

FIGURE 2.4 Part of an "evolutionary tree" for rhodopsin-like 7TM receptors. Only a few branches of the tree are shown to highlight certain principles. The sequence similarity scale starting at the center of the tree is not linear and does not start at zero. All rhodopsin-like receptors are at least 15 to 20% homologous — for example, rhodopsin vs. the monamine receptors or rhodopsin vs. peptide receptors. The shaded area indicates more than 70% sequence identity, which covers most receptor subtypes such as the, muscarinic receptors and the endothelin receptors. However, note that for other ligand subtypes, such as in the neuropeptide Y and angiotensin receptors, the sequence identity can be very limited, although they bind the same endogenous hormone or transmitter with nanomolar affinity. Also note that certain receptor subtypes appear to originate from different branches (here, histamin, dopamine, and angiotensin), indicating a possible convergent evolution during which receptors may have "picked up" ligands.

new potential drug targets will have to be clarified. In this connection, it should be noted that the physiological role and the pharmacological potential have as yet only been characterized to a reasonable degree for a few receptors, mainly due to a lack of useful, selective pharmacological tools. This is the case even for many of the subtypes of the well-known monoamine receptors.

2.3.2 Subtypes of Receptors that Bind the Same Ligand May Have Evolved for Several Reasons, Some of which Are Still Unclear

Many hormones and transmitters have several subtypes of receptors — and more subtypes than expected from classical physiological and pharmacological studies. Structurally, these subtypes of receptors may or may not be very similar. For example, most subtypes in the monoamine systems or, for example, the endothelin ET-A and ET-B receptors are more than 70 or 80% identical in their amino-acid sequence (Figure 2.4). On the other hand, some members of the four different histamine receptors and the five different neuropeptide Y (NPY) receptors are almost as distantly related to each other as they are to any other rhodopsin-like 7TM receptor (i.e., around 25–30% identity), which relates to the occurrence of generally conserved residues in the transmembrane regions. However, the different receptor subtypes, whether or not they are closely related in primary amino-acid sequence, usually all bind their natural ligand with high and similar affinity, and originally they were identified primarily by means of their different reactions with synthetic agonists or antagonists. In some cases, the functional significance of receptor subtypes is rather obvious; for example, receptor subtypes frequently give the transmitter or hormone the opportunity to couple through different G-proteins and thereby activate different effector systems. However, in many cases, the functional significance of receptor subclasses is more subtle — for example, where subtypes only display slight differences in desensitization properties or differences in their ability to be constitutively active (see discussion below).

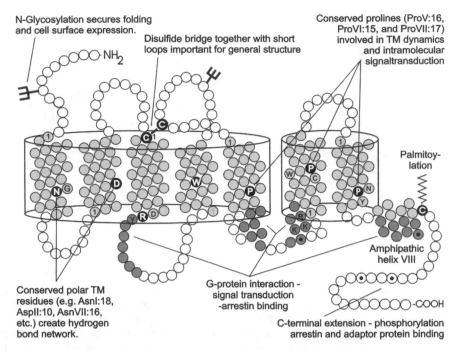

FIGURE 2.5 Some structural characteristics of the rhodopsin-like family A of 7TM receptors. Residues located in the transmembrane helices are shaded light gray. The subunits of the heterotrimeric G-proteins are believed to interact mainly with residues located in the intracellular segments, which are shaded dark gray. In each of the transmembrane segments, one or more residue is conserved among nearly all of the family members. These key transmembrane fingerprint residues are highlighted: AsnI:18, AspII:10, CysIII:01, ArgIII:26, TrpIV:06, ProV:16, ProVI:15, and ProVII:17. The structural and/or functional importance of selected parts of the receptor structure is indicated in the figure.

2.4 RHODOPSIN-LIKE 7TM RECEPTORS ARE THE QUANTITATIVELY DOMINANT FAMILY

The archetypal G-protein-coupled receptor is rhodopsin. A series of "fingerprint" residues, most of which are located within the transmembrane segments, have been conserved among the rhodopsin-like receptors, as indicated in Figure 2.5. These fingerprint residues are conserved in 95 to 98% of the receptors, and any given receptor will contain most of them.* Nevertheless, among all rhodopsin-like G-protein-coupled receptors there is no totally conserved residue. The most conserved one is ArgIII:26 located at the intracellular pole of TM-III in the DRY sequence (only lacking in a couple of receptors). This residue is believed to be involved in the signaling to the G-protein (see discussion below). Nevertheless, some structural features discriminate between subfamilies, for example, chemokine receptors from other rhodopsin-like receptors.

2.4.1 A CONSERVED DISULFIDE BRIDGE CREATES TWO EXTRA LOOPS FROM THE TOP OF TM-III

One of the most highly conserved features among 7TM receptors is the disulfide bridge between the Cys at the top of TM-III and a Cys situated somewhere in the middle of the second extracellular loop. This loop is thereby transformed into two loops connecting the top of TM-III with the top

---

* In this chapter, we are using a generic numbering/nomenclature system in which residues are referred to by a generic number corresponding to their position (for example, residue no. 10) in a given transmembrane helix (for example, TM-II:AspII:10) as suggested by Baldwin and modified slightly by Schwartz (see Further Reading).

of both TM-IV and TM-V. These two extra loops tie TM-IV and TM-V closely to TM-III, which generally is considered to be the central column in the seven-helical bundle. In rhodopsin, these loops form a β-sheet "lid" over the ligand-binding pocket where retinal is located (see Figures 2.1 and 2.2). In the MSH/adrenocorticotrophic hormone (ACTH) and the cannabinoid CB1 and CB2 receptors, this disulfide bridge is absent. However, in the case of the MSH/ACTH receptors, only two hydrophilic residues separate TM-IV and TM-V, which is just another way of holding TM-V closely together with the rest of the A-domain.

2.4.2 A NETWORK OF RELATIVELY SHORT AND WELL-CONSERVED LOOPS APPEARS TO DEFINE TWO INTRAMOLECULAR DOMAINS

Despite the fact that the amino-acid sequence of 7TM receptors is rather poorly conserved, especially outside the transmembrane segments, the *length* of most of the loops is surprisingly well conserved. The loops connecting TM-I and TM-II and those connecting TM-II and TM-III are short and of almost the same length in all rhodopsin-like receptors, despite great variance in actual amino-acid sequence (Figure 2.6). As discussed above, the conserved disulfide bridge creates two short

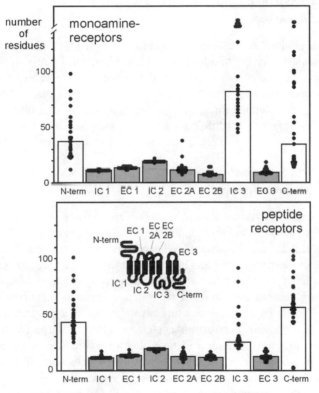

FIGURE 2.6 Length of the intra- and extracellular segments of rhodopsin-like family A receptors. The columns indicate the median length of intra- and extracellular segments from 29 human monoamine and 29 human peptide hormone or neuropeptide receptors. N-term, N-terminal extracellular extension; IC, intracellular loop; EC, extracellular loop; C-term, C-terminal intracellular extension. The highly conserved disulfide bridge from the extracellular end of TM-III to the middle of extracellular loop-2 (see Figure 2.2) divides this loop into two loops, designated EC2A and EC2B. Note how well-conserved most of the loops are in respect of the number of amino-acid residues, which is not the case for sequence identity, except for intracellular loop-3, which is longer than the rest and which varies highly in length among the receptors. This could indicate that the receptors are structurally and perhaps functionally composed of two domains: an A domain consisting of TM-I to TM-V and a B domain consisting of TM-VI and –VII, each connected by short, and in length but not sequence, well-conserved loops. (The figure is based on data presented in Nielsen, S. M. et al., *Eur. J. Biochem.*, 251, 217–226, 1998.)

loops, which tether TM-IV and TM-V closely together with the first three transmembrane segments. The two C-terminal transmembrane segments, TM-VI and TM-VII, are also connected by a short intracellular loop of approximately ten residues (Figure 2.6). However, the loop connecting TM-V and TM-VI is remarkably poorly conserved in respect to both sequence and length and is often relatively long, in some cases up to several hundred residues. Thus, it appears that the rhodopsin-like receptors are structurally composed of two intramolecular domains held together by a network of relatively short loops: an A-domain consisting of TM-I through TM-V and a B-domain consisting of TM-VI and TM-VII. In fact, the two hypothetical domains can form a fully functional split-receptor upon co-expression of two plasmids, each of which codes for one of the domains.

In rhodopsin, EPR studies have demonstrated a clear helical periodicity in most of intracellular loop-3, except for a couple of residues in the middle (indicated in Figure 2.5). This would suggest that TM-V and TM-VI extend way into the cytosol and that only a very short loop connects these two helical extensions. However, in the three-dimensional crystals, most of intracellular loop-3 is a rather unstructured loop. Thus, in this case, it is likely that the EPR studies tell us something about the "solution" structure of the receptor, which may not be clear in the x-ray structure.

2.4.3 SOME RECEPTORS HAVE DISULFIDE-RICH, LIGAND-BINDING, N-TERMINAL DOMAINS

The N-terminal extracellular segment is quite variable both in length and sequence. In the subfamily of receptors that binds the glycoprotein hormones TSH, FSH, and LH/chorionic gonadotropin, this segment is very long and contains a set of conserved cysteines, which are expected to form a network of disulfide bridges, thus creating a well-defined, globular domain that is homologous to a transcription factor with a well-defined three-dimensional structure. In this subfamily of receptors, the glycoprotein hormones obtain most of their binding energy by interaction with the large N-terminal domain, which in some cases, even in a truncated soluble form, is capable of binding the hormone.

2.4.4 GLYCOSYLATION IS IMPORTANT FOR PROTEIN FOLDING AND INTRACELLULAR TRANSPORT

Nearly all 7TM receptors are glycosylated. Usually several Asn–X–Thr/Ser recognition sequences for N-linked glycosylation are found in the amino-terminal segment but occasionally also elsewhere. The glycosylation is not directly important for ligand binding or receptor function. However, as is the case for most other membrane proteins expressed at the cell surface, the glycosylation appears to be a post-translational modification, which through recognition by a specific protein in the endoplasmic reticulum, calnexin, ensures that the protein is retained in the cellular export machinery until it is correctly folded. To what degree calnexin functions as a chaperone, "foldase," or just a retention protein is still unclear. For many receptors, a relatively large fraction of the molecules never make it to the plasma membrane in heterologous expression systems. Certain synthetic ligands, referred to as molecular or pharmacological chaperones, can, through diffusion into the endoplasmic reticulum, bind and stabilize such newly synthesized receptors and help bring them to the cell surface. Such compounds could become useful (orphan) drugs to treat diseases caused by mutations in 7TM receptors leading to malfolding and lack of surface expression of otherwise functional receptors, such as, for example, in the case of diabetes insipidus.

2.4.5 CONSERVED PROLINE RESIDUES IN THE TRANSMEMBRANES MAY BE OF FUNCTIONAL IMPORTANCE

Because the pyrolidine ring of the amino acid proline involves the backbone nitrogen, it prevents the formation of one of the stabilizing hydrogen bonds in the α-helix backbone. Thus, prolines rarely occur in α-helices in globular proteins. Nevertheless, proline residues are among the well-conserved fingerprint residues in several of the transmembrane helices. In bacteriorhodopsin,

rhodopsin, and other membrane proteins, prolines in several but not all cases cause a kink in the transmembrane helix. The conserved prolines in TM-V, TM-VI, and TM-VII of the 7TM receptors will create "weak points" in these helices. Thus, it may be speculated that the conserved proline residues serve an important role in the dynamic function of the receptors, possibly by facilitating the interchange between different conformations and/or by allowing the otherwise very stable transmembrane helices to "wobble" in order for ligands and G-protein subunits to associate and dissociate. In this respect, particular attention has been paid to ProVI:15 in TM-VI in regard to its crucial involvement in the activation process. However, the highly conserved ProVII:17 in TM-VII is very likely also to be involved in this process.

2.4.6   Interhelical Constrains through Hydrogen-Bond Networks and Other Nonhydrophobic Interactions

Just like soluble proteins, the packing of rhodopsin and membrane proteins generally occurs through hydrophobic interactions in the core of the molecule. However, the x-ray structure of rhodopsin confirmed the assumption that a series of relatively well-conserved polar residues (for example, AsnI:18, AspII:10, and AsnVII:18), often together with intercalated water molecules, form a hydrogen-bond network in the center of the receptor. In several receptors, cations (especially Na^+) will modulate the binding affinity of the agonist, presumably through an interaction with this hydrogen-bond network located relatively deep in the middle of the receptor, facing toward the intracellular surface of the membrane. As most ligands bind either to the exterior part of the receptor or in between the outer parts of the transmembrane segments, depending on the size and chemical structure of the ligand (see below), the effect of the cations is considered to be allosteric in nature.

2.4.7   An Intracellular Amphipathic Helix Connects TM-VII to the Palmitoylation Site

In the x-ray structure of rhodopsin, an amphipathic helix runs parallel to the membrane from the intracellular end of TM-VII beneath the seven-helical bundle to the other side of TM-I and TM-II. At this point, one or more Cys residues are often found and are known to be subject to a dynamic posttranslational modification with palmitic acid residues. Like the phosphorylation event, the palmitoylation process appears to be dynamically regulated by receptor occupancy and is also involved in the desensitization phenomenon. The two posttranslational modifications can influence each other. For example, the conformational constraint induced by palmitoylation may alter the accessibility of certain phosphorylation sites. Like the phosphorylation process, the functional consequences of palmitoylation also appear to vary from receptor to receptor.

2.4.8   Agonist-Dependent Phosphorylation Alters Interaction with Intracellular Proteins

As described in more detail below, agonist binding will lead to signaling as well as phosphorylation of Ser and Thr residues, especially, but also, in selected cases, Tyr residues located in intracellular loop-3 and in the C-terminal extension. This post-translational modification alters the affinity of the receptor for various intracellular proteins, including arrestin, which sterically prevents further G-protein binding and functions as an adaptor protein. Also, interaction with other types of scaffolding proteins such as PSD-95-like proteins, is influenced by the phosphorylation state of the receptor.

2.5   FAMILY B IS A DISTINCT FAMILY OF GLUCAGON/VIP/CALCITONIN 7TM RECEPTORS

Receptors for a series of peptide hormones and neuropeptides constitute a separate family of G-protein-coupled receptors often called family B, members of which are devoid of the classical

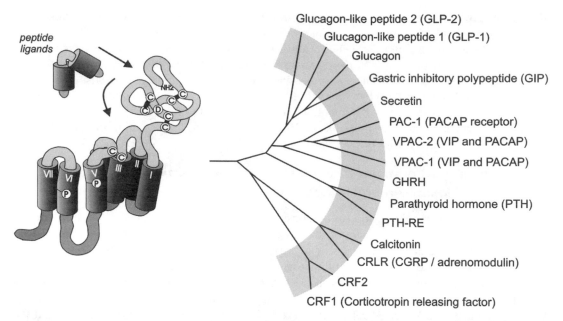

FIGURE 2.7 The glucagon/VIP/calcitonin family B of 7TM receptors. To the right is an evolutionary tree for the receptors of this family. The shaded area indicates 70% sequence identity. The two-helical conformation of the ligand indicates that several of the peptide ligands for family B receptors appear to have a common secondary structure at low water activity, as determined by NMR experiments. Only a few of the common fingerprint residues of this family are indicated in the serpentine model. Note that members of this family do not share any of the transmembrane fingerprint residues of the rhodopsin-like family; however, they do have the potential to form a disulfide bridge from the top of TM-III and the middle of extracellular loop-2. As rhodopsin-like receptors, members of family B also have conserved prolines in their transmembranes, but not at positions corresponding to the prolines of family A.

fingerprint residues of rhodopsin-like receptors. This family includes receptors for hormones involved in calcium metabolism (calcitonin and parathyroid hormone [PTH]), glucose metabolism (glucagon, glucagon-like peptide I [GLP-I]), gastrointestinal-tract function (secretin, gastric inhibitory polypeptide [GIP], GLP-II), as well as neurohormones involved in pituitary function (growth-hormone-releasing factor [GHRH], ACTH-releasing factor [CRF]), and important neuropeptides (vasoactive intestinal polypeptide [VIP], pituitary adenylate cyclase stimulatory peptide [PACAP]) (Figure 2.7). In view of the physiological importance of these peptides, it is likely that receptors of this family will become major targets for the development of nonpeptide drugs in the years to come.

Besides their seven transmembrane segments, the most conspicuous common feature among these receptors is their large extracellular N-terminal domain. This segment contains a set of six conserved Cys residues, conceivably interconnected by a number of disulfide bridges, thus forming a globular domain supposedly involved in ligand binding. Two more Cys residues, at the top of TM-III and in the middle of extracellular loop-2, are also conserved and could form a disulfide bridge similar to the one found in the rhodopsin-like receptors. The first extracellular loop is variable in length and can be up to 30 residues long. As in the large rhodopsin-like family, a number of proline residues are conserved in the transmembrane segments of family B receptors (Figure 2.7). However, in this family the prolines are located in TM-IV, TM-V, and TM-VI and not in TM-VII. In TM-V and TM-VI, the prolines are located at different positions from the conserved prolines of the rhodopsin-like receptors. All receptors from this family stimulate adenylate cyclase and, therefore, couple through a G_s protein. The coupling mechanism including the G_s molecule appears to be shared with rhodopsin-like receptors, despite the lack of sequence homology.

2.5.1 THE PHARMACOLOGICAL PHENOTYPE OF CERTAIN FAMILY B RECEPTORS IS DETERMINED BY INTERACTION WITH RAMPs

Members of a small family of one-transmembrane proteins function as receptor activity modifying proteins (RAMPs), which interact with certain receptors from family B: the calcitonin receptor and the calcitonin receptor-like receptor (CRLR). RAMPs serve two purposes. In the case of CRLR, they function as chaperones, ensuring that the receptor is targeted at the cell membrane instead of accumulating in the endoplasmic reticulum. Second, CRLR in complex with RAMP-1 functions as a calcitonin gene-related peptide (CGRP) receptor, whereas CRLR in complex with RAMP-2 functions as a receptor for another messenger peptide, adrenomodulin. The calcitonin receptor arrives at the cell surface on its own and here binds the hormone calcitonin. However, when it is expressed in cells that also express RAMP-1, the calcitonin receptor instead functions as an amylin receptor. For the moment, it appears that the RAMPs we know today are rather selective for the calcitonin and the CRLR receptors. However, observations of these receptors clearly demonstrate that the molecular, pharmacological phenotype of a given receptor can be dramatically influenced by its interaction with other protein partners (see later discussion on dimerization and scaffolding/adaptor proteins).

2.5.2 MEMBERS OF A SUBFAMILY OF FAMILY B RECEPTORS ARE STRUCTURALLY SIMILAR TO CELL ADHESION MOLECULES

A large number of orphan receptors (approximately 40), due to the occurrence of conserved residues in their seven-helical domains, clearly belong to family B and are characterized by having very large N-terminal extracellular domains. Instead of the characteristic peptide–hormone/neuropeptide-binding domain, the N-terminal segments of these receptors are classically composed of, for example, a number of epidermal growth factor (EGF) domains placed on a mucin-like stalk, as in the EMR-1, EMR-2, and EMR-3 and CD97 receptors. However, the N-terminal extension of lactophilin, for example, is decorated by other cell adhesion domains such as lectin-like domains. Only in a few cases has the ligand or partner for these presumed cell adhesion/receptor molecules been identified. For example, the CD97 receptor has been shown to specifically interact with CD55, which is not the case for the homologous EMRs. Many of these cell adhesion/receptor molecules are expressed on leukocytes, but some are also expressed, for example, in the CNS.

2.6 A THIRD FAMILY OF METABOTROPIC GLUTAMATE RECEPTORS AND CHEMOSENSORS

Members of a third, structurally distinct family of G-protein-coupled receptors, family C, bind either glutamate or GABA, or they act as chemical sensors for calcium ions or taste components (Figure 2.3). Glutamate and GABA are important amino-acid transmitters in the nervous system, reacting both with ligand-gated ion channels (see Chapters 3 and 6) and with a series of G-protein-coupled receptors called metabotropic glutamate receptors and GABA$_B$ receptors. Among the chemical sensors known to couple through G-proteins, the calcium sensors of the parathyroid and the kidney are homologous to the metabotropic glutamate receptors. Structurally, these receptors are characterized by having a very large N-terminal extracellular segment (500 to 600 residues) and frequently also a similarly large intracellular C-terminal domain separated by the seven transmembrane segments. The transmembrane segments are connected by short loops and differ in sequence totally from the two other families presented above. Interestingly, some of the most detailed information available concerns the structure of members of family C as compared to other 7TM receptors, in respect to ligand binding, receptor activation, receptor dimerization, and interaction with scaffolding/adaptor proteins (see later discussion).

2.6.1 THE X-RAY STRUCTURE OF THE LIGAND-BINDING EXTRACELLULAR DOMAIN OF mGLUR1 IS KNOWN WITH AND WITHOUT GLUTAMATE

The large extracellular domain of family C receptors is structurally related to a family of bacterial binding proteins that function as transporters for amino acids and other small molecules across the periplasmic space. X-ray structural analysis has demonstrated that glutamate in the mGluR1 binds in an interdomain crevice between the so-called LB1 and LB2 domains in a manner similar to, for example, amino acids binding in the bacterial transport proteins (Figure 2.8). The binding is dominated by interaction with polar residues in LB1 and LB2, which are brought into close proximity by closure of the crevice between LB1 and LB2 — the two domains "sandwich" the ligand. In the disulfide-connected dimer, each monomer binds a glutamate. Not only is ligand binding associated with a conformational change within each monomer (the closure of the ligand binding crevice in the bi-lobed extracellular domain), but a major conformational change also occurs between the two protomers as the two LB2s are brought, on average, 26 Å closer to each other upon ligand binding. Due to concomitant rotation, residues are present in the two LB2s that, in the inactive, unliganded form, are 43 Å apart and, in the glutamate-bound form, are found almost touching each other (Figure 2.8). In fact, two unligated crystal structures were determined, and one of these was almost identical to the glutamate-bound form in respect to interdomain and intersubunit interactions, indicating that the receptor can adopt the active conformation by itself. Thus, it appears that the receptor is in a dynamic equilibrium between an open and a closed form, between the ligand-binding domains within each monomer, and between the two monomers of the disulfide-linked dimer. The agonist ligand appears to act merely by stabilizing the closed, active conformation, which the receptor adopts by itself (see discussion below concerning generality of this theme). It could be envisioned that the two seven-helical bundles of each monomer (which are not yet part of the x-ray structure) are being held apart in the unligated open form but are brought close to each other in the active, closed form. Such a structural rearrangement of monomers within a preformed dimer is also found in the one-transmembrane cytokine receptor system as described for the erythropoietin receptor, where ligand binding in a very similar manner results in a closure of a spatial gap between the transmembrane segments and conceivably the intracellular, enzyme-linked domains.

2.7 7TM RECEPTORS UNDERGO DIMER- AND OLIGOMERIZATION

Much biochemical evidence shows that many if not all 7TM receptors have a strong tendency to aggregate both with themselves and with other 7TM receptors, as most clearly seen in multiple high-molecular-weight bands on sodium dodecyl sulfate (SDS) gels. These bands are by no means restricted to dimers as, in most cases, several higher order oligomeric structures are observed. This is an important point to consider when the functional correlation of dimer formation is addressed in non-family C receptors.

2.7.1 FAMILY C RECEPTORS FUNCTION AS HOMO- OR HETERODIMERS

Structural and functional evidence clearly demonstrates that family C receptors function as dimers, either as homodimers or as heterodimers. The metabotropic glutamate receptors and the calcium sensors, as discussed in Section 2.6.1, are found as covalently connected dimers in which there is a disulfide bridge between a Cys residue located in a loop in the N-terminal extracellular domain of each monomer. This disulfide bridge apparently serves only to hold the monomers in close proximity, as the loop is so unstructured that it does not resolve in the x-ray structure.

The GABA$_B$ receptor is not a single 7TM receptor but rather a heterodimer formed by two 7TM receptors from family C. The GABA$_B$-R1 receptor, which was initially cloned, binds the ligand GABA, but when expressed alone it is to a large extent retained in the endoplasmic reticulum,

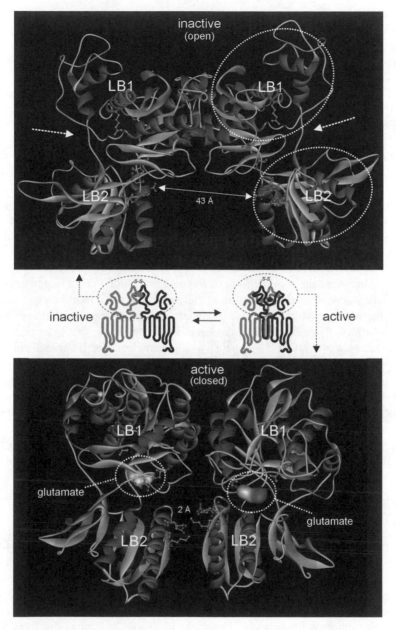

FIGURE 2.8 The active (bottom) and inactive (top) structure of the extracellular domain of the metabotropic glutamate mGluR1 receptor from family C. A schematic serpentine diagram indicates the basic equilibrium of the full receptor between active and inactive conformations and the location of the part of the receptor that has been structurally characterized with and without the bound ligand, glutamate. Family B receptors generally function as dimers — in the case of the mGluRs, as disulfide-linked dimers, as indicated. The ligand-binding domain of each is a "fly-trap" made up of two smaller domains, LB1 and LB2, which are found in an open configuration in the inactive state but close around and are stabilized by the glutamate ligand in the active state. Note the considerable conformational changes, which occur not only within but also between the two extracellular domains of the dimer. A few residues that are more than 40 Å apart in the inactive state but which face each other directly in the active state are indicated. The conformational change between the two parts of the dimer in the mGluR1 is rather similar to the conformational change that occurs between the monomers of the erythropoietin receptor upon activation, which brings the transmembrane and intracellular domains into closer contact.

it signals poorly, and it does not give the appropriate pharmacological profile. In contrast, the GABA$_B$-R2 receptor does not bind the ligand by itself, but this receptor functions as a chaperone that secures the cell-surface expression of the GABA$_B$-R1 subunit. The heterodimer displays the correct pharmacological profile corresponding to the GABA$_B$ receptor from the CNS and it signals as the natural GABA$_B$ receptor through potassium channels, which is not the case for the monomer. This signaling is, interestingly, mediated through the R2 subunit. The structural basis for dimer formation in the GABA$_B$ receptor is mainly a coil–coil structure formed between segments of the C-terminal tails of the R1 and R2 subunits

2.7.2 THE FUNCTIONAL SIGNIFICANCE OF DIMERIZATION IS MORE UNCLEAR AMONG RHODOPSIN-LIKE RECEPTORS

For most members of family A, in contrast to family C receptors, it has been difficult to prove that dimerization, or rather oligomerization, has a functional consequence and that it is, as a general phenomenon, closely associated with the activation process as such. There is no doubt that homo- and hetero-oligomerization of 7TM receptors is a common phenomenon as demonstrated by, for example, co-immunoprecipitation using various appropriate controls. Several studies using light-resonance energy transfer (either in the form of fluorescence [FRET] or bioluminescence [BRET]) have convincingly shown that such homo- and hetero-oligomers are found on the surface of intact living cells in the absence of ligands; that is, dimers/oligomers are constitutively formed. Note, however, that no effect of inverse agonists has been demonstrated for this phenomenon. The effect of agonists on the constitutive FRET or BRET signals is unclear, and it varies from study to study and from receptor system to receptor system. Nevertheless, in several receptor systems, heterodimerization/-oligomerization has been observed, with pharmacological profiles being different from the profiles observed in homo-oligomers expressed in the same heterologous expression system.

The prototype family A receptor, rhodopsin itself, clearly functions as a monomer despite its occurrence in very high density in the light-sensitive membranes; however, it could be argued that rhodopsin should not be used as an example for receptors in general as it has very special requirements in respect to signaling due to its function as an ultra-rapid light sensor.

2.8 7TM RECEPTORS ARE IN A DYNAMIC EQUILIBRIUM BETWEEN ACTIVE AND INACTIVE CONFORMATIONS

The crystal structures of the mGluR1 clearly demonstrate that activation of a 7TM receptor can occur through a major conformational interchange between two protomers within a preformed dimer. This could possibly represent the activation mechanism for 7TM receptors in general. But, it is believed that a conformational change within the seven-helical bundle is associated with receptor activation, which obviously is essential in those receptors that function as monomers, which could be the majority. Importantly, the series of mGluR1 structures did show that the active conformation is not induced by ligand binding *per se*, but that even very substantial conformational changes can occur spontaneously. Thus, the active conformation of the receptor is not induced by the ligand; the receptor can fold into the active conformation by itself. The receptor is a dynamic membrane protein that exists naturally in equilibrium between inactive and active conformations.

If a fraction of the receptor population at any given time is in the active conformation without any ligand present, then 7TM receptors should display some degree of constitutive signaling activity. That is, in fact, the case. In cells transfected with 7TM receptors, the level of the appropriate intracellular second messenger is generally increased, without any agonist present (Figure 2.9). Furthermore, the higher the expression level of the receptor, the higher is the intracellular level of second messenger. The degree of constitutive activity varies from receptor to receptor. Some receptors, such as the virally encoded 7TM oncogene ORF74, can show up to 50% constitutive activity. In other receptors, the degree of constitutive activity is so low that it is

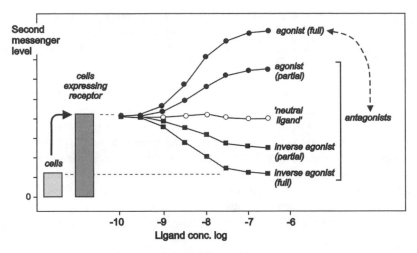

FIGURE 2.9 Agonism vs. inverse agonism and antagonism. The increased level of second messenger in cells expressing a 7TM receptor is shown. This constitutive signaling activity can range from unmeasurable to 50% or more of the maximal signaling capacity, depending upon the receptor and the number of receptors expressed by the cells. Agonism and inverse agonism are properties of the ligand itself in its interaction with the receptor. *Agonists* will increase the level of second messenger further, whereas *inverse agonists* will decrease the spontaneously increased level of second messenger back to the level of untransfected cells. Ligands that show less signaling efficacy than the full agonist (i.e., partial agonists and inverse agonists) will function as *antagonists* in competition for receptor occupancy with the full agonist (note that antagonism is not a property of a ligand by itself on the receptor). Neutral ligands are often, but not necessarily, also antagonists.

almost impossible to demonstrate. In the nicotinic acetylcholine receptor, a ligand-gated ion channel, it is estimated that only one in a million receptors at a given time is in the active conformation without ligand present. Such a low degree of constitutive activity would not be detectable in a 7TM receptor. Nevertheless, 7TM receptors are, like ligand-gated ion channels and most other proteins, allosteric proteins that obey the basic principle of the concerted type of allostery of Monod, Wyman, and Changeux; that is, they interchange between different conformations which can be stabilized by ligands.

2.8.1 AGONISM AND INVERSE AGONISM ARE THE BASIC PROPERTIES OF LIGANDS ALONE ON THE RECEPTOR

In a system where the receptor is in a dynamic equilibrium between an active and an inactive form, a ligand that binds to the receptor will shift this equilibrium to one side, depending on the relative affinity of the compound for either the active or the inactive conformation. Thus, a ligand called an *agonist* will either increase the signaling if it has highest affinity for the active conformation or decrease the signaling activity if it has highest affinity for an inactive conformation; the ligand is then called an *inverse agonist* (Figure 2.9). A ligand that has equal affinity for the active and inactive conformation, which is not very often observed, will not shift the equilibrium and will accordingly not change the signaling and is called a *neutral ligand* (or *neutral antagonist*). Thus, agonism and inverse agonism are properties of a ligand alone on the receptor, whereas antagonism is a property observed with a ligand in the presence of an agonist. In the presence of a full agonist, inverse agonists, neutral ligands, and partial agonists will, when competing for occupancy of the receptor with the full agonist, bring the signaling down to the activity observed with these ligands alone, and they will accordingly all function as antagonists. In fact, neutral ligands, in general, will also antagonize the effect of inverse agonists and bring the signaling back up to the normal constitutive level.

It should be noted that inverse agonism can only be appreciated in receptor systems where the constitutive activity is measurable and therefore can be observed to decrease. Thus, neutral antagonists and inverse agonists can only be differentiated in a system where the receptor demonstrates constitutive activity. In the *in vivo* setting, the natural agonist will most often be present, and for all practical purposes it is difficult to differentiate between inverse agonism and the effect on spontaneous activity caused by a tone of the endogenous ligand on the receptor.

In mathematical models used to explain observed binding and activity relationships, these phenomena are described in the so-called allosteric ternary complex model of Lefkowitz and Costa and subsequent versions of this. According to these models, the principal signaling form of the receptor is the one that occurs in the ternary complex consisting of the agonist, the receptor, and the G-protein. Both agonist and G-protein will have high affinity for an "isomerized" form of the receptor. It is important to note that in 7TM receptors, agonists will have a significantly lower affinity for the G-protein-uncoupled form of the receptor; that is, they bind in a G-protein-dependent way. It is becoming increasingly clear that antagonists, in fact, have the highest affinity for the G-protein-uncoupled conformation of the receptor. In other words, agonists and antagonists bind preferentially to distinct and complementary conformational populations of their common receptor target.

2.8.2 MUTATIONS OFTEN SHIFT THE EQUILIBRIUM TOWARD THE ACTIVE CONFORMATION

Apparently, structural constraints keep the 7TM receptor in an inactive conformation that prevents the productive interaction between sequences in the cytoplasmic parts of the transmembrane segments and intracellular loops and the G-protein. Disruption of these constraints will shift the equilibrium toward the active conformation and cause spontaneous or constitutive activity. Thus, in some receptors it is clear that the receptor is very easily shifted toward the active, signaling conformation, as many different experimentally induced mutations will result in increased constitutive signaling. For example, in some monoamine receptors introduction at certain positions just below TM-VI of any of the 19 amino-acid residues other than the one chosen by evolution will increase the constitutive activity above the normal level. Although certain hot spots for the location of mutations lead to high constitutive activity (for example, the Asp in the DRY sequence), such activating mutations have been found all over the 7TM receptor structure, including the extracellular loops. In general, the active signaling form of the receptor is rather unstable, which has been observed directly in fluorescently labeled receptors and is also reflected in the low surface expression levels of constitutively active mutants.

Mutations that shift the equilibrium toward the constitutively active form will often cause disease. For example, activating mutations in the TSH or LH receptors are responsible for the development of thyroid adenomas and the development of puberty in small children, respectively. In the case of the thyroid adenomas, a normal TSH receptor is expressed in the surrounding normal thyroid tissue.

2.8.3 TM-VI ESPECIALLY APPEARS TO UNDERGO MAJOR CONFORMATIONAL CHANGES UPON RECEPTOR ACTIVATION

Several different types of biochemical and biophysical evidence indicate that TM-VI is performing the most crucial conformational change during agonist-induced receptor activation. For example, EPR experiments using systematically introduced spin labels have demonstrated that the intracellular end of TM-VI moves out and away from the center of the receptor. Evidence also indicates that helix VI may undergo a counterclockwise rotation during this movement. TM-VI only interacts with TM-II, TM-III, and TM-V through van der Waals interactions and not hydrogen-bond interactions. Moreover, the cytoplasmic part of TM-VI below the well-conserved ProVI:15 is not packed very efficiently to the neighboring transmembrane segments. Thus, the energy barrier for a rigid-body movement of this part of TM-VI away from the helical bundle is not as large as generally imagined in a densely packed protein. It has been suggested that ProVI:15 is crucial for the

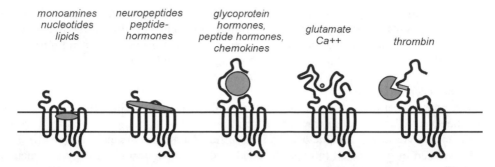

FIGURE 2.10 Overview of different patterns of ligand binding to 7TM receptors shown schematically in two-dimensional serpentine models. There appear to be multiple different ways for ligands to bind and activate 7TM receptors, conceivably because these agonists primarily serve only to stabilize an active conformation, which the receptor can fold into by itself (see Figure 2.8 and the text). In the thrombin receptor, shown to the right, the enzyme cleaves the N-terminal segment and thereby reveals an oligopeptide (gray box), which then activates the receptor while it is still covalently tethered to the transmembrane domain.

activation mechanism and that the movement of TM-VI occurs around this weak point, or joint, in the helix.

Through the suggested movement of TM-VI, a space is generated between TM-III and TM-VI that could be envisioned to be an important interaction site for part of the G-protein, which interacts with the intracellular ends of TM-III, TM-V, and TM-VI, as well as the horizontal helix VIII (see Figure 2.5). Binding of the G-protein is obviously known to induce the high-affinity agonist binding state of 7TM receptors in general. The binding of arrestin, somewhat surprisingly, like the G-protein, also induces a high-affinity agonist-binding state, and so it could be envisioned that arrestin is able to occupy some of the same space in the intracellular part of the receptor as the G-protein. This space could be between TM-III and TM-VI, thereby stabilizing a similar active conformation of the receptor, which nevertheless cannot signal because the G-protein is prevented from binding by the presence of arrestin.

2.9 7TM RECEPTORS Have Multiple Agonist Binding Modes

It was initially believed that there would be a common "lock" in all the homologous 7TM receptors, corresponding to the initially identified monoamine-binding site, into which all agonists in some way would fit. It was envisioned that in the different 7TM receptors this lock had, during evolution, been specifically equipped to recognize the specific agonists. However, as shown schematically in Figure 2.10, mutational analysis and cross-linking experiments have demonstrated that the chemically very different ligands apparently bind in rather different fashions. Unfortunately, most of our knowledge on ligand–receptor interactions is still based on loss-of-function experiments (i.e., mutations or substitutions that impair binding or coupling). Very few of these presumed points of interaction have in fact been studied in greater detail using alternative, supplementary methods.

2.9.1 RETINAL, MONOAMINES, AND OTHER SMALL MESSENGERS BIND BETWEEN THE TRANSMEMBRANE SEGMENTS

Binding of these ligands does not occur in a "concave groove" located on the surface of the receptor protein as otherwise often imagined. As described in Section 2.2.1, the x-ray structure of rhodopsin showed that retinal is bound deep in the seven-helical structure with major interaction points in TM-III and TM-VI, as well as the covalent attachment point in TM-VII. In fact, rhodopsin interacts with basically all transmembrane segments. Importantly, side-chains from the transmembrane helices cover the retinal molecule on all sides, and its binding site is found deep in the middle of the protein, covered by a plug of well-ordered extracellular loops (Figures 2.1 and 2.2). Thus, major movements of significant parts of the receptor will have to occur in order for the ligand to move in or out of its binding site, which does occurs because the "back-isomerization" of retinal occurs in another cell. This is rather analogous to the binding of steroid hormones and other ligands in nuclear receptors, where a long, well-ordered helix covers the binding pocket located almost in the middle of the receptor protein.

Monoamines appear to bind in a manner rather similar to that of retinal. In the catecholamine systems, the specific and direct interaction of the amine group of the ligand with the carboxylic group of a totally conserved aspartic acid residue in transmembrane segment III (AspIII:08) has been substantiated in great detail through the combined use of molecular biology and medicinal chemistry. The interaction was probed both by destroying the binding and activation of the receptor by mutating the Asp to a Ser (converting the carboxylic acid to a hydroxyl group) and by destroying the binding of the ligand by changing the amine to a ketone or an ester. In contrast to the wild-type receptor, the mutant receptor, which had a serine residue introduced in place of the aspartate in TM-III, bound ligands with high affinity when ketones or esters replaced the amine. In other words, the specific interaction between the amine and the carboxylic-acid group of the receptor can be exchanged by another type of chemical interaction through an intelligent, complementary modification of both the ligand and the receptor.

Thus, the currently favored picture of the binding of isoproterenol to the β-adrenergic receptor is that the ligand binds in a pocket centered between TM-III, TM-V, and TM-VI. The amine of the ligand interacts with the carboxylic-acid group of the conserved Asp in TM-III, whereas the catechol ring is oriented through hydrogen-bond interactions with two serine residues at the extracellular end of TM-V. The ring itself undergoes an aromatic–aromatic interaction with a phenylalanine residue in TM-VI located one helical turn below an Asn, which leads to hydrogen-bond interaction with the β-hydroxy group (Figure 2.11). Acetylcholine, histamine, dopamine, serotonin, and the other amines are believed to bind in a similar fashion by interacting with residues located at corresponding and/or neighboring positions in their target receptors. The amine interaction point, AspIII:08, is conserved among all monoamine receptors and is also found in, for example, opioid, somatostatin, and MCH receptors.

2.9.2 PEPTIDES BIND IN SEVERAL MODES WITH MAJOR INTERACTION SITES IN THE EXTERIOR SEGMENTS

The large glycoprotein hormones, such as TSH and LH, achieve most of their binding energy by interaction with the large N-terminal segment of their receptors. Medium- and small-size neuropeptides and peptide hormones such as substance P and angiotensin usually also have major points of interaction located in the N-terminal segment of their receptors, but with additional essential contact points in the loops and in the outer portion of the transmembrane segments. These contact points, which are scattered in the primary structure, appear to be located in relatively close spatial proximity in a folded model of the receptor (Figure 2.12). In some cases, contact points for peptides are also located more deeply in the receptor. For example, angiotensin appears to interact with a Lys residue in position V:05. Mutations have in some studies indicated that large peptides such as NPY should interact with residues deep in the middle of the receptor, even more deeply located than the monoamine-binding pocket; however, it is likely that such mutational hits are influencing the binding of the peptide indirectly. For smaller peptides such as TRH, it appears that most of their interaction points are located more closely to where the contact points for the monoamines are found: in the same deep pocket part of the main ligand-binding crevice of the receptor.

The protease activated receptors PAR-1 to PAR-4, of which PAR-1 is the thrombin receptor and PAR-2 conceivably a Factor-VIIa receptor, are particularly interesting cases. The ligands for these receptors are part of the N-terminal extension of the receptor. The enzyme (for example, thrombin) will bind and cleave off most of this extracellular segment and thereby reveal a new,

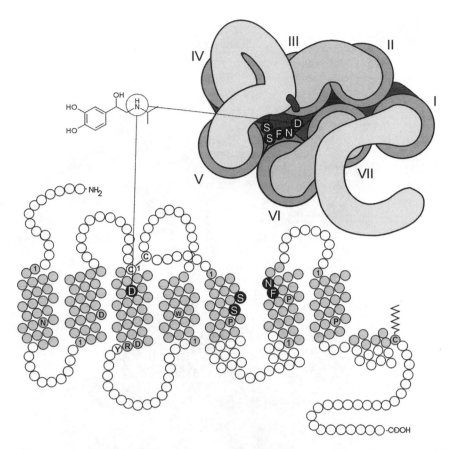

FIGURE 2.11 Binding site for catecholamines in the adrenergic receptors. The main contact residues for the agonist isoproterenol are indicated in white on black The monoamine *agonist* is believed to interact mainly with AspIII:08, SerV:09, SerV:12, PheVI:17, and AsnVI:20. The indicated interaction between the amine group of the ligand and the carboxylic-acid group of AspIII:08 has convincingly been demonstrated by combined modifications of the receptor by mutagenesis and complementary modifications of the ligand performed by medicinal chemistry. (From Strader, C. D. et al., *J. Biol. Chem.,* 266, 5–8, 1991. With permission.)

free N-terminus, a small pentapeptide of which is still covalently bound to the rest of the receptor. This small, tethered peptide "ligand" will activate the receptor by binding primarily to other parts of the exterior domain of the receptor, including the rest of the now-truncated N-terminal segment (Figure 2.10). Thus, this receptor has a shielded or caged peptide ligand already covalently tethered to the N-terminal extension. It could be imagined that several other peptide ligands (for example, in the chemokine family or the glucagon GLP-1 family) act as "pseudo-tethered" ligands. They would, through an initial binding to the N-terminal segment of their target receptors, become tethered and then, through secondary interactions with the main domain of the receptor, complete the activation process.

2.9.3 Nonpeptide Agonists Bind in the Deep Part of the Main Ligand-Binding Crevice

Not many nonpeptide agonists are yet available, but such compounds have been described — for example, in the angiotensin, CCK, and opioid receptor systems. In fact, for a few receptors, such as the somatostatin, ghrelin, and complement C5A receptors, basically all compounds found by screening using binding assays are agonists. In contrast, for the majority of receptors for which

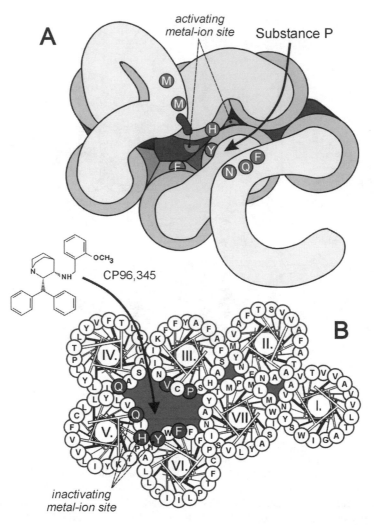

FIGURE 2.12 Different binding site for agonists and nonpeptide antagonist in the NK-1 (substance P) receptor. (A) The presumed contact points for the natural *agonist,* substance P, are indicated in white on gray circles located in the more extracellular part of the main ligand-binding crevice. The location of two residues, which when mutated into metal-ion binding residues can form an activating metal-ion switch, are pointed out to be located one helical turn below two interaction points for the peptide agonist in TM-III and TM-VII, respectively. Thus, agonism by ligands appears to be obtained mainly through stabilization of an active conformation between the outer segments of TM-III, TM-VI, and TM-VII. (B) The helical wheel diagram shows the presumed contact residues for the quinuclidine nonpeptide antagonist CP96,345 in white on gray located in the deep pocket of the main ligand-binding crevice. This binding site can structurally and functionally also be turned into an antagonistic metal-ion switch through introduction of metal-ion binding residues, as indicated. Note the considerable difference in the binding site for the agonists and antagonists, which in the case of the antagonistic metal-ion site has no overlap. This indicates that the ligands act as "allosteric competitive" ligands, competing for binding to the receptor by binding to different sites displayed in different conformations of the receptor: an active conformation and one of the many inactive conformations, respectively (see also Figure 2.8). In this way, binding of one ligand excludes the binding of the other type. (Part A from Holst, B. et al., *Mol. Pharmacol.*, 58, 263–270, 2000. With permission. Part B from Elling, C. E. et al., *Nature*, 374, 74–77, 1995. With permission.)

compounds are found in this way, they are antagonists. The reason for this is not known. No detailed mapping studies of nonpeptide agonists have demonstrated the actual binding pocket, but it is clear that the map of mutational hits is far from coinciding with that of the corresponding peptide agonist and that the nonpeptide agonists appear to bind in the seven-helical bundle. Such an allosteric binding and activation mechanism has most clearly been demonstrated for nonpeptide agonists for metabotropic glutamate receptors and calcium sensors, where glutamate or calcium binds out in the extracellular domain, whereas the small nonpeptide agonists activate these receptors by binding in the seven-helical bundle. For the substance P NK-1 receptor, an activating metal-ion switch has been built between TM-III and TM-VII (residues III:08 and VII:06) without affecting substance P binding and activation (Figure 2.12). In this case, it is also clear that the same receptor can be activated either by binding of the peptide up at the loops and extracellular ends of the helices or by the small, well-defined metal-ion binding deep between the helices, which fits well with the allosteric activation mechanism described above.

2.10 ANTAGONIST MAY BIND LIKE THE AGONISTS OR THEY MAY BIND VERY DIFFERENTLY

Originally it was believed that competitive antagonists would bind to the same site as the agonists and function simply by hindering the binding of the agonist to the receptor; however, it is clear today that antagonists, whether or not they behave in a classical competitive manner, may act independently of the agonist. Most if not all antagonists are inverse agonists, which is a property in itself independent of the presence of an agonist, as the ligand inhibits the constitutive activity of the receptor and therefore does not just hinder the access of the agonist to the receptor. In agreement with this, it is not surprising that antagonists often have binding sites of their own, which may or may not coincide with that of the corresponding agonist.

2.10.1 MONOAMINE ANTAGONISTS OFTEN BIND CLOSE TO WHERE THE AGONIST BINDS (ISOSTERICALLY)

Many antagonists for monoamine receptors are chemically similar to the corresponding agonists in respect to exposing a positively charged nitrogen. In these receptor systems, the agonist can often be converted into an antagonist through relatively small chemical modifications. In most of these systems, it has been demonstrated or it is assumed that the antagonists, like the agonists, are interacting with the conserved Asp in TM-III and that they occupy much of the same space, which the agonists normally occupy, in the pocket between TM-III, TM-V, and TM-VI. However, several antagonists, many of which are partial agonists, have been shown to have additional interaction points — for example, at the top of TM-VII. Thus, antagonists for monoamines, which in many cases are also classical competitive antagonists, bind to a large extent to the same site as the corresponding agonists and function as *isosteric competitive antagonists*.

2.10.2 NONPEPTIDE ANTAGONISTS MAY BIND RATHER DIFFERENTLY FROM THE AGONIST

For many years, analogs of peptides have been known that act as antagonists or partial agonists. The antagonist property was obtained by substitutions with D-amino acids, introduction of reduced peptide bonds, or substitution with conformationally constrained amino-acid analogs. Such peptide antagonists share much of their binding site with the natural peptide agonist and are therefore also isosteric competitive antagonists.

Recently, nonpeptide compounds have been developed for many peptide receptor systems. These compounds, which usually are discovered through screening of chemical files, generally do not resemble the corresponding peptide ligands chemically. Nevertheless, they act as specific and often competitive antagonists for the peptide ligand on the peptide receptor. Mapping of binding sites for nonpeptide antagonists has revealed that they often bind rather differently from the peptide agonists. The nonpeptide compounds typically have interaction points located relatively deep in the pocket between TM-III, TM-V, TM-VI, and TM-VII, corresponding to where agonists and antagonists for the monoamine receptors bind (Figure 2.12). As discussed above, many of the peptide agonists apparently do not reach into the lower part of this pocket. Thus, in some cases, nonpeptide antagonists for peptide receptors can act as *allosteric competitive antagonists*, binding to a different epitope from the agonist; however, the two ligands still compete for occupancy of the receptor. The competitive kinetics in such cases is a result of the phenomenon that binding of one ligand excludes the binding of the other ligand. The peptide agonist and the nonpeptide antagonist bind mutually exclusively and thereby compete for the entire receptor, though not necessarily a common binding site. Mathematically, this is similar to a classical competitive binding model. The mutually exclusive binding pattern is probably a result of the fact that the agonist and antagonist preferentially bind to different conformational states of the receptor (i.e., an active and an inactive conformation, respectively). In the substance P receptor, the binding site for a nonpeptide antagonist has even been exchanged by a metal-ion binding site without any effect on the binding of the agonist. In the mutant receptor, zinc ions have replaced the nonpeptide antagonist in antagonizing both the binding and the function of substance P. It is believed that the nonpeptide compound and the zinc ions act as antagonists by selecting and stabilizing an inactive conformation and that they thereby prevent the binding and action of the agonist.

Although binding pockets have been identified for several ligands, it is only in very few cases that specific interactions between a particular chemical moiety on the ligand and a particular side-chain of the receptor have been identified by hard biochemical evidence. As discussed above, the mapping of such interactions should be based on real gain-of-function experiments. Thus, we are still surprisingly far away from knowing the actual orientation of the natural messengers and drugs within their binding pockets.

2.11　7TM RECEPTORS APPEAR TO FUNCTION IN PROTEIN COMPLEXES TOGETHER WITH OTHER SIGNAL-TRANSDUCTION PROTEINS

It is often imagined that 7TM receptors float around in the membrane waiting for a hormone to bind and that the hormone-receptor complexes then have to collide with an appropriate G-protein. The active G-protein subunit will then diffuse away to encounter a down-stream effector molecule, which for example will generate a second messenger, which in turn is believed to diffuse deep into the cell to eventually encounter a further down-stream effector molecule. However, it appears that most of these processes occur within preformed complexes of signal-transduction proteins, including the hormone receptor held in close proximity by special scaffolding or adaptor proteins. An example of such a protein is the so-called multi-PDZ protein, which expresses a number of different PDZ domains, each of which binds a different signal-transduction protein, usually through the far C-terminal oligopeptide sequence. By bringing sequential signaling proteins close together, speed, selectivity, and efficiency are achieved because diffusional limitations are eliminated. This proximity is especially important in neuronal communication, where adaptor proteins create the synapse in which 7TM receptors, ion channels, and cytoplasmic signaling proteins are localized in a discrete focal structure in the membrane, tightly linked to the cytoskeleton. A large number of proteins are involved in creating synapses, including multi-PDZ proteins such as PSD-95 (postsynaptic density-95) (Figure 2.13).

For family C receptors, the importance of and structural basis for interaction with intracellular adaptor or scaffolding proteins have been characterized in great detail, just as the issue of dimer formation is rather clear for these receptors. The main family of adaptor proteins, which ensures the cellular targeting and correct signaling function for the metabotropic glutamate receptors, appear

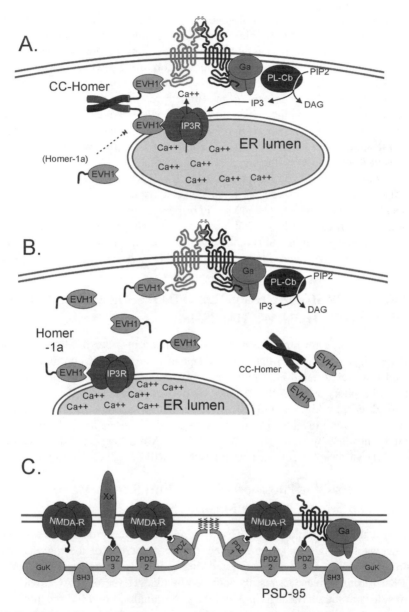

FIGURE 2.13 Examples of interaction of receptors with adaptor and scaffolding proteins. (A) Interaction of metabotropic glutamate receptors with Homer proteins, which through their EVH1 domain bind both the tail of the receptor located in the cell membrane and the IP3 receptor located in the membranes of the calcium stores of the endoplasmic reticulum. Through the leucine zipper domain of the Homer protein, dimerization of Homers in a coil–coil structure occurs. In this way, major components of the signal-transduction machinery are held in close proximity to create an efficient signaling mechanism through the G protein, phospholipase C, and IP3. (B) The same system showing that upregulation of a Homer-1a protein, which only has a single EVH1 domain and no leucine zipper domain, will, through competition, break the close association between the receptor and the downstream signal-transduction molecule, in this case the IP3 receptor. (C) Illustration of how PSD-95 (postsynaptic density protein 95) through PDZ domains can hold both 7TM receptors and ligand-gated ion channels in the synaptic area. As with many other scaffolding proteins, PSD-95 has several different binding domains, in this case three different PDZ domains, an SH3 domain, and a GuK domain. As PSD-95 can interact both with other PSD-95 proteins as well as with other scaffolding proteins and with proteins in the cytoskeleton, the micro-architecture of signal-transduction complexes can be built.

to be the so-called Homer proteins, most of which consist of two domains: (1) an N-terminal EHV domain that can bind to either the C-terminal end of the mGluRs or to the inositol-1,4,5-phosphate (IP_3) receptor/ryanodine receptor on the endoplasmic reticulum membranes, and (2) a C-terminal leucine zipper motif responsible for coil–coil interaction. As shown in Figure 2.13, the EHV domains will bind to the C-terminal tail of the mGluR receptor and to the IP3 receptor, and homodimerization of the coil–coil domains of the Homer proteins will then ensure a close proximity between these two signaling proteins, which otherwise would be located far away from each other in the cell. This is a dynamic system, as upregulation of a Homer-1a protein, which importantly does not have a leucine zipper motif domain, will compete for binding with the bifunctional Homer proteins and result in disruption of the signal transductosomes.

It is expected that a given 7TM receptor in a given cell will be able to participate in not only a single but also more than one type of signal transductosome. Thus, the receptor will display different molecular pharmacological phenotypes in respect to signaling and probably also in respect to ligand-binding properties. It is likely that it will not be a simple process for a receptor to move from one type of signaling complex to another, and it can be envisioned that the receptor may even have to go through a cycle of internalization and recycling in order to change signaling partners.

2.12   7TM RECEPTOR SIGNALING IS TURNED OFF, OR SWITCHED, BY DESENSITIZATION MECHANISMS

Seven-transmembrane receptor signaling is tightly regulated in order to allow for adjustments to changes in the environment and so that it can adapt to a situation of continued stimulation and protect the cell from overstimulation. A number of different processes are involved in 7TM receptor desensitization. Phosphorylation of the receptor by both second-messenger kinases and so-called G-protein-coupled receptor kinases (GRKs) will occur within seconds, followed within minutes by binding of arrestin, which prevents G-protein binding and functions as an adaptor for subsequent clathrin binding, and then by endocytosis (Figure 2.14). More long-term downregulation is controlled through altered receptor gene expression, which will occur within hours.

2.12.1   7TM RECEPTORS ARE PHOSPHORYLATED BY BOTH SECOND-MESSENGER KINASES AND SPECIFIC RECEPTOR KINASES

Phosphorylation is the most rapid way of desensitizing a 7TM receptor by uncoupling it from the G-protein, conceivably through altering the electrostatic properties of the regions involved in G-protein binding. The second-messenger-activated kinases PKA (protein kinase A, cAMP-dependent kinase) and PKC (protein kinase C, mainly activated by diacylglycerol [DAG]) will phosphorylate Ser and Thr residues in intracellular loop-3 and the C-terminal tail of 7TM receptors close to TM-VII regardless of the activation state of the receptor. The second-messenger kinases are therefore mainly involved in so-called heterologous desensitization, where stimulation of one type of 7TM receptor can desensitize a number of other receptors in the same cell. Interestingly, at least for the β_2-adrenoreceptor, the $G\alpha_s$-mediated PKA phosphorylation not only uncouples the receptor from G_s but apparently at the same time shifts the signaling to G_i.

In contrast to the second-messenger-regulated kinases, the GRKs selectively phosphorylate agonist-activated 7TM receptors and thereby increase the affinity of the receptors for the signal-blocking protein, arrestin. The target residues for GRKs are located in intracellular loop-3, especially in the C-terminal tail and often in an acidic sequence. GRKs constitute a family of at least seven proteins that consist of (1) an N-terminal receptor binding domain (often including an RGS domain involved in shutting off the G_i and G_q protein function); (2) a middle, catalytic kinase domain; and (3) a C-terminal membrane anchoring domain. Dynamic and regulated membrane association is an important part of the function of most GRKs, as it brings them into close proximity with their

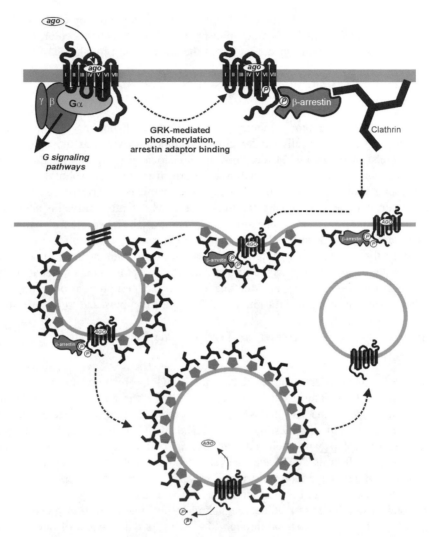

FIGURE 2.14 Agonist-induced receptor desensitization and internalization. Agonist binding will stabilize an active conformation of the receptor which will interact with a heterotrimeric G-protein, leading to signal transduction (top left corner). This signaling is turned off by receptor phosphorylation by GRK and perhaps PKA, which increases the affinity for β-arrestin. β-Arrestin functions as an adaptor protein coupling to clathrin and AP2 (symbolized by the gray pentamers), and this induces the formation of coated pits (in the middle of the figure), which are pinched off by the GTPase, dynamin, resulting in a coated vesicle. The vesicles move intracellularly through the endocytotic pathway, where changes in the environment (including, for example, acidification) lead to ligand dissociation and to detachment of β-arrestin. The agonist is passaged for degradation, and the receptor is dephosphorylated. Depending on the type of receptor, it is subsequently either degraded or, more often, recycled back to the cell surface, ready for a new encounter with an agonist.

substrates, the receptors. In GRK1 and GRK7 (visual GRKs), membrane association is achieved through farnesylation of their C-terminal CAAX sequence. In GRK2 and GRK3, which historically are called β-adrenergic receptor kinases (or βARKs) but which in fact are widely distributed and act on a multitude of 7TM receptors, the C-terminal 125-amino-acid pleckstrin homology domain will specifically bind to the β-γ subunit of the heterotrimeric G-protein and thereby secure a close proximity to the membrane-associated receptor–G-protein complex. GRK4 and GRK6 are membrane associated even in the absence of activated 7TM receptors through palmitoylation, which is a regulated posttranslational modification. The effect of phosphorylation by GRKs is not identical, as both GRK2 and GRK5 will bind to and phosphorylate the β_1-adrenoceptor, but only GRK5 phosphorylation leads to receptor uncoupling from the scaffolding protein PSD-95.

2.12.2 Arrestin Blocks Signaling and Functions as an Adaptor Protein to Clathrin

Full inactivation of 7TM receptor signaling is achieved through binding of one of a family of arrestin molecules, which sterically hinder G-protein binding. Arrestins are cytosolic proteins, which, upon agonist binding to 7TM receptors, are translocated to the activated, phosphorylated receptor within minutes. The difference in affinity of arrestin for the phosphorylated vs. nonphosphorylated receptor is only 10- to 30-fold. Although key elements for arrestin binding are believed to be located mainly in the C-terminal extension of the 7TM receptors, arrestins interact also with intracellular loop-2 and -3. Arrestins are structurally composed of two main domains, each consisting of a seven-stranded β-sandwich followed by a C-terminal extension. Receptor binding is mediated mainly through the most N-terminal β-sandwich domain of arrestin, whereas the C-terminal part of the protein is responsible for bringing the receptor to clathrin-coated pits and the subsequent endocytotic events. Thus, arrestin functions as an adaptor protein connecting the receptor to the β_2-adaptin subunit of the heterotrimeric AP-2 adaptor complex and to clathrin itself.

2.12.3 Internalization Is Followed by Targeting to Lysosomes or by Recycling

Receptor internalization through clathrin-coated pits brings the receptor through the endocytotic compartments where the ligand usually will dissociate from the receptor due to the low pH to eventually be degraded in the late endosomes and lysosomes. The sequestered receptor either follows the same route and fatal destiny as the ligand, which is the case, for example, for the protease-activated receptors with their tethered ligands, or the receptor is dephosphorylated by receptor-specific phosphatases and is then recycled to the membrane in recycling vesicles. The degree and speed of resensitization and recycling vary among 7TM receptors. In some cases, signaling of 7TM receptors can be switched from G-protein-mediated signaling to a microtubule-associated protein (MAP)-kinase-mediated signaling by the internalization process; however, in other cases, 7TM receptors may signal through MAP kinases independent of internalization.

2.13 FURTHER READING

Rhodopsin-like 7TM receptor structure

Ballesteros, J. A., Shi, L., and Javitch, J. A., Structural mimicry in G-protein-coupled receptors: implications of the high-resolution structure of rhodopsin for structure–function analysis of rhodopsin-like receptors, *Mol. Pharmacol.*, 60(1), 1–19, 2001.

Palczewski, K., Kumasaka, T., Hori, T., Behnke, C. A., Motoshima, H., Fox, B. A., Le, T. I., Teller, D. C., Okada, T., Stenkamp, R. E., Yamamoto, M., and Miyano, M., Crystal structure of rhodopsin: a G-protein-coupled receptor, *Science*, 289(5480), 739–745, 2000.

Teller, D. C., Okada, T., Behnke, C. A., Palczewski, K., and Stenkamp, R. E., Advances in determination of a high-resolution three-dimensional structure of rhodopsin, a model of G-protein-coupled receptors (GPCRs), *Biochemistry*, 40(26), 7761–7772, 2001.

Orphan 7TM receptor

Stadel, J. M., Wilson, S., and Bergsma, D. J., Orphan G-protein-coupled receptors: a neglected opportunity for pioneer drug discovery, *Trends Pharmacol. Sci.*, 18(11), 430–437, 1997.

Wilson, S., Bergsma, D. J., Chambers, J. K., Muir, A. I., Fantom, K. G., Ellis, C., Murdock, P. R., Herrity, N. C., and Stadel, J. M., Orphan G-protein-coupled receptors: the next generation of drug targets?, *Br. J. Pharmacol.*, 125(7), 1387–1392, 1998.

Family B and C 7TM receptors

Bockaert, J. and Pin, J. P., Molecular tinkering of G-protein-coupled receptors: an evolutionary success, *EMBO J.*, 18(7), 1723–1729, 1999.

7TM receptor dimerization

Bouvier, M., Oligomerization of G-protein-coupled transmitter receptors, *Nat. Rev. Neurosci.*, 2(4), 274–286, 2001.
Milligan, G., Oligomerisation of G-protein-coupled receptors, *J. Cell. Sci.*, 114(pt. 7), 1265–1271, 2001.

7TM receptors in equilibrium between active and inactive conformations

Elling, C. E., Thirstrup, K., Holst, B., and Schwartz, T. W., Conversion of agonist site to metal-ion chelator site in the beta(2)-adrenergic receptor, *Proc. Natl. Acad. Sci. USA*, 96(22), 12322–12327, 1999.
Gether, U., Uncovering molecular mechanisms involved in activation of G-protein-coupled receptors, *Endocr. Rev.*, 21(1), 90–113, 2000.
Gether, U. and Kobilka, B. K., G-protein-coupled receptors. II. Mechanism of agonist activation, *J. Biol. Chem.*, 273(29), 17979–17982, 1998.
Kenakin T., Inverse, protean, and ligand-selective agonism: matters of receptor conformation, *FASEB J.*, 15(3), 598–611, 2001.
Lefkowitz, R. J., Cotecchia, S., Samama, P. S., and Costa, T., Constitutive activity of receptors coupled to guanine nucleotide regulatory proteins, *Trends Pharmacol. Sci.*, 14, 303–307, 1993.

Ligand binding in 7TM receptors

Elling, C. E., Nielsen, S. M., and Schwartz, T. W., Conversion of antagonist-binding site to metal-ion site in the tachykinin Nk-1 receptor, *Nature*, 374(2), 74–77, 1995.
Kunishima, N., Shimada, Y., Tsuji, Y., Sato, T., Yamamoto, M., Kumasaka, T., Nakanishi, S., Jingami, H., and Morikawa, K., Structural basis of glutamate recognition by a dimeric metabotropic glutamate receptor, *Nature*, 407(6807), 971–977, 2000.
Schwartz, T. W., Locating ligand-binding sites in 7TM receptors by protein engineering, *Curr. Opin. Biotechnol.*, 5, 434–444, 1994.
Schwartz, T. W. and Rosenkilde, M. M., Is there a "lock" for all "keys" in 7TM receptors?, *Trends Pharmacol. Sci.*, 17, 213–216, 1996.
Strader, C. D., Gaffney, T., Sugg, E. E., Candelore, M. R., Keys, R., Patchett, A. A., and Dixon, R. A. F., Allele-specific activation of genetically engineered receptors, *J. Biol. Chem.*, 266, 5–8, 1991.

7TM scaffolding and adaptor proteins

Milligan, G. and White, J. H., Protein–protein interactions at G-protein-coupled receptors, *Trends Pharmacol. Sci.*, 22(10), 513–518, 2001.
Xiao, B., Tu, J. C., and Worley, P. F., Homer: a link between neural activity and glutamate receptor function, *Curr. Opin. Neurobiol.*, 10(3), 370–374, 2000.

7TM receptor desensitization

Ferguson, S. S., Evolving concepts in G-protein-coupled receptor endocytosis: the role in receptor desensitization and signaling, *Pharmacol. Rev.*, 53(1), 1–24, 2001.
Krupnick, J. G. and Benovic, J. L., The role of receptor kinases and arrestins in G-protein-coupled receptor regulation, *Annu. Rev. Pharmacol. Toxicol.*, 38, 289–319, 1998.
Pierce, K. L., Lefkowitz, R. J., and Lefkowitz, R. J., Classical and new roles of beta-arrestin in the regulation of G-protein-coupled receptors, *Nat. Rev. Neurosci.*, 2(10), 727–733, 2001.

3 The Structure of Ligand-Gated Ion Channels

Jan Egebjerg

CONTENTS

3.1 INTRODUCTION

Ligand-gated ion channels are integral glycoproteins that transverse the cell membrane. All molecularly characterized ligand-gated ion channels are multisubunit complexes. Ligand-gated ion channels generally exist in one of three functional states: resting (or closed), open, or desensitized. Each functional state may reflect many discrete conformational states with different pharmacological properties. Receptors in the resting state, upon application of agonist, will undergo a fast transition to the open state, called *gating*, and most agonists will also undergo a transition to the desensitized state. Because the desensitized state often exhibits higher agonist affinity than the open state, most of the receptors will be in the desensitized state after prolonged agonist exposure.

Receptors have three important properties: (1) they are activated in response to specific ligands, (2) they conduct ions through the otherwise impermeable cell membrane, and (3) they select among different ions.

Molecular cloning, combined with a variety of different techniques, has revealed the existence of at least three structurally different families of ligand-gated channels. These families can be classified as the four-transmembrane receptors (4TM), the excitatory amino-acid receptors (3TM), and the adenosine triphosphate (ATP) receptors (2TM). These receptors constitute the major classes of ligand-gated ion channels in the plasma membrane. Other receptors, such as the capsaicin-activated vallinoid receptor (6TM), for which no endogenous ligand has been identified; the intracellular Ca^{2+}-activated ryanodine receptor; and the inositol 1,4,5-triphosphate (IP_3)-activated receptor, are also ligand-gated ion channels but will not be discussed in this chapter.

3.2 THE 4TM RECEPTORS

The 4TM family of receptors consists of the nicotinic acetylcholine receptor (nAChR), serotonin receptor ($5HT_3$), glycine receptor, and γ-aminobutyric acid receptors ($GABA_A$ and $GABA_C$). The nAChRs are the primary excitatory receptors in the skeletal muscle and the peripheral nervous system of vertebrates. In the central nervous system, nAChRs are present in much smaller number than the glutamate receptors. $5HT_3$ receptors are also cation-selective but are located exclusively on neurons. Glycine and GABA are the major inhibitory neurotransmitters. GABA predominates in the cortex and cerebellum, whereas glycine is most abundant in the spinal cord and brainstem. Both ligands activate a chloride current. Most of the agonists also activate G-protein-coupled receptors.

3.2.1 MOLECULAR CLONING

The 4TM receptors are pentameric complexes composed of subunits of 420 to 550 amino acids. The subunits exhibit sequence identities from 25 to 75%, with a similar distribution of hydrophobic and hydrophilic domains (Table 3.1). The hydrophilic 210 to 230 amino-acid N-terminal domain is followed by three closely spaced hydrophobic and putative transmembrane domains, then a variable-length intracellular loop, and finally a fourth putative transmembrane region shortly before the C-terminus (Figure 3.1). Of the four candidate transmembrane regions, evidence suggests that TM2 forms an α-helix, while the other hydrophobic regions more likely are folded as β-sheets.

Molecular cloning has resulted in the identification of the muscle nAChR subunits $\alpha_1, \beta_1, \gamma, \delta$, and ε and the structurally related neuronal α_2 to α_{10} and β_2 to β_4. The neuronal nAChR subunits α_2 to α_4 can assemble with β_2 or β_4 and generate functional heteromeric receptors; the α_7 to α_9

TABLE 3.1
Subunits of the 4TM Superfamily

nAChR					$5HT_3$	Glycine Receptors		$GABA_A$ Receptors							
α_1	β_1	γ	δ	ε	A	α_1	β	α_1	γ_1	ε	β_1	ρ_1	δ	π	θ
α_2	β_2					α_2		α_2	γ_2		β_2	ρ_2			
α_3	β_3					α_3		α_3	γ_3		β_3	ρ_3			
α_4	β_4							α_4	(γ_4)		β_4				
α_5								α_5							
α_6								α_6							
α_7															
(α_8)															
α_9															
α_{10}															

Note: Mammalian orthologs for the avian α_8 and γ_4 subunits have not yet been identified. The ρ 1–3 subunit constitutes the $GABA_C$ receptors.

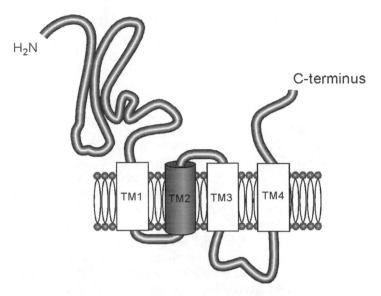

FIGURE 3.1 Schematic representation of the transmembrane topology of the 4TM receptor family. Only TM2 show an α-helical structure in electron microscopic studies; the remaining TM regions may fold in β-sheet structures. Both the N-terminus (indicated by NH_2) and the C-terminus are located extracellularly. The cytoplasmic loops between TM3 and TM4 are variable in size and contain putative phosphorylation sites.

subunits can generate functional homomeric receptors; and the α_{10} subunit only forms functional channels in combination with α_9 subunits. The neuronal nAChRs assemble according to the general stoichiometry $\alpha_2\beta_3$ with a β subunit between the α subunits (Figure 3.2). Obviously, the properties of the receptor depend on the subunit composition. An assembly process that was not controlled in cells expressing more than two different subunits would result in a very large number of different receptor types. At least in muscle cells where four different subunits are expressed at the same time, the subunits are assembled in an ordered sequence to achieve the correct stoichiometry and neighborhood relationship.

Four glycine receptor subunits have been identified: three α subunits and one β subunit. When expressed in heterologous systems, homomeric α receptors generate functional channels, and strychnine and picrotoxin inhibit the current. A more detailed analysis has revealed that the β subunit, probably in the stoichiometry $\alpha_3\beta_2$, is necessary to generate channel properties similar to

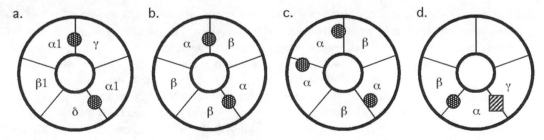

FIGURE 3.2 Schematic representation of the subunit organization in the most abundant heteromeric receptor complex: (a) embryonic muscle nicotinic AChR muscle nAChR has the stoichiometry $(\alpha_1)_2\beta\gamma\epsilon$ (adult), (b) neuronal nicotinic AChR, (c) glycine receptors, and (d) GABA$_A$ receptors. The circles indicate the location of the agonist binding site at the interface between the subunits in nAChR and GABA$_A$ receptors. The square indicates the location of the benzodiazepine binding site. The depicted GABA$_A$ receptor model is the general model with at least one GABA and one benzodiazepine binding site. The number of different binding sites on the GABA$_A$ receptor depends on the final stoichiometry of the pentameric complex.

the channels studied in adult spinal cord neurons, while the embryonic glycine receptors are more like homomeric α receptors.

The diversity of the $GABA_A$ subunits (Figure 3.2d) is reflected in a very complex pharmacology. Expression of the subunits in heterologous systems shows that the combinations α, β, and γ can yield functional receptors, indicating that the limitation in subunit combination is defined by expression levels and most likely cell-dependent assembly mechanisms also. The ρ_1 to ρ_3 subunits mainly co-assemble with each other to form the $GABA_C$ receptors.

The GABA receptors can be modulated, in a subtype-selective manner, by a number of agents that either enhance the current (benzodiazepines, barbiturates) or reduce the current (bicuculline, β-carbolines, picrotoxin). The GABA binding site is strongly influenced by the β subunit, but co-expression with an α subunit is necessary for significant functional expression. The complexity of the benzodiazepine pharmacology is illustrated by the observation that heteromeric α/β receptors are not potentiated by benzodiazepine. This is surprising, because cross-linking experiments assigned the benzodiazepine binding site to the α subunit. Only co-expression of the α and β subunits with a γ subunit generates receptors that are potentiated by benzodiazepine. Thus, benzodiazepine pharmacology depends on the α subunit; but in order to have any functional implications, the receptor complex must also contain a γ subunit. The majority of $GABA_A$ receptors contain the α, β, and γ subunits with the GABA and benzodiazepine binding sites at the α–β and α–γ interfaces, respectively. The pharmacology of the receptor will depend not only on these three subunits but also on the remaining two subunits.

The contribution of the different receptor subtypes in neuronal activity is an overwhelmingly complex problem. Recent advances in mouse genetics have provided methods to use the detailed information obtained by studies of the recombinant receptors in heterologous systems. An elegant example has been the elucidation of the contributions from the different $GABA_A$ α subunits on the wide spectrum of actions elicited by the clinically used benzodiazepines. As mentioned, the benzodiazepines bind at the interface between the α and γ subunits, but the known benzodiazepines exhibit low selectivity among the α_1, α_2, α_3, and α_5 subunits. Molecular studies have demonstrated that a histidine-to-arginine substitution in the α subunit abolishes benzodiazepine interaction. Substituting part of the gene encoding the α_1 subunit with the His-to-Arg mutant in mice resulted in mice for which the benzodiazepine effects on the α_1-containing receptors were eliminated. In the mutant mice, the known effects of benzodiazepine such as myorelaxation, motor impairments, anxiolysis, and ethanol potentiation remained, while other benzodiazepine effects such as sedation and amnesia were not induced, indicating that the α_1-containing receptors contribute to these behaviors.

3.2.2 THE THREE-DIMENSIONAL STRUCTURE

The nAChRs of skeletal muscles and fish electric organs are the best characterized 4TM ligand-gated ion channels. The receptor is a 290 kDa complex composed of four distinct subunits assembled into a heterologous $(\alpha_1)_2\beta_1\gamma\delta$ pentameric complex. In skeletal muscles, the embryonic γ subunit is replaced by the ε subunit in adult tissue. In electron micrographs from the synaptic site, viewed perpendicular to the plane of the membrane, the receptor complex, in the resting state, appears as a ring-like particle with an outer diameter of 80 Å and an inner tube of 20 to 25 Å. Viewed from the side (Figure 3.3), the receptor looks like a 125-Å-long cylinder protruding 60 Å into the synaptic cleft and 20 Å into the cytoplasm, with a square-like density located beneath the cytoplasmatic vestibule. The cation-conducting pathway consists of three parts. In the synaptic portion, it forms a water-filled tube 20 Å in diameter and 60 Å long. The next part, across the membrane, is formed by a more constricted region about 30 Å long (the pore). Near the middle of the membrane, the pathway becomes constricted in a region where the pathway is blocked when the channel is closed (the gate). The cytoplasmic part of the pathway forms a cylinder 20 Å in diameter and 20 Å long. Close inspection of the electron micrographs reveals that each subunit has an α-helical-like segment lining the pore. This segment consists of two α helices separated by a kink around the midpoint

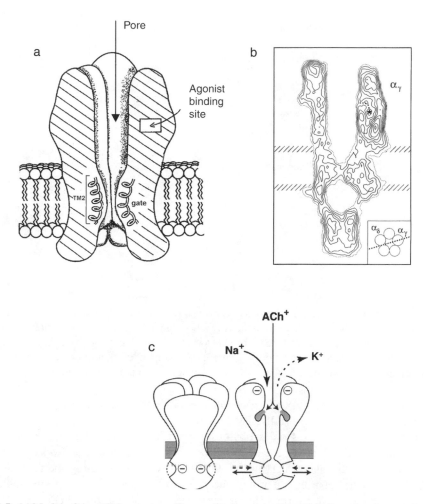

FIGURE 3.3 (a) Model of the 4TM receptors. The model shows the ligand binding site, the membrane bilayer, and the position of the channel gate. (b) Electron density map of the nAChR in profile at 4.6 Å data. The electron density is shown through a cross section of an α subunit and the interface between the other α subunit and the δ subunit. The asterisk indicates the proposed ACh binding site. (c) Model of the AChR suggesting: (1) that ACh enters the extracellular vestibule before binding to the binding site; (2) that entering cations will pass through the extracellular vestibule, the pore, and at the cytoplasmic site will be filtered through a negatively charged opening in the receptor (courtesy of N. Unwin).

pointing into the pore (in the resting state), giving the pore an "hourglass" shape with the kink located at the most constricted point. When the receptor is activated by acetylcholine, each of the helical segments rotates, opening the gate. In the open state, the pore narrows from the outside to the cytoplasmic site, where the diameter is roughly 11 Å. Thus, the flexure between the two α helices provides an effective way of altering the shape and size of the pore (Figure 3.4).

3.2.3 THE RECEPTOR PORE

The ability of a receptor channel to conduct ions, which is measured as the conductance (the reciprocal of resistance) of the channel, depends on TM2. The experiments that showed this were based on the observation that receptors made of *Torpedo* α, β, γ, and δ subunits had a different conductance from receptors made of *Torpedo* α, β, γ, and calf δ subunits. When chimeric δ subunits in which parts of the *Torpedo* sequences were replaced by the corresponding calf sequence, were

Closed state

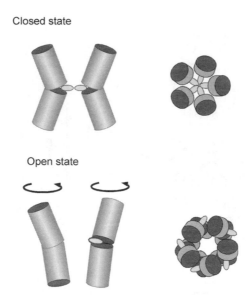

Open state

FIGURE 3.4 The orientation of the TM2 helical segment in the closed and open states of the channel. On the left is a view of two of the five helices from the side, where the helical segment is illustrated as two helices (rods) separated by a kink where the leucine (ellipse) is located. On the right, the five helices are viewed from the synaptic side, where the leucines will block the pore. The binding of an agonist causes the helical segments to rotate, and the narrowest region is then in the open state at the cytoplasmic part of the pore.

co-expressed with the *Torpedo* α, β, and γ subunits, it was demonstrated that the entire difference in conductance could be attributed to the TM2 region.

The structure of the TM2 region is obviously not a perfect α helix; however, assuming a symmetric pentameric distribution of α helices gives us a useful structural model to describe the molecular environment through which an ion must pass when permeating the receptor channel. Because of the symmetric distribution around the pore, amino acids assigned to the same position in the sequence alignments will form a ring in the three-dimensional model (Figure 3.5).

Important clues as to how the pore is structurally organized were obtained by examining the distribution of the charged and uncharged residues in the *Torpedo* nAChR subunits. As expected for hydrophobic segments, the TM2 bears no charged residues; however, a number of charged and polar residues were located at both ends of TM2 (Figure 3.5). According to the 4TM model, the charged residues in the TM1–TM2 loop will be located at the entrance to the pore from the cytoplasmatic side, while the charged residues in the TM2–TM3 loop are located at the pore entrance from the extracellular side. Because nAChR conducts cations, the negatively charged rings were expected to line the channel and attract permeant cations to the pore. Indeed, when the number of charged amino acids in the intermediate ring was reduced from the four negative charges in the native *Torpedo* receptor, a clear reduction in the conductance of the channel was observed. Mutations that altered the charge of the inner and outer rings also changed the conductance but to a much lesser extent. Thus, these residues must be exposed to the lumen of the pore, although additional experiments suggest that the inner and outer rings are more involved in regulating the access of the cations to the channel than being in direct contact with the permeating ions. The optimal effect of the negatively charged rings on the current is a subtle balance between attracting monovalent ions and boosting the current, on the one hand, and, on the other hand, attracting divalent ions that bind to the residues in the charged rings with higher affinity, thereby reducing the current. These counteracting effects might explain why some functional nAChR subunits encode positively charged amino acids at the ring positions.

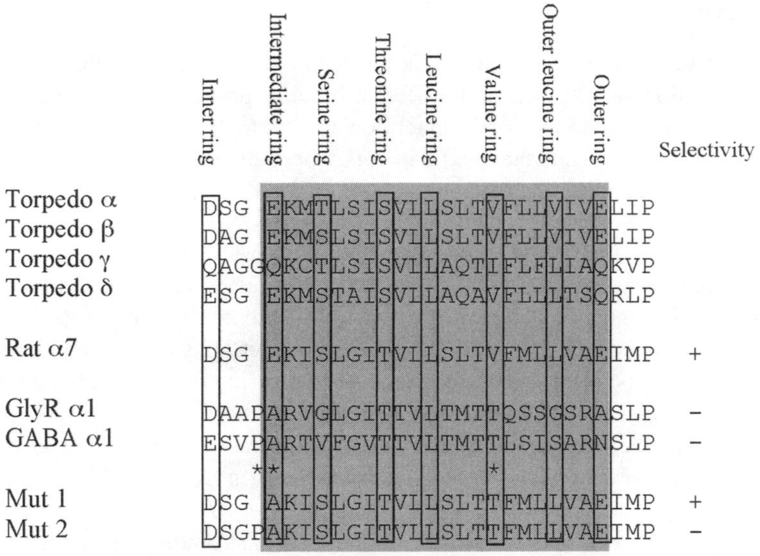

Inner ring / Intermediate ring / Serine ring / Threonine ring / Leucine ring / Valine ring / Outer leucine ring / Outer ring / Selectivity

		Selectivity
Torpedo α	DSG EKMTLSISVILSLTVFLLVIVELIP	
Torpedo β	DAG EKMSLSISVLLSLTVFLLVIVELIP	
Torpedo γ	QAGGQKCTLSISVLLAQTIFLFLIAQKVP	
Torpedo δ	ESG EKMSTAISVLLAQAVFLLLTSQRLP	
Rat α7	DSG EKISLGITVILSLTVFMLLVAEIMP	+
GlyR α1	DAAPARVGLGITTVLTMTTQSSGSRASLP	−
GABA α1	ESVPARTVFGVTTVLTMTTLSISARNSLP	−
	** *	
Mut 1	DSG AKISLGITVILSLTTFMLLVAEIMP	+
Mut 2	DSGPAKISLGITVILSLTTFMLLVAEIMP	−

FIGURE 3.5 Alignment of the TM2 amino acid sequences. The nomenclature of the rings is based on the α_7 sequence. Selectivity indicates the charge of the permeant ions. Mut1 and Mut2 are site-directed mutants (indicated by the asterisks) of the α_7 subunit (see text).

In the GABA and glycine receptors, where the permeant ion is negatively charged, the inner ring remains negatively charged, and the outer is either negative or neutral. The question, then, is what determines the ion selectivity of the channel? An alignment of the TM2 region between the nAChR α_7 subunit and glycine and GABA subunits revealed amino-acid differences at five of the positions lining the pore; in addition, an extra amino acid was present at the N-terminal end of the TM2 segment in the anion-selective channels (Figure 3.5). Mutagenesis studies showed that substitutions of the amino acids lining the pore did not influence the cation selectivity of α_7 nAChR (Figure 3.5, Mut1); however, insertion of a proline into Mut1 at the N-terminus of TM-II, as for the GABA receptors, changed the channel to be anion selective. Thus, the pore can be permeable to both cations and anions; consequently, the ion selectivity is not directly related to the amino-acid sequence within the pore. Slight changes in the position of the TM2 or the surrounding amino acids, however, apparently determines the ion selectivity.

It is important that conclusions based on mutagenesis studies are confirmed by other experiments, as mutations involving residues in key positions for structure or for function may have an effect not only as a result of changes at the site of substitution but also as a result of nonlocalized structural perturbations created to accommodate that change. In fact, most of the residues facing the lumen of the pore were also identified in labeling experiments using noncompetitive antagonists known to bind in the pore. When the noncompetitive antagonist [3H]chlorpromazine was photolabeled to the receptor, the cross-linked amino acids were located in the serine, threonine, and leucine rings (Figure 3.5). Evidence for structural changes in the pore were obtained by the antagonist trifluoromethyl-iodophenyldiazirine which, in the absence of agonist, cross-linked to amino acids equivalent to the valine and the leucine ring. However, in the presence of agonist, the labeling pattern extends down to the threonine and serine rings, indicating that the central valine, leucine, and threonine rings may correspond to the constricted region observed in the electron micrographs. The leucine is suggested to be the gate-forming residue pointing into the pore from the kink in TM-II. This is supported by mutagenesis studies, which demonstrated that a substitution of the leucine with a smaller amino acid affects the ability of the receptor to close in the desensitized state.

3.2.4   THE LIGAND-BINDING SITE

To study the properties of the binding site, it is important to keep in mind that receptors exist in a number of conformations that may exhibit different binding properties. As mentioned, the affinity for the ligand in the open state is usually much lower (10- to 1000-fold) than the affinity for the desensitized state. Thus, in biochemical experiments where the receptor is exposed to a ligand for prolonged time periods, agonist–receptor interactions will reflect the receptor conformations of the desensitized state, while antagonist interaction may reflect conformation of either the resting state or the desensitized states. In contrast, electrophysiological evaluations of the agonist interactions reflect the low-affinity binding conformation of the open state except for certain mutants. As an example, in studies of a mutant α_7 subunit for which the leucine ring (at the gate) was substituted for a smaller amino acid, the potency for ACh measured in electrophysiological recordings increased 150-fold. The data might be interpreted as the leucine interfering directly with the binding of ACh; however, the single-channel conductance state activated at low ACh concentrations was different from the states activated at higher concentrations. An alternative explanation is that the leucine mutation at the gate cannot close in one of the conformations in the desensitized state, which binds ACh with high affinity.

Insights into the three-dimensional structure of the agonist binding site of the 4TM receptors have been obtained from comparisons with the crystal structure of a soluble acetylcholine-binding protein (AChBP) found in the snail *Lymnaea stagnalis*. The AChBP exhibits the highest sequence identity with the N-terminal domain of the nAChR α_7 subunit (24%). Obviously, comparisons among proteins with low sequence identity should be treated with caution. However, residues that are conserved between the members of the 4TM superfamily are nearly all conserved in the AChBP, and a number of competitive agonists and antagonists also bind to the AChBP, suggesting that the overall structure might be similar. Examination of the three-dimensional structure supports the structural similarity (see below).

Acetylcholine-binding proteins crystallize as a pentameric complex, with dimensions similar to the extracellular part of the nicotinic receptor (Figure 3.6). The subunits form a ring, thereby generating a central hydrophilic pore, observed as the extracellular vestibule in the electron microscopic studies. The central part of each subunit is formed by ten β-sheets, forming a β-sandwich (Figure 3.6). The five ligand-binding sites in the pentameric complex are situated between subunits,

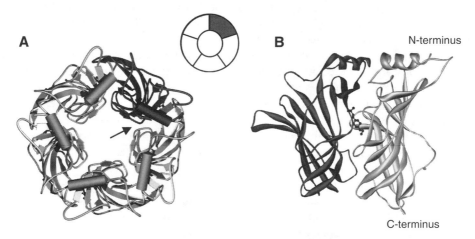

FIGURE 3.6 Crystal structure of the acetylcholine-binding protein (AChBP). (A) The complex, as viewed in the pore formed by the subunits. The complex consists of five identical subunits. One of the subunits is highlighted (as shown in the insert), and the arrow indicates the agonist binding site. (B) View of the proposed agonist binding from the pore site (along the arrow in A). The structure is due to the crystallization condition, crystallized with HEPES at the binding site.

where loop regions, between the β-strands, form one side of the binding interface. Residues from the adjacent subunit line the other part of the binding site, which are located both in the loop regions and in the β-sheets. All the residues involved in the ligand binding have also been identified in mutagenesis or cross-linking experiments on the nAChR. Apart from one residue, all the potential ligand-interacting residues are conserved among the nAChR; however, as might be expected, these residues are variable between pharmacologically different classes within the 4TM superfamily. The formation of the ligand-binding site at the interface between adjacent subunits provides a simple explanation for the pharmacological diversity observed in receptors formed from different subunits. Interestingly, the conserved residues, which mostly are hydrophobic, are involved in maintaining the overall structure of the subunits, further supporting the similar three-dimensional structure of the members of the 4TM superfamily.

The ACh binding cavity is located approximately 30 Å above the membrane. It is still not clear how the agonist binding might activate the receptor. At least two different models have been proposed: (1) agonist binding promotes an "intersubunit sliding," where the relative positioning of the subunits changes; and (2) agonist-induced changes occur within the subunit (intrasubunit), possibly as perturbations of the loops between the β-sheets, which might be transmitted directly to the pore region or indirectly through changes in the β-sheet regions. Currently, evidence is insufficient to decide between these or additional models; however, chimeric receptor subunits containing the agonist binding site from the $5HT_3$ subunit and the pore region from the nAChR α_7 subunit can be activated by 5HT. This supports the notion that the overall structure and the conformational changes during activation of the members of the 4TM superfamily are highly conserved. In addition, each receptor subunit might be envisioned as a two-domain protein, with an N-terminal agonist binding site and a C-terminal pore region.

3.3 EXCITATORY AMINO-ACID RECEPTORS: 3TM RECEPTORS

L-Glutamate acts as an excitatory neurotransmitter at many synapses in the mammalian central nervous system. Electrophysiological measurements and the use of various selective agonists and antagonists indicate that different glutamate receptors co-exist on many neurons.

The exogenous agonist N-methyl-D-aspartate (NMDA) activates receptors that are characterized by slow kinetics and a high Ca^{2+} permeability (see Figure 3.8). In addition to glutamate (or NMDA), these receptors require glycine as a co-agonist. The currents conducted by NMDA receptors are blocked by extracellular Mg^{2+} in a voltage-dependent mode (Figure 3.7). At resting membrane potential (–70 mV), activation of the channel will result only in a low current because entry of Mg^{2+} ions into the channel will block the current. The affinity for the Mg^{2+} ions will decrease at less negative membrane potentials as the electric driving force for Mg^{2+} is reduced and the block becomes ineffective (Figure 3.7).

Another class of ionotropic glutamate receptors exhibits fast kinetics and, in most neurons, a low Ca^{2+} permeability when activated by glutamate. The selective agonist α-amino-3-hydroxy-5-methyl-4-isoxazole propionate (AMPA) activates a fast desensitizing current, as does glutamate, in the majority of these receptors. Consequently, this subtype is referred to as AMPA receptors. Kainate activates a nondesensitizing current when applied to AMPA receptors, but it activates a fast-desensitizing current on another receptor type, the kainate receptor. This type of glutamate receptor binds kainate with high affinity (Figure 3.8). In addition to the three groups of ionotropic receptors, glutamate also activates G-protein-coupled receptors called *metabotropic glutamate receptors*.

The AMPA receptors mediate the majority of fast excitatory neurotransmission in the mammalian brain. The rapid kinetics and the low Ca permeability make these receptors ideal for fast neurotransmission without sufficient changes in the intracellular calcium concentration to activate Ca^{2+}-dependent processes. The NMDA receptors are co-localized with the AMPA receptors on many synapses, but the slow kinetics of the NMDA receptor minimize the receptor activation after a single presynaptic glutamate release where the neuron quickly repolarizes, resulting in Mg^{2+} block

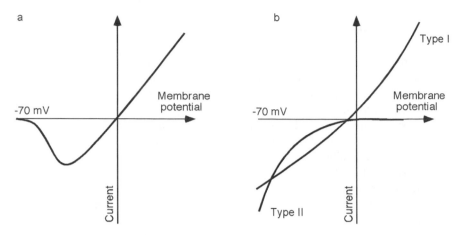

FIGURE 3.7 Current–voltage relationships for the *N*-methyl-ᴅ-aspartate (NMDA) and non-NMDA glutamate receptors. (a) Current–voltage relationship of the NMDA receptor recorded in the presence of Mg^{2+}. The current through the channel becomes progressively smaller at negative membrane potentials due to the Mg^{2+} block. (b) Expression of the AMPA and kainate receptor subunits generates either a linear (type I) or an inwardly rectifying (type II) current–voltage relationship, depending on the subunit composition of the receptor. If the receptor contains subunits edited at the Q/R site (i.e., GluR2 for the AMPA receptors, GluR5R or GluR6R for the kainate receptors), the current–voltage relationship is linear. Receptors made of unedited subunits alone or in combination with each other exhibit inwardly rectifying current–voltage relationships.

of the NMDA receptor. However, the NMDA receptor will be fully activated after extensive stimulation of the synapse when repetitive activation of the AMPA receptors evokes sufficient depolarization of the postsynaptic membrane to relieve the NMDA receptors of the Mg^{2+} block. This use-dependent Ca^{2+} influx has been interpreted to be one of the underlying mechanisms for many different neuronal processes, including learning and memory.

3.3.1 MOLECULAR CLONING

Seventeen genes encoding glutamate receptor subunits have been identified (Table 3.2). These subunits are based on sequence identities grouped into seven different classes. All the subunits have similar profiles in hydrophobicity plots and presumably the same topology with a 400- to 500-amino-acid extracellular N-terminal part followed by a 400-amino-acid region encoding the trans-membrane domains (Figure 3.9). The C-terminus is intracellular and varies in size from 50 to 750 amino acids. The glutamate receptor subunits exhibit, in contrast to the 4TM receptors, the highest sequence variability between the subunits at the N-terminal region, while the transmembrane domain is highly conserved.

There is still not solid evidence on the stoichiometry of the receptor complex. Various approaches have indicated either a pentameric or tetrameric structure; however, more recent data favor the tetrameric configuration (Figure 3.10d), and some evidence implies that the receptor may be organized as two pairs.

3.3.1.1 AMPA Receptors

The GluR1 to GluR4 subunits (also named GluRA–GluRD) co-assemble with one another but not with subunits from the other classes. The functional profile of these cloned receptors demonstrated a desensitizing response to AMPA, or glutamate, but a nondesensitizing response to kainate (EC_{50} > 30 μM), features similar to studies of AMPA receptors from the brain. The affinity for AMPA in binding experiments also resembles the affinities observed in brain tissue.

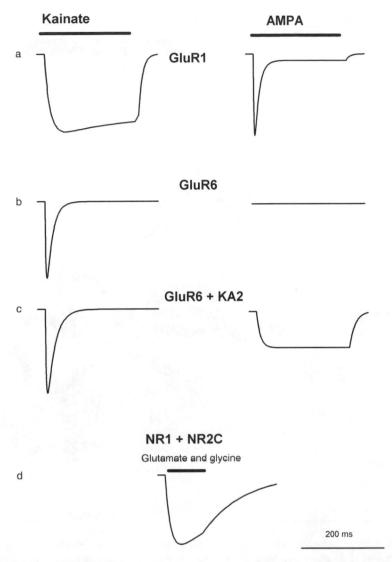

FIGURE 3.8 Kainate and AMPA activate different current responses in the different classes of kainate and AMPA receptors: (a) the AMPA receptor, GluR1; (b) and (c) kainate receptors; (d) glutamate + glycine activation of the NMDA receptor. The current response is characterized by a slow onset and offset compared to the kainate and AMPA receptors.

TABLE 3.2
Subunits of the 3TM Superfamily

NMDA Receptors			AMPA Receptors	Kainate Receptors		Orphan Receptors
NR1	NR2A	NR3A	GluR1 (A)	GluR5	KA1	δ_1
	NR2B		GluR2 (B)	GluR6	KA2	δ_2
	NR2C		GluR3 (C)	GluR7		
	N2D		GluR4 (D)			

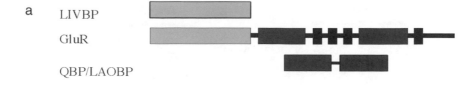

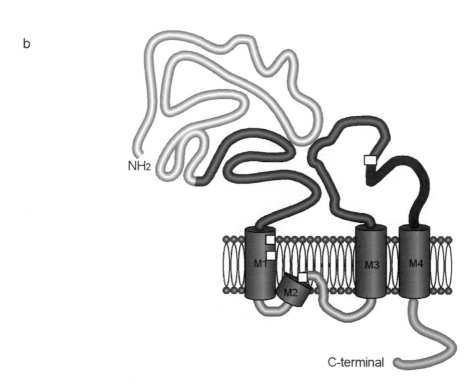

FIGURE 3.9 (a) Diagram showing the regions of glutamate receptors that exhibit sequence homology to bacterial peri-plasmatic 2 amino acid binding proteins. (b) Schematic representation of the transmembrane topology of the excitatory amino-acid receptors. The dark extracellular regions indicate the two lobes forming the agonist binding site. The darkest region represents the alternatively spliced element (flip/flop) in the AMPA class of receptors. The edited sites are indicated by squares.

3.3.1.2 Kainate Receptors

The kainate receptors are composed of subunits from the GluR5–GluR7 class and the KA1–KA2 class of subunits. Homomeric receptors of the former class generate functional receptors and bind kainate with an affinity of 50 to 100 nM. KA1 or KA2 do not generate functional channels, but the receptors bind kainate with an affinity of 5 to 10 nM. Homomeric GluR6 and KA2 receptors are neither activated by AMPA, nor do they bind AMPA. Interestingly, when they are co-expressed, heteromeric receptors respond to AMPA.

3.3.1.3 NMDA Receptors

Functional NMDA receptor complexes contain at least one NR1 and one NR2 subunit. The heteromeric composition demands two agonists for activation because glycine binds to the NR1

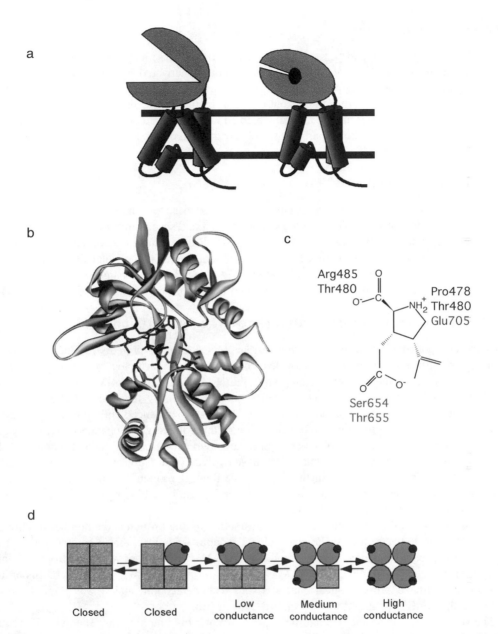

FIGURE 3.10 (a) Schematic illustration of the proposed model for subunit activation. Agonist binding stabilizes a closed conformation of the lobes in the binding domain. (b) Structure of the co-crystal of kainate and the soluble form of the GluR2 ligand-binding domain. The backbone is shown in a "ribbon" format, and the residues of the amino acids interacting with kainate are shown. (c) Illustration of the agonist bridging between the lobes. Arg485, Thr480, Pro478, and Thr480 are located in lobe A, while Glu705, Ser654, and Thr655 are located in lobe B. (d) Model for receptor activation. Activation of the receptor is proposed to require activation of two subunits, and activation of more subunits opens the channels to higher conductance levels.

subunit and glutamate binds to the NR2 subunit. The NR2 subunits have the same basic structure as the other glutamate subunits, except for a large 400- to 630-amino-acid C-terminal domain. Many of the receptor features such as the Mg^{2+} block, glycine sensitivity, deactivation kinetics, and the single-channel conductance differ, depending on which NR2 subunit co-assembles with NR1.

3.3.1.4   Orphan Receptors

Two additional subunits, δ_1 and δ_2, have been identified. Based on sequence similarities, they belong to the glutamate receptor family, although they cannot be activated by glutamate or any of the common glutamate receptor agonists. At least two lines of evidence support the functional importance of these channels: (1) genetic knockout of the δ_2 results in impaired cerebellar Purkinje cell function, and (2) the Lurcher mutant mouse, which shows significant cerebellar atrophy, is a result of a mutation in the extracellular part of the second transmembrane segment which renders the receptor constitutively active.

3.3.2   RECEPTOR TOPOLOGY

Results from a number of biochemical and mutagenesis studies support a three-transmembrane topology of the glutamate receptor. The region between the first and second transmembrane region forms a re-entrant loop, with a proposed structural similarity to the P-loop found in the voltage-gated channels. However, the loop enters the membrane from the cytoplasmic side in the glutamate receptors, while it is located at the extracellular side of the voltage-gated channels. The transmembrane nomenclature in the literature is dominated by the initially proposed four-transmembrane topology (Figure 3.9).

3.3.3   THE EXTRACELLULAR PART OF THE RECEPTOR: The Agonist Binding Site

Sequence comparisons between the glutamate receptors and other proteins revealed that the N-terminal part of the receptor exhibited a low level of sequence similarity to a bacterial periplasmic leucine–isoleucine–valine binding protein, while the N-terminal region of M1 (130 amino acids) and the region between M3 and M4 showed sequence similarity to another bacterial protein: lysine–arginine–ornithine binding protein (Figure 3.9). These sequence similarities and the resemblance of the M1–M3 segment with the pore region of the voltage-gated channels suggest that the glutamate receptor might have evolved as a chimera of two evolutionarily ancient modules. It has been proposed that the receptor subunits might have evolved from an insertion of a gene encoding the pore segment into a gene encoding a periplasmic binding protein. Identification of a bacterial potassium-selective glutamate receptor, GluR0, containing only the binding domain intersected by the pore region, strongly supports the evolutionary model.

The sequence similarity to the soluble periplasmic binding protein and a number of chimeric receptors formed between the AMPA and kainate receptors suggests that a soluble form of the binding domain could be engineered by replacing the M1–M3 segment with a hydrophilic linker and by truncating the N-terminal part and M4 and the C-terminal tail. When examined, this protein exhibited the same pharmacological characteristics as the receptor, and it was possible to co-crystallize the GluR2 binding domain with different ligands.

The structure is remarkably similar to the periplasmic binding proteins. The overall structure of the binding domain is two regions (called lobe A and B) where the agonist binds between the lobes. In the unbound condition (apo form), the lobes are separated. Binding of an agonist stabilizes the closure of the domains, which can be described as a rotation of the domains relative to each other, where the degree of rotation depends on the agonist. Kainate induces a rotation of 8 degrees, while agonists such as glutamate and AMPA induce a tighter closure resulting from a rotation of 20 degrees. Interestingly, an antagonist such as DNQX also induces a closure of the lobes but only by 3 degrees, apparently insufficient to open the pore. The forces that stabilize the closure can, for simplicity, be divided into three different categories of contributions. First, the glutamate-like moiety found in all the agonists forms a bridge between the lobes (Figure 3.10), and, second, the unique structures of the agonists, such as the pyrrolidine ring and isopropenyl in kainate (Figure 3.10c), contribute to the selective binding either by direct interactions with the binding domain or by confining the conformation of the glutamate moiety. Finally, the proximity of the lobes in the closed form promotes direct interactions between the lobes.

The residues located in the agonist binding pocket are highly conserved. Competitive antagonists and agonists selecting between the NMDA receptors and the AMPA/kainate receptors have been identified, where AP–V and NBQX or CNQX are the most commonly used selective NMDA and AMPA/kainate receptor antagonists, respectively. However, the high degree of conservation in the binding pocket has made identification of subtype-selective competitive antagonists very difficult. As a result, nearly all the known selective compounds act through noncompetitive mechanisms — for example, the AMPA receptor-selective GYKI-53655, cyclothiazide, which potentiates AMPA receptors in a splice-variant-dependent manner, or the polyamines, which block AMPA and kainate receptors depending on the presence of an edited subunit (see below).

An important question is how changes in the agonist binding domain might be transmitted to the pore region and induce channel opening. Our knowledge is very limited, and studying isolated ligand-binding domains has obvious limitations; however, there are some striking correlations between the degree of closure and the mode of activation. Kainate, which induces a minor closure, activates a nondesensitizing current, while AMPA activates a larger but transient current before entering into a desensitized state (Figure 3.8). This has prompted the hypothesis that a partially closed binding domain will induce a full opening of the channel while the closed binding domain (20-degree twist) will result in a desensitized state. According to this model, the brief opening induced by AMPA or glutamate reflects the fast molecular transition from the open conformation of the binding state to the tightly closed form. An alternative model proposes that the channel opening (conductance) increases as the binding domain closes, and the desensitization is a result of structural rearrangements between the subunits. The latter hypothesis is supported by a single mutation (L507Y in GluR3), which completely abolishes desensitization. In this mutant, the maximal currents elicited by glutamate or AMPA are threefold larger than the kainate-induced currents. In the crystal structure, L507 is located at the interface between the subunits. In addition, the action of compounds that reduce the rate of desensitization, such as cyclothiazide, are affected by mutations at the subunit interface. It should be kept in mind, however, that the affinity between the soluble binding domains is very low in solution, in contrast to the AChBP. Therefore, the interfaces observed in the crystal might be slightly different from the interactions within the receptor.

Because glutamate receptors can form homomeric receptors, an obvious question is how many subunits should bind a ligand in order to activate the channel? Studies on a nondesensitizing chimera have indicated that receptor activation requires binding of two agonists. Interestingly, binding of additional agonists resulted in an increased conductance, suggesting that each subunit could be activated independently and thereby alter the channel opening (Figure 3.10d). In order to resolve the different conductance states, the experiments have been performed in the presence of a slowly dissociating antagonist. More studies are required to evaluate the importance of the subconductance states in the absence of antagonist. If, indeed, the subunits are activated independently and the binding of more agonists results in increasing conductance, the dose–response curves should be interpreted with caution (see Problems).

The size of the agonist-activated current is not solely dependent on the degree of domain closure, as, particularly for the NMDA receptor, a number of modulatory sites have been located in the N-terminal part of the receptor. Zinc ions inhibit NR2A-containing receptors, while a number of compounds, such as ifenprodil, selectively inhibit NR2B-containing receptors. A splice variant in the N-terminal part of NR1 affects the pH and spermidine-sensitivity of the receptor. The mode of action of these noncompetitive inhibitors is not clear, although some studies suggest that they might share a common mechanism.

3.3.4 POSTTRANSCRIPTIONAL MODIFICATIONS

One important form of regulation is achieved by splice variants exhibiting functional differences and differential regulation. For instance, a 38-amino-acid segment preceding TM-IV is present in one of two alternative spliced forms (called "flip" or "flop") in GluR1–GluR4. The current amplitude is smaller in the flop receptors compared with the flip receptors. This might be a mechanism that could enable the neurons to switch from a low-gain flop version to a high-gain flip receptor, simply by alternative splicing of the transcripts.

Another form of regulation is editing of the RNA transcript. When GluR1, GluR3, or GluR4 is expressed individually or in combination, the current–voltage relationship exhibits an inwardly rectifying form, and the receptor channel is permeable to Ca^{2+}. However, if the GluR2 subunit is part of the receptor, the current–voltage relationship is linear, and the channel is impermeable to Ca^{2+}. Site-directed mutagenesis demonstrated that the channel properties were determined by a single amino acid difference in the putative M2. GluR2 encodes an arginine (R) at that position, while the other AMPA receptor subunits encode a glutamine (Q), hence the name Q/R site. Analysis of the genomic sequences revealed that GluR2, as in the other AMPA receptor subunits, encodes a glutamine (codon GAC), but the cDNA encodes an arginine (GGC) at that position. The A-to-G transition is catalyzed by an enzyme that recognizes an RNA structural element in the GluR2 transcript and then specifically deaminates the adenosine to an inosine (which is equivalent to a G). The presence of an edited subunit in the receptor complex prevents interaction with channel blockers such as Joro spider toxin and philantotoxins. In addition to the editing at the Q/R site in M2, GluR6 edits at two sites in M2 which also influence the Ca^{2+} permeability. This suggests that M1 might contribute to the pore in the glutamate receptors.

Another A-to-G editing, at a site designated the R/G site, can occur immediately preceding the flip–flop segment in GluR2–GluR4. The flip–flop segment influences the rate of desensitization, while the rate of recovery from the desensitized state depends on the R/G site where the edited form, G, recovers faster than the unedited form, R.

3.3.5 THE PORE REGION

The pore region has been studied extensively using mutagenesis and the substituted cysteine accessibility method (SCAM) in combination with electrophysiological measurements. These studies have provided some insight into the architecture of the glutamate receptor pore, and the data are to a large extent compatible with an overall structure similar to the three-dimensional structure of the crystallized potassium channel KcsA. The pore forms a cone-like structure, where the tip is located at the extracellular surface and the M2 region is inserted from the cytoplasmatic side. The reactivity of the residues located just at the N-terminal of M1 changes, depending on the activation of the receptor, and mutations in the C-terminal part of M3 make the receptor constitutively active, suggesting that the gate might be located at the cytoplasmatic surface, between M1 and M3.

The experimental data also support a similar structure for the M2 region and the P-element in KcsA, where the N-terminal part of M2 forms an α-helical structure located parallel to the wall of the cone formed by the transmembrane regions. The α-helical structure is followed by a random coiled structure pointing toward the center of the pore. That region forms the selective filter for potassium in the KcsA channel; however, the lack of discrimination between potassium and sodium currents in the glutamate receptor channel argues for a different structure. The Q/R site (see above) is located at the tip of the reentry loop. That position determines the permeability of divalent ions relative to monovalent ions. The equivalent position at the NMDA receptor is occupied by an aspargine, which is involved in the discrimination between the impermeable Mg^{2+} and the permeable Ca^{2+} ions. Additional amino acids are also involved, but they are not located at equivalent positions on the NR1 and the NR2 subunits, suggesting an asymmetry in the pore at that position.

The regions involved in the cation vs. anion selectivity are not well defined, as they are for the nAChR. However, in contrast to the nAChR, the residues within the pore contribute to the selectivity, as receptors formed from fully edited AMPA or kainate receptors (e.g., having an R at the Q/R site) are also permeable to chloride.

3.3.6 THE INTRACELLULAR SITE OF THE RECEPTOR

Long-term potentiation and depression of glutamatergic synapses are involved in many models for brain function and development. A key factor in the plasticity is a change in the AMPA and kainate receptor activities induced after NMDA receptor-dependent elevations of the intracellular Ca^{2+} concentration. Strong evidence exists for the involvement of two receptor-dependent mechanisms in the changes in the receptor activity. Glutamate receptors are, as for most ion channels, regulated by phosphorylation. Phosphorylation and dephosphorylation have been shown to alter both the probability for opening and the distribution of various conductance states. The second mechanism involves the dynamic change in the number of AMPA receptors at the synapse. The four amino acids at the very C-terminal of GluR1–GluR3 bind a number of anchoring proteins; in addition, GluR2 binds, at its cytoplasmatic tail, an ATPase (NSF) involved in membrane fusion. As a result, AMPA receptor trafficking exhibits a subtype-specific kinetics, depending on the presence of GluR2 in the receptor complex.

3.4 ATP RECEPTORS: 2TM RECEPTORS

Extracellular ATP has been demonstrated to activate a depolarizing current in different neuronal and non-neuronal cell types. These receptors are also referred to as P2 receptors. The receptors can further be divided into the G-protein-coupled P2Y receptors and the ligand-gated ion channels P2X. Currently, seven P2X receptors ($P2X_1$–$P2X_7$) have been cloned (Table 3.3). The receptors exhibit between 26 and 50% overall amino-acid identities, with the highest level of conservation in the extracellular and transmembrane regions. $P2X_7$ (also called P2Z) is the most distant member of the family.

The receptors range in size from 379 to 595 amino acids. The receptors have two transmembrane regions with intracellular N- and C-termini (Figure 3.11). Extensive SCAM analysis suggests that TM2 forms the pore, and a conserved glycine residue in the middle of TM2 lines the narrowest part of the channel. The structure of the pore and the location of the gate have still not been determined.

Different approaches have been employed to determine the receptor stoichiometry. Currently, a trimer is the favored model. All the subunits except $P2X_6$ can form functional homomeric receptors, and, except for $P2X_7$, all (currently tested) subunits can form a heteromeric complex. However, *in vivo*, the assembly seems to be guided by mechanisms that restrict the number of combinations compared to the theoretical possibilities.

The number of selective compounds acting on the different P2X subtypes is very limited. P2X channels can be distinguished from the P2Y receptors by their much faster kinetics. Kinetic properties, such as desensitization, can also be used in electrophysiological recordings to distinguish among the different subtypes. For example, $P2X_1$ and $P2X_3$ desensitize fast at saturating ATP concentrations, while $P2X_2$ and $P2X_4$ desensitize only very slowly. However, desensitization generally is not an optimal criterion for characterization of the receptors. First, different receptor-independent mechanisms (phosphorylation, binding proteins, etc.) might influence the desensitization. Second, desensitization is difficult to measure accurately in multicellular systems and with

TABLE 3.3
Subunits of the 2TM Superfamily

P2X Receptors	P2Z Receptor
$P2X_1$	$P2X_7$
$P2X_2$	
$P2X_3$	
$P2X_4$	
$P2X_5$	
$P2X_6$	

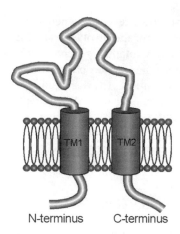

FIGURE 3.11 Schematic representation of the transmembrane topology of the adenosine triphosphate (ATP) receptors.

methods other than electrophysiology. Third, different channel substates may have different desensitization properties.

The P2X receptors are cation-selective channels, and it is generally assumed that ion selectivity is conserved for a given channel. Studies on the $P2X_2$, $P2X_4$, and the $P2X_7$ receptors, however, have revealed a shift in the ion selectivity after prolonged receptor activation. A short agonist application opens the channel pore to be permeable only for small cations, while longer activation (hundreds of milliseconds to seconds) induces a pore conformation permeable to large dyes (>630 Da). The larger pore conformation can be obtained by sustained application or by repetitive pulse. Interestingly, despite the change in pore size, the channel remains cation selective. Similar changes in conductance levels have been observed for a few other channels, but it remains to be shown how general the phenomenon is and whether it exhibits agonist specificity.

3.5 PROBLEMS

Problem 3.1

The prevalent receptor model for the excitatory amino acid is a tetrameric complex. As mentioned in the text, there is evidence that the channel conductance depends on the number of subunits that bind a ligand. Estimate the EC_{50} value and Hill coefficient for a dose–response curve assuming that the occupation at each subunit has a K_d value of 1 μM, an n_H of 1, and that activation induces a transition to an active state independent of the state of the other subunits:

    a. Binding of two or more agonists activates a state that conducts the same current.
    b. Binding at two adjacent subunits is required for channel opening.
    c. As proposed, the receptor consists of two dimers and only binding at both subunits in a dimer results in receptor activation.
    d. Binding at two subunits conducts a current I; at three subunits, a current $2 \times I$; and binding all four subunits, a current of $3 \times I$.

Problem 3.2

Assume the assembly of nicotine acetylcholine receptor (nAChR) subunits is completely permissive. How many different receptors can be assembled in a cell expressing α_3, β_2, and β_4? Group the receptors according to which ones are likely to have similar single-channel conductance and/or activation kinetics.

3.6 FURTHER READING

Armstrong, N. and Gouaux, E., Mechanisms for activation and antagonism of the AMPA-sensitive glutamate receptor: crystal structures of the GluR2 ligand binding core, *Neuron*, 28, 165–181, 2000.

Brejc, K., van Dijk, W. J., Klassen, R. V., Schuurmans, M., van der Oost, J., Smit, A. B., and Sixma, T. K., Crystal structures of an ACh-binding protein reveal the ligand-binding domain of nicotinic receptors, *Nature*, 411, 269–276, 2001.

Corringer, P. J., Le Novere, N., and Changeux, J. P., Nicotic receptors at the aminoacid level, *Annu. Rev. Phamacol. Toxicol.*, 40, 431–458, 2000.

Dingledine, R., Borges, K., Bowie, D., and Traynelis, S. F., The glutamate receptor ion channels, *Pharmacol. Rev.*, 51, 7–61, 1999.

Egebjerg, Schousboe, and Krogsgaard-Larsen, Eds., *Glutamate and GABA Receptors and Transporters: Structure, Function and Pharmacology*, Taylor & Francis, London, 2001.

Khakh, B. S., Molecular physiology of P2X receptors and ATP signalling at synapses, *Nat. Rev. Neurosci.*, 2, 165–174, 2001.

Khakh, B. S., Burnstock, G., Kennedy, C., King, B. F., North, R. A., Seguela, P., Voigt, M., and Humphrey, P. P., International union of pharmacology. XXIVC. Current status of the nomenclature and the properties of P2X receptors and their subunits, *Pharmacol. Rev.*, 53, 107–118, 2001.

Kuner, T., Beck, C., Sakmann, B., and Seeburg, P. H., Channel-lining residues of the AMPA receptor M2 segment: structural environment of the Q7R site and identification of the selective filter, *J. Neurosci.*, 21, 4162–4172, 2001.

North, R. A. and Surprenant, A., Pharmacology of cloned P2X receptors, *Annu. Rev. Pharmacol. Toxicol.*, 40, 563–580, 2000

Rudolph, U., Crestani, F., and Mohler, H., $GABA_A$ receptor subtypes: dissecting their pharmacological functions. *Trends Pharmacol. Sci.*, 22, 188–194, 2001.

Sheng, M. and Lee, S. H., AMPA receptor trafficking and the control of synaptic transmission, *Cell*, 105, 825–828, 2001.

3.7 SOLUTIONS TO PROBLEMS

Problem 3.1

The occupancy at each subunit is $p = [L]/K_d + [L]$, where $[L]$ is the ligand concentration. If activation of the subunits is independent, as assumed, the number of activated subunits at the receptor complex will follow a binomial distribution; that is, the likelihood for activation of n subunits is $K_{4,n}p^{4-n}(1 - p)^n$. The current will be proportional to:

a. $6 * p^2(1 - p)^2 + 4 * (p)^3(1 - p) + p^4$, $K_d = 0.62$; $n_H = 1.70$
b. $4 * p^2(1 - p)^2 + 4 * (p)^3(1 - p) + p^4$, $K_d = 0.84$; $n_H = 1.57$
c. $2 * p^2(1 - p)^2 + 4 * (p)^3(1 - p) + p^4$, $K_d = 1.17$; $n_H = 1.56$
d. $1/3 * (6*p^2(1 - p)^2 + 2 * 4 * (p)^3(1 - p) + 3 * p^4)$; $K_d = 1.67$; $n_H = 1.23$

The K_d and n_H values are obtained using a normal fitting procedure.

Problem 3.2

The answer is eight. In linear representation:

1. $\alpha_3–\beta_2–\alpha_3–\beta_2–\beta_2$
2. $\alpha_3–\beta_2–\alpha_3–\beta_2–\beta_4$

3. $\alpha_3-\beta_2-\alpha_3-\beta_4-\beta_2$
4. $\alpha_3-\beta_4-\alpha_3-\beta_2-\beta_2$
5. $\alpha_3-\beta_2-\alpha_3-\beta_4-\beta_4$
6. $\alpha_3-\beta_4-\alpha_3-\beta_2-\beta_4$
7. $\alpha_3-\beta_4-\alpha_3-\beta_4-\beta_2$
8. $\alpha_3-\beta_4-\alpha_3-\beta_4-\beta_4$

Combinations with similar stoichiometry would be likely to have similar conductance (i.e., four groups of 1, 2–4, 5–7, and 8), while the subunit arrangement may be more important for the receptor kinetics because the agonist binding site is located between an α and a β subunit. If the binding site is assumed to be between the α subunit and the β subunit on the right (in this linear representation), there are three groups: (1) 1–2, $2 \times (\alpha_3 - \beta_2)$; (2) 3–6, $(\alpha_3 - \beta_2)(\alpha_3 - \beta_4)$; and (3) 7–8, $2 \times (\alpha_3 - \beta_2)$.

4 Molecular Structure of Receptor Tyrosine Kinases

Steen Gammeltoft

CONTENTS

4.1 INTRODUCTION

Cell-surface receptors are involved in transmission of extracellular signals across the plasma membrane and regulation of intracellular signal-transduction pathways mediating development and multicellular communication in all living organisms. These receptors bind a large variety of water-soluble ligands, including amines, amino acids, lipids, peptides, and proteins. For convenience, they can be sorted into four major classes with different signaling mechanisms: G-protein-coupled receptors, ion-channel receptors, cytoplasmic tyrosine kinase (CTK)-linked receptors, and receptors with intrinsic enzymatic activity. In the latter class, receptor tyrosine kinases (RTKs) are predominant, whereas guanylate cyclase receptors and serine/threonine kinase receptors are minor groups. CTK-linked receptors mediate the responses to cytokines and hormones such as erythropoietin (EPO), interferon, and growth hormone (GH). RTKs bind a variety of growth factors and hormones, such as epidermal growth factor (EGF), fibroblast growth factor (FGF), and insulin. Although RTKs and CTK-linked receptors formally belong to different classes, the signaling mechanism shows similarities regarding receptor dimerization and tyrosine phosphorylation.

The RTKs catalyze the transfer of the γ-phosphate of adenosine triphosphate (ATP) to hydroxyl groups of tyrosines on target proteins. RTKs play an important role in the control of most fundamental processes, including the cell cycle, cell migration, cell metabolism, and survival, as well as cell proliferation and differentiation. All RTKs contain an extracellular ligand-binding domain that is usually glycosylated. The ligand-binding domain is connected to the cytoplasmic domain by a single transmembrane helix. In receptors with intrinsic enzymatic activity, the cytoplasmic domain contains a conserved protein tyrosine kinase (PTK) core and additional regulatory sequences that are subjected to autophosphorylation and phosphorylation by heterologous protein kinases. In CTK-

0-8493-1029-6/03/$0.00+$1.50

linked receptors, the relatively short cytoplasmic domains interact through noncovalent interactions with members of the Janus kinase (JAK) family of CTKs. Apart from the lack of covalent linkage to a kinase, the mechanism of action of these binary receptors largely resembles that of RTKs. The purpose of this review is to describe the molecular structure of RTKs with an emphasis on the general concepts underlying the receptor activation and signal transduction of growth factors, cytokines, and hormones.

4.2   RECEPTOR TYROSINE KINASE FAMILIES

The sequencing effort of the genomes of eukaryotic organisms has revealed that up to about 20% of the 6200 to 32,000 coding genes in *Saccharomyces cerevisiae, Caenorhabditis elegans, Drosophila melanogaster, Arabidopsis thaliana*, and *Homo sapiens* encode proteins involved in signal transduction, including transmembrane receptors, G-protein subunits, and signal-generating enzymes. In the human genome, more than 520 protein kinases and 130 protein phosphatases exert reversible control of protein phosphorylation. Both of these enzyme categories can be subdivided into tyrosine- or serine/threonine-specific, based on their catalytic specificity. In addition, some possess dual specificity for both tyrosine and serine/threonine, and a few members of the phosphatidylinositol kinase family also exhibit protein kinase activity. There are more than 90 known PTK genes in the human genome; 59 encode transmembrane RTKs distributed among 20 subfamilies, and 32 encode cytoplasmic, nonreceptor PTKs in 10 subfamilies. It is important to note that of the 30 growth-suppresser genes and more than 100 dominant oncogenes, protein kinases, in particular PTKs, comprise a large fraction of the latter group. PTKs evolved to mediate aspects of multicellular communication and development in metazoans, where they comprise about 0.3% of genes. Somatic mutations in this very small group of genes cause a significant fraction of human cancers, emphasizing the inverse relationship between normal developmental regulation and oncogenesis.

The PTK group includes a large number of enzymes with closely related kinase domains that specifically phosphorylate tyrosine residues and do not phosphorylate serine or threonine. These enzymes, first recognized among retroviral oncoproteins, have been found only in metazoan cells, where they are widely recognized for their role in transducing growth and differentiation signals. Included in this group are more than 20 distinct receptor families made up of membrane-spanning molecules that share similar overall structural topologies. All members of the RTK superfamily have a large extracellular domain with a high degree of diversity in the primary sequence and tertiary structure. The single-chain membrane-spanning domain shows no conservation among the various RTKs. The cytoplasmic domain contains the catalytic entity consisting of the well-conserved PTK. The amino-acid sequence shows significant homology reflecting the conserved protein kinase fold, in general, and the PTK structure, in particular. The eukaryotic protein kinase superfamily can be subdivided into distinct families that share structural and functional properties. Phylogenetic trees derived from an alignment of kinase-domain, amino-acid sequences serve as the basis for the classification. Thus, the sole consideration is similarity in kinase-domain, amino-acid sequence.

The specificity determinants surrounding the tyrosine phospho-acceptor sites have been determined by various procedures. In PTK assays using various substrates, it was determined that glutamic residues of the N-terminal or C-terminal side of the acceptor are often preferred. The substrate specificity of PTK catalytic domains has been analyzed by peptide library screening for prediction of the optimal peptide substrates. Finally, bioinformatics has been applied to identify phospho-acceptor sites in proteins of PTKs by application of a neural network algorithm.

4.3   IDENTIFICATION OF RECEPTOR TYROSINE KINASES

Thirty years ago, receptors for polypeptide hormones such as insulin and GH were identified as binding activity in cells, membranes, or solubilized membrane proteins using radiolabeled proteins as ligand. However, the signal transduction of these receptors remained a "black box" for about 10 years before their PTK activity was demonstrated. The first RTK to be identified functionally and structurally was the epidermal growth factor (EGF) receptor. Stanley Cohen and co-workers isolated the EGF receptor and demonstrated that it was an intrinsic membrane glycoprotein of 170 kDa, that it contained a specific binding site for EGF, and that the EGF-activated PTK activity was intrinsic to the receptor. The primary structure of the EGF receptor, determined by cDNA cloning and sequencing of receptor mRNA, localized PTK sequences in the cytoplasmic portion of the receptor polypeptide chain. Ligand binding induces dimerization of the EGF receptor and rapid activation of PTK with autophosphorylation of several tyrosine residues located in the C-terminus of the receptor. These phosphotyrosine residues act as binding sites for Src homology 2 (SH2) domains or phosphotyrosine-binding (PTB) domains of a variety of signaling proteins.

Subsequently, RTKs belonging to 20 subfamilies have been cloned (Figure 4.1). These structures are highly conserved in the catalytic PTK domain but show large variations in the extracellular domain as well as the juxtamembrane and C-terminal portions of the cytoplasmic domain. The classification of RTK subfamilies is based on primary-sequence homology and similarities in secondary structure. Cysteine-rich domains, immunoglobulin-like (Ig-like) domains, leucine-rich domains, cadherin-like domains, fibronectin type III domains, EGF-like domains, and kringle-like domains characterize the extracellular portions of RTKs (Figure 4.1).

4.4 PARADIGMS FOR RECEPTOR TYROSINE KINASE ACTIVATION

Studies of EGF receptor function defined two general paradigms in RTK activation and signal transduction. First, RTKs are activated by dimerization induced by ligand binding. With the exception of the insulin receptor family of RTKs, all known RTKs (e.g., EGF receptor or platelet-derived growth factor [PDGF] receptor) are monomers in the membrane. Ligand binding induces dimerization of these receptors, resulting in autophosphorylation of their cytoplasmic domains. Insulin receptor is a disulfide-linked dimer of two polypeptide chains forming a $\alpha_2\beta_2$ heterotetramer. Insulin binding to the extracellular α subunits induces a rearrangement in the quaternary heterotetrameric structure that leads to activation of the intracellular PTK and increased autophosphorylation of the cytoplasmic domain. The active forms of insulin receptor and monomeric RTK are both dimeric, and the activation mechanisms of the receptors are likely to be very similar. Second, receptor autophosphorylation generates phosphotyrosine sites in the cytoplasmic portion of the receptor that act as docking sites for binding of SH2 domains and PTB domains. In addition to its central role in the control of PTK activity, tyrosine autophosphorylation of RTK is crucial for recruitment and activation of a variety of signaling proteins. Most tyrosine autophosphorylated sites are located in noncatalytic regions of the cytoplasmic portion of the receptor molecule. These regions include the C-terminal tail, as in the EGF receptor, and the kinase insert region, as in the PDGF receptor. The interaction between SH2 domains and phosphotyrosine motifs provides a mechanism for assembly and recruitment of signaling complexes by activated RTK. Accordingly, every RTK should be considered not only as a receptor with PTK activity but also as a platform for the recognition and recruitment of a specific complement of signaling proteins.

4.4.1 ACTIVATION BY DIMERIZATION

During the last decade, significant progress has been made in understanding the molecular basis for dimerization of RTKs. Biochemical studies of ligand binding and activation of RTK have led to the hypothesis that RTKs are activated by dimerization (Figure 4.2). The exact molecular basis for the formation of the oligomer remained unclear, however. Structural studies of ligands in complex with the receptor-binding domain have provided insight into the nature of the dimerization mechanism. Several crystal structures of receptors in complex with their ligand have been solved, including cytokine as well as growth factor receptors. Different ligands employ different mechanisms for inducing the active dimeric state of RTK.

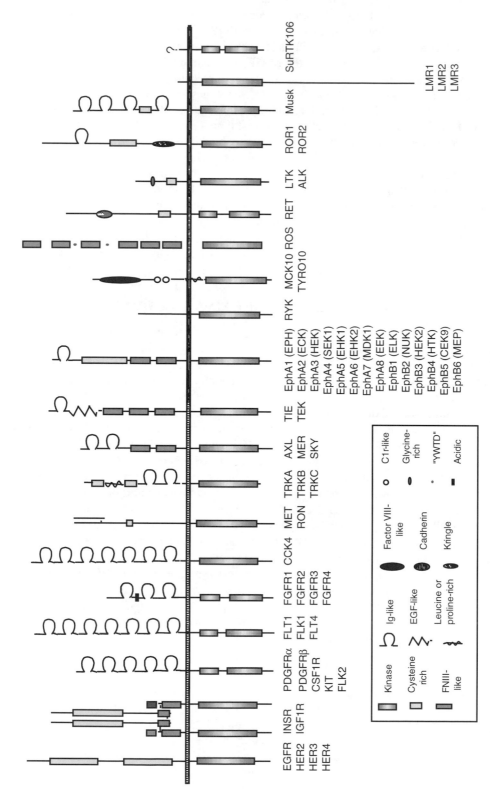

FIGURE 4.1 RTK superfamily. Figure shows a schematic representation of the domain structure of 20 RTK families. (Courtesy of SUGEN, Inc.)

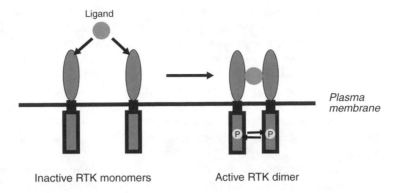

FIGURE 4.2 Receptor tyrosine kinase dimerization. Binding of monomeric or dimeric ligands to RTK monomers leads to formation and stabilization of activated RTK dimers. Cytoplasmic domains of RTK are *trans*-phosphorylated by active PTK.

The crystal structures of monomeric ligands such as GH and EPO in complex with their respective receptors show that these hormones are bivalent and one ligand binds simultaneously to two receptor molecules to form a 1:2 (ligand:receptor) complex. Receptor dimerization is further stabilized by additional receptor–receptor interactions.

Several growth factors are homodimers, such as vascular endothelial growth factor (VEGF) and PDGF, and provide a simple basis for ligand-induced receptor dimerization. The VEGF receptor contains seven Ig-like domains in their extracellular domain, of which only Ig domains 2 and 3 are required for ligand binding. The crystal structure of VEGF in complex with the Ig-like domain 2 of the Flt-1 VEGF receptor provides a view of ligand-induced receptor dimerization. The structure shows that one receptor molecule binds to each of the two junctions between VEGF protomers to yield a complex that is close to twofold symmetric and contains two VEGF protomers plus the two Ig-like domains.

The fibroblast growth factor (FGF) is a monomeric ligand that activates FGF receptors with the cooperation of the accessory molecule, heparin sulfate proteoglycan. The crystal structures of FGF in complex with the ligand-binding domain of FGF receptor (consisting of Ig-like domains 2 and 3) provide a molecular view of FGF receptor dimerization. Each structure shows a 2:2 FGF:FGF receptor complex, in which FGF interacts extensively with Ig-like domains 2 and 3 and with the linker that connects these two domains within one receptor. The dimer is stabilized by a secondary binding site involving interactions between FGF and D2 of the second receptor in the complex as well as receptor–receptor interactions. In contrast to the disulfide-linked VEGF homodimer, the two FGF molecules in the 2:2 FGF:FGF receptor complex do not make any contact. FGF and FGF receptor are not sufficient for stabilizing FGF receptor dimers at the cell surface. Heparin or heparan sulfate proteoglycans are essential for stable dimerization of FGF:FGF receptor complexes. Heparin binds to a positively charged canyon formed by a cluster of exposed Lys and Arg residues that extends across the D2 domains of the two receptors in the dimer and the adjoining bound FGF molecules.

4.4.2 Tyrosine Autophosphorylation

Activation of RTKs is accomplished by autophosphorylation on tyrosine residues, a consequence of ligand-mediated dimerization (Figure 4.2). Two processes are involved: enhancement of catalytic activity of PTK and creation of binding sites in the cytoplasmic domain to recruit downstream signaling proteins. In general, autophosphorylation of tyrosines in the activation loop within the PTK domain results in stimulation of kinase activity, and autophosphorylation of tyrosines in the juxtamembrane, kinase insert, and carboxyl-terminal regions generates docking sites for modular domains that recognize phosphotyrosine in specific contexts. The two well-established phosphoty-rosine-binding modules present within signaling proteins are the SH2 domain and the PTB domain.

All RTKs contain between one and three tyrosines in the kinase activation loop, which is composed of subdomains VII and VIII of the protein kinase catalytic core. Phosphorylation of these tyrosines has been shown to be critical for stimulation of catalytic activity and biological function for a number of RTKs, including insulin receptor, FGF receptor, VEGF receptor, PDGF receptor, Met (hepatocyte growth factor receptor), and TrkA (NGF receptor). A major exception is the EGF receptor, for which autophosphorylation of a conserved tyrosine in the activation loop does not seem to be involved in signaling. Substitution of tyrosine with phenylalanine has no effect on RTK activity or downstream signals.

In principle, RTK autophosphorylation could occur in *cis* (within a receptor monomer) or in *trans* (between two receptors in a dimer). In the first case, ligand binding would cause a change in receptor conformation that would facilitate *cis*-autophosphorylation of tyrosine residues located within or outside the PTK domain. In the second case, no conformational change must occur upon dimerization. The simple proximity effect would provide sufficient opportunity for *trans*-phospho-rylation of tyrosines in the cytoplasmic domain by a second RTK.

The crystal structure of the unphosphorylated forms of the insulin receptor has provided details on the molecular mechanisms by which RTKs are kept in a low activity state prior to autophos-phorylation of tyrosines in the activation loop. In the insulin receptor structure, one of the three tyrosines in the activation loop, Tyr^{1162}, is bound in the active site, seemingly in position to be autophosphorylated (in *cis*). However, Asp^{1150} of the PTK-conserved Asp–Phe–Gly sequence in the beginning of the activation loop is not in the proper position to coordinate MgATP but interferes with ATP binding. This is consistent with biochemical data for phosphorylation of Tyr^{1162} (and Tyr^{1158} and Tyr^{1163}) occurring in *trans* (by a second insulin receptor molecule). Moreover, substi-tution of Tyr^{1162} with phenylalanine results in an increase in basal kinase activity consistent with an autoinhibitory role for Tyr^{1162}.

The crystal structure of the tris-phosphorylated PTK domain of the insulin receptor reveals the role of activation loop phosphorylation in the stimulation of catalytic activity. Autophosphorylation of the insulin receptor brings about a dramatic repositioning of the activation loop. The conformation of the tris-phosphorylated insulin RTK activation loop is stabilized in part by interactions involving the phosphotyrosines, particularly phosphorylated Tyr^{1162}, which is hydrogen-bonded to a conserved arginine in the beginning of the activation loop (Arg^{1155}) and to a backbone amide nitrogen in the latter half of the loop. Accordingly, the insulin receptor is *cis*-inhibited by the binding of Tyr^{1162} in the active site that competes with protein substrates but is not *cis*-autophosphorylated because of steric constraints that prevent binding of MgATP. The insulin receptor is *trans*-activated by a second receptor molecule that phosphorylates Tyr^{1162}. The temperature factors (B-factors) derived during crystallographic refinement indicate that portions of the phosphorylated insulin RTK acti-vation loop are quite mobile, suggesting that an equilibrium between multiple conformations exists in solution. A subset of these (e.g., observed in the crystal structure of inactive insulin RTK) will hinder substrate (protein and ATP) binding, whereas other conformations (e.g., observed in the active insulin RTK crystal structure) will facilitate substrate binding and phosphorylation.

4.5 STRUCTURAL STUDIES OF RECEPTOR TYROSINE KINASES

4.5.1 LIGAND-BINDING DOMAINS

Several structures of ligand-binding domains of RTKs have been reported in the last 10 years, providing a basis for understanding dimerization mechanisms and ligand-receptor specificity (Table 4.1). The structures include receptors for cytokines such as growth hormone, prolactin, and eryth-ropoietin, as well as receptors for growth factors such as insulin-like growth factor I, fibroblast growth factor, nerve growth factor, and vascular endothelial growth factor. In general, only a subset

TABLE 4.1
Crystal Structures of RTK Extracellular Binding Domains

Ligand	Receptor	Domain	Ligand	Stoichiometry (ligand:receptor)
Growth hormone (GH)	GH receptor	Extracellular domain	Monomeric	1:2
GH	Prolactin receptor	Extracellular domain	Monomeric	1:2
Placental lactogen	Prolactin receptor	Extracellular domain	Monomeric	1:2
Erythropoietin (EPO)	EPO receptor	Extracellular domain	Monomeric	1:2
Vascular endothelial growth factor (VEGF)	Flt-1 receptor	Immunoglobulin (Ig) domains 2 and 3	Dimeric	1:1
Fibroblast growth factor 2 (FGF2)	FGF receptor 1	Ig domains 2 and 3	Monomeric	1:1
FGF1	FGF receptor 1	Ig domains 2 and 3	Monomeric	1:1
FGF2	FGF receptor 2	Ig domains 2 and 3	Monomeric	1:1
FGF2 and heparin	FGF receptor1	Ig domains 2 and 3	Monomeric	1:1:1
No ligand	EphB2 receptor	N-terminal globular domain	—	—
Nerve growth factor (NGF)	TrkA	Ig domain 5	Dimeric	1:2
No ligand	IGF-I receptor	Domains 1, 2, and 3	—	—

of domains in the extracellular portion of an RTK is involved in ligand binding. All RTKs consist of multiple extracellular domains that represent common protein folds such as cysteine-rich, fibronectin-III-like, Ig-like, and EGF-like domains (Figure 4.1).

Binding of GH to its receptor is required for regulation of normal human growth and development, including growth and differentiation of muscle, bone, and cartilage cells. The GH receptor, a member of the class 1 hematopoietic receptor superfamily is a single-pass transmembrane receptor that lacks a kinase region. This classification is based on sequence similarity in the extracellular domains, notably a highly conserved pentapeptide, the so-called "WSXWS box," the function of which is controversial. Signaling occurs through the JAK/signal transducer and activator of transcription (STAT) pathway, where ligand-induced homodimerization has been proposed to promote stable association of JAK2, with phosphorylation of JAK2, receptor, and STAT (Figure 4.3). In the case of GH, activation involves receptor homodimerization in a sequential process. The association of the hormone and one receptor molecule to an intermediary 1:1 complex forms the active ternary

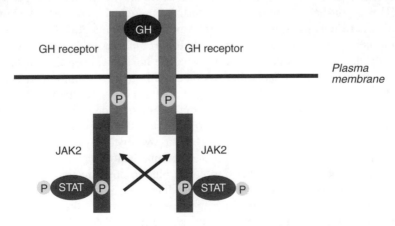

FIGURE 4.3 Growth hormone receptor. Monomeric GH associates with two receptor monomers. Activated JAK2 kinases *trans*-phosphorylate JAK2 and GH receptors, and STAT transcription factors are phosphorylated by JAK2.

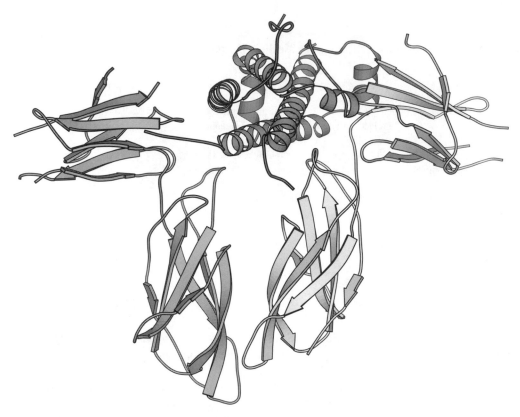

FIGURE 4.4 Structure of the complex between human GH and extracellular domain of its receptor. GH is composed of four tightly packed α helices that are shown in dark gray. The two binding proteins are composed of β sheets and they are shown in light and medium gray, respectively. PDB id: DHHR. The figures with molecular structures were created using the program Molscript. (Vos, A. M. et al., *Science*, 255, 306–312, 1992.)

complex consisting of one ligand and two receptor molecules. GH binds both to the GH receptor and the prolactin receptor.

Examination of the crystal structure of the complex between the hormone and the extracellular domain of its receptor has shown that the complex consists of one molecule of GH per two molecules of receptor. GH is a four-helix bundle with an unusual topology (Figure 4.4). The binding protein contains two distinct domains, similar in some respects to immunoglobulin domains. Both GH binding domains contribute residues that participate in GH binding. In the complex, both receptors donate essentially the same residues to interact with the hormone, even though the two binding sites on GH have no structural similarity. In addition to the hormone-receptor interfaces, substantial surface contact is present between carboxyl-terminal domains of the receptors. The relative extents of the contact areas support a sequential mechanism for dimerization that may be crucial for signal transduction. The structure of the 1:1 complex of GH bound to the extracellular domain of the prolactin receptor revealed how the hormone can bind to two distinctly different receptors. Finally, the structure of the ternary complex between ovine placental lactogen and the extracellular domain of the rat prolactin receptor showed that two receptors bind to opposite sides of placental lactogen with pseudo twofold symmetry. The two receptor binding sites differ significantly in their topography and electrostatic character. The binding interfaces also involve different hydrogen bonding and hydrophobic packing patterns compared to the structurally related GH receptor complexes.

Erythropoietin is a glycoprotein hormone that regulates the proliferation, differentiation, and maturation of erythroid cells. The EPO receptor is a member of the class 1 cytokine receptor superfamily. The crystal structure of an EPO-mimetic peptide and the extracellular portion of the

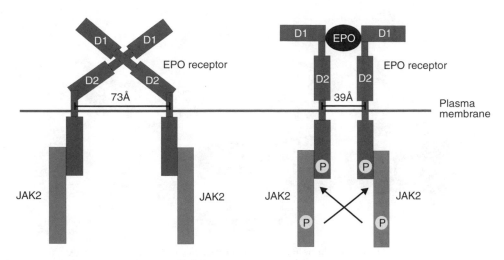

FIGURE 4.5 Unligated and ligated erythropoietin receptor dimer configurations. In the absence of the ligand, the D2 domains and consequently the cytoplasmic domains of the two EPO receptor monomers are oriented with 73-Å separation between them. In the presence of ligand, the distance between the two EPO receptor monomers is reduced to 39 Å so activation of JAK2 and *trans*-phosphorylation of JAK2 and the cytoplasmic domains of EPO receptor can occur. (Modified after Livnah, O. et al., *Science*, 273, 464–471, 1996. With permission.)

EPO receptor revealed an asymmetric dimer with two EPO binding proteins. Each EPO binding protein monomer consists of two fibronectin-III folds (D1 and D2) connected approximately at right angles, as in other cytokine receptors (Figure 4.5). In the ligand–receptor complex, the ligand induces a close dimer formation of both the D1 and D2 domains separated by 39 Å, so that their intracellular regions become substrates for phosphorylation by two JAK2 molecules. In contrast, the structure of native, unligated EPO binding protein showed a cross-shaped dimer where the membrane-proximal ends of D2 domains are separated by 73 Å, and the D1 domains of each monomer point in opposite directions. The scissors-like dimer configuration keeps the intracellular ends far enough apart so that autophosphorylation of JAK2 cannot occur. Accordingly, other phosphorylation events, such as on the cytoplasmic domain of EPO receptor, do not occur. The two structures of EPO receptors suggest that unligated receptors would self-associate on the cell surface and form inactive dimers. Binding of EPO to the receptor dimer induces the active conformation. A self-associated dimer would explain how EPO could activate efficiently on the cell surface where relatively few receptors (<1000) are present. Without some clustering of receptors, even transitory, monomeric receptor–erythropoietin complexes would be prevalent, especially in an excess of EPO.

Vascular endothelial growth factor is a homodimeric hormone that induces proliferation of endothelial cells and angiogenesis through binding to specific RTKs. Two RTKs have been described: the kinase domain receptor (KDR) and the Fms-like tyrosine kinase (Flt-1), both of which are located on the surface of vascular endothelial cells. The extracellular portions consist of seven Ig domains, and the second and third domains of Flt-1 are necessary and sufficient for binding of VEGF with near-native affinity; domain 2 alone binds only 60-fold less tightly than wild-type. The crystal structure of the complex between VEGF and the second domain of Flt-1 shows that domain 2 interacts with the "poles" of the VEGF dimer in a predominantly hydrophobic manner (Figure 4.6).

The mammalian FGF receptor family includes at least four different gene products, with additional diversity generated by alternative splicing. To date, 18 mammalian FGFs have been identified and have been shown to be involved in the control of a variety of biological responses

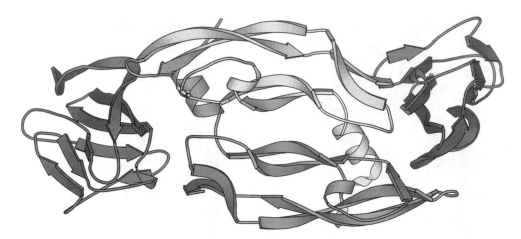

FIGURE 4.6 Structure of the complex between VEGF and Flt-1. The two monomers of VEGF are composed of parallel β sheets and they are shown in light and medium gray, respectively. The two copies of Flt-1 are in dark gray. PDB id: 1FLT. (Wiesmann, C. et al., *Cell,* 91, 641, 1997.)

that are crucial for development and survival. The four high-affinity receptors, FGF receptors 1 to 4, are composed of an extracellular ligand-binding domain that contains three Ig-like domains (D1 to D3), a single transmembrane helix, and a cytoplasmic domain that contains PTK activity. Receptor dimerization is an essential step in FGF signaling and requires heparan sulfate proteoglycans. The crystal structure of FGF2 bound to a naturally occurring variant of FGF receptor 1 consisting of Ig-like domains D2 and D3 showed that FGF2 interacts extensively with the two D domains as well as with the linker between the two domains. The dimer is stabilized by interactions between FGF2 and D2 of the adjoining complex and by a direct interaction between D2 of each receptor (Figure 4.7). The crystal structures of FGF1 and FGF2 complexed with the ligand-binding domains D2 and D3 of FGF receptor 1 and 2 reveal the determinants of ligand–receptor specificity. Highly conserved regions of FGF receptors including D2 and the linker between D2 and D3 define a common binding site for all FGFs. Specificity is achieved through interactions between the N-terminal and central regions of FGFs and two loop regions in D3 that are subject to alternative splicing.

The crystal structure of a ternary FGF2–FGF receptor 1–heparin complex is composed of a dimer with 2:2:2 stoichiometry. Within each 1:1 FGF:FGF receptor complex, heparin makes numerous contacts with both FGF and FGF receptor, thereby augmenting FGF–FGF receptor binding. Heparin also interacts with FGF receptor in the adjoining 1:1 FGF:FGF receptor complex to promote FGF receptor dimerization. The 6-O-sulfate group of heparin plays a pivotal role in mediating both interactions. On the basis of the crystal structure it is possible to design heparin analogs capable of modulating FGF activity. Given the important roles FGF plays in angiogenesis and cellular growth, synthetic heparin agonists and antagonists may have potential therapeutic value.

The ephrin (Eph) receptors fall into two groups, A and B, based on their ability to bind ligands (ephrins), which are themselves cell-surface proteins anchored to the plasma membrane either through a glycosylphosphatidylinositol (GPI) linkage (A type) or a transmembrane region (B type). Signaling between Eph receptors and ephrins generally involves direct cell–cell interactions and frequently results in cell repulsion. Vertebrate Eph receptors have numerous functions in cell movement, formation of cell boundaries, and morphogenesis of complex tissues such as the brain and cardiovascular system. The Eph receptors are RTKs with an extracellular region, a single-chain membrane-spanning region, and a cytoplasmic region with a PTK domain. The extracellular region consists of two fibronectin type III repeats: a cysteine-rich region and a conserved 180-amino acid N-terminal globular domain, which is both necessary and sufficient for binding of the receptors to their ephrin ligands. Eph receptors bind their ephrin ligands with high affinity and with one-to-one stoichiometry. The crystal structure of the amino-terminal domain of the EphB2

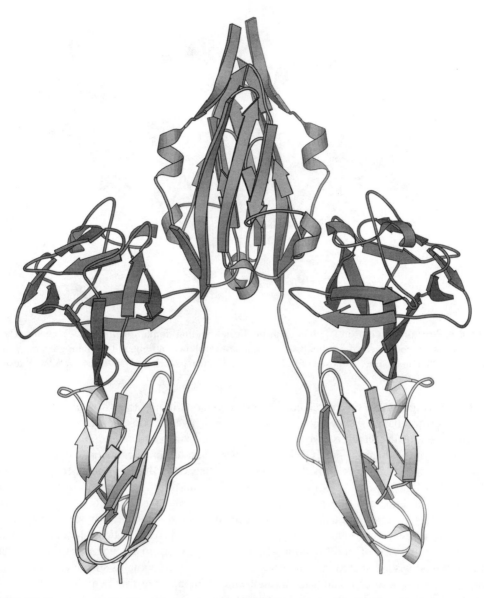

FIGURE 4.7 Structure of the dimeric complex between FGF2 and FGF receptor 1. The Ig-like domains 2 and 3 of the two FGF receptor 1 molecules are composed of parallel β sheets and they are shown in medium and light gray, respectively. The two FGF2 molecules are composed of a bundle of β sheets that are shown in dark gray. PDB id: 1CVS. (Plotnikov, A. N. et al., *Cell*, 98, 641, 1999.)

receptor folds into a compact jellyroll β-sandwich composed of 11 antiparallel β-strands. Using structure-based mutagenesis, an extended loop that is important for ligand binding and class specificity has been identified.

Nerve growth factor is involved in a variety of processes involving signaling, such as cell differentiation and survival, growth cessation, and apoptosis of neurons. These events are mediated by NGF as a result of its binding to its two cell-surface receptors, TrkA and p75. TrkA is a receptor with PTK activity that forms a high-affinity binding site for NGF. Of the five domains comprising its extracellular portion, the Ig-like D5 domain proximal to the membrane is necessary and sufficient for NGF binding. The crystal structure of human NGF in complex with the D5 domain of human TrkA shows that the NGF dimer binds two receptors with an interface consisting of two patches

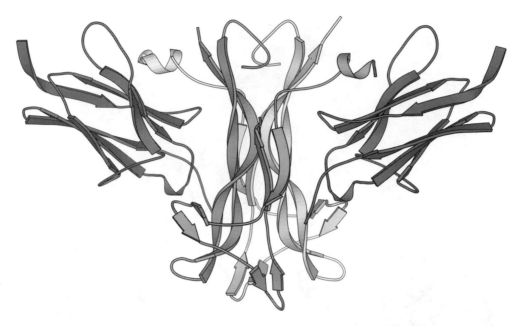

FIGURE 4.8 Structure of NGF in complex with the ligand-binding domain of the TrkA receptor. The two NGF monomers are composed of parallel β sheets and they are shown in light and medium gray, respectively. The two TrkA D5 domains are composed of β sheets that are shown in dark gray. PDB id: 1WWW. (Wiesmann, C. et al., *Nature*, 401, 184, 1999.)

of similar size (Figure 4.8). One patch constitutes a common binding motif for all family members, whereas the second patch is specific for the interaction between NGF and TrkA.

Insulin-like growth factor I is involved in both normal growth and development of many tissues and malignant transformation. The IGF-I receptor is a heterotetrameric molecule consisting of two α chains and two β chains linked by disulfide bonds. The extracellular α chains consist of several domains with a ligand-binding region located at the amino-terminus. The β chains consist of a short extracellular domain, a transmembrane domain, and a cytoplasmic PTK domain. The crystal structure of the first three domains of IGF-I receptor, including the L1, cysteine-rich, and L2 domains, show that each L domain consists of a single-stranded right-handed β helix. The cysteine-rich region is composed of eight disulfide-bonded modules, seven of which form a rod-shaped domain with modules associated in an unusual manner. The three domains surround a central space of sufficient size to accommodate a ligand molecule. Although the fragment (residues 1 to 462) does not bind ligand, many of the determinants responsible for hormone binding and ligand specificity map to this central site.

4.5.2 PROTEIN KINASE DOMAINS

Crystal structures of the PTK domains from several RTKs have been reported (Table 4.2). These followed the structure determinations of several related protein serine/threonine kinases, the first of which was cyclic AMP-dependent protein kinase (PKA). The overall PTK domain is similar to that of the serine/threonine kinases (Figure 4.9). It is composed of an amino-terminal lobe, composed of a five-strand β-sheet and one α helix, and a larger C-terminal lobe that is mainly α helical. ATP binds in the cleft between the two lobes, and the tyrosine-containing peptide substrate binds to the C-terminal lobe. Several residues are highly conserved in all PTKs, including several glycines in the nucleotide-binding loop, a lysine in β-strand 3, a glutamic acid in α helix C, an aspartic acid and asparagine in the catalytic loop, and an Asp-Phe-Gly motif at the beginning of the activation loop. Protein kinases are capable of a range of conformations owing to an inherent interlobe flexibility that allows for both

TABLE 4.2
Crystal Structures of RTK Intracellular Catalytic Domains

Receptor	Activity	Structure	Inhibition/Activation
Insulin	Inactive	Catalytic domain	Activation loop Tyr[1162] in catalytic site
Insulin	Active	tris-Phosphorylated catalytic domain	Release of activation loop by pTyr[1162]
Fibroblast growth factor (FGF) receptor 1	Inactive	Catalytic domain	Activation loop Pro[663] in catalytic site
FGF receptor 1	Inhibited	Catalytic domain	Indolinone in ATP binding site
FGF receptor1	Inhibited	Catalytic domain	Pyrimidine in ATP binding site
Vascular endothelial growth factor (VEGF) receptor	Inactive	Catalytic domain lacking kinase insert	Activation loop Pro[1168] in catalytic site
Tie2 receptor	Inactive	Catalytic domain, kinase insert, and C-terminal tail	ATP binding site blocked
Ephrin receptor B2 (EphB2)	Inactive	Juxtamembrane and catalytic domain	N-terminal lobe inhibited by juxtamembrane region
Insulin-like growth factor I (IGF-I) receptor	Active	tris-Phosphorylated catalytic domain	Activation loop released by pTyr[1135]
IGF-I receptor	Partially active	bis-Phosphorylated catalytic domain	Activation loop Tyr[1135] disordered

open and closed conformations. However, the catalytically competent conformation is generally a closed structure in which the two lobes clamp together to form an interfacial nucleotide binding site and catalytic cleft. The N-terminal lobe of protein kinases consists minimally of a twisted five-strand β-sheet (denoted β1 to β5) and a single helix αC. The N-terminal lobe functions to assist in the binding and coordination of ATP for the productive transfer of the γ-phosphate to a substrate oriented by the C-terminal lobe. In this regard, β-strands 1 and 2 and the glycine-rich connecting segment form a flexible flap that interacts with the adenine base, ribose sugar, and the nonhydrolyzable phosphate groups of ATP. Furthermore, an invariant salt bridge between a lysine side-chain in β-strand 3 and a glutamic acid side-chain in helix αC coordinates the β-phosphate of ATP.

The C-terminal lobe of protein kinases consists minimally of two β-strands (β7 and β8) and a series of α helices (αD to αI). Strands β7 and β8 locate to the cleft region between the N- and C-terminal lobes where they contribute side-chains that participate in catalysis and the binding of magnesium for the coordination of ATP phosphate groups. The activation segment, which is also located in the large catalytic lobe, is disordered in protein kinase structures in which the activation segment is not phosphorylated. The remaining C-terminal lobe elements, including the α helices αD to αI, are well ordered, and the kinase terminates with a short αJ. The catalytic activity of RTK is stimulated by autophosphorylation of tyrosines in the activation loop. In the unphosphorylated state, RTK is inactive.

Crystal structures of the unphosphorylated forms of RTK domains of insulin receptor, FGF receptor, VEGF receptor 2, Tie2 receptor, and EphB2 receptor provide the molecular basis for an understanding of how catalytic activity is repressed before receptor activation. Each of the five RTK structures reveals different mechanisms of inactivation. The activation loop of the insulin receptor contains three tyrosine autophosphorylation sites. In the crystal structure of unphosphorylated insulin receptor, one of the tyrosines is bound in the active site, hydrogen-bonded to a conserved aspartic acid and arginine in the catalytic loop. Tyr[1162] is seemingly in the position to be autophosphorylated in *cis*, but the conserved aspartic acid of the DFG motif (Asp[1150]) at the beginning of the activation loop, which is involved in Mg-ATP binding, is not properly positioned for catalysis (Figure 4.9). The structural data indicate that before autophosphorylation, Tyr[1162] competes with the protein substrates for the active site. Biochemical studies support a *trans-*

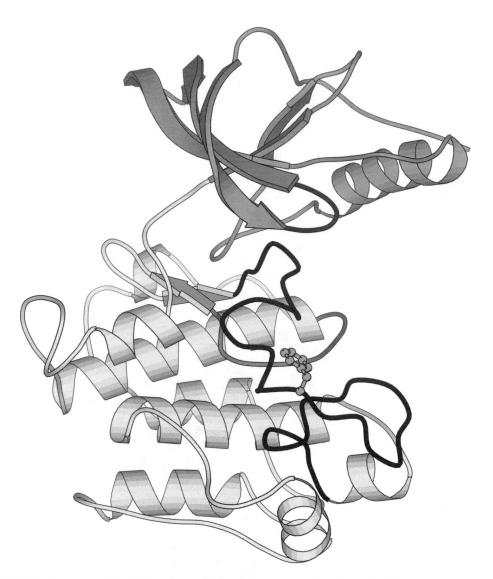

FIGURE 4.9 Structure of the PTK domain of the insulin receptor. The N-terminal kinase lobe is composed of one α helix and five β sheets that are shown in medium gray with the nucleotide-binding loop in dark gray. The C-terminal kinase lobe is composed of α helices and β sheets that are shown in light gray with the catalytic loop in medium gray. The activation loop is shown in dark gray with Tyr[1162] in medium gray. PDB id: 1IRK. (Hubbard, S. R. et al., *Nature,* 372, 746, 1994.)

phosphorylation mechanism for Tyr[1162] as well as Tyr[1158] and Tyr[1163] in the activation loop. Phenylalanine substitution of Tyr[1162] results in an increase in catalytic activity of RTK in the absence of insulin supporting the autoinhibitory role for Tyr[1162].

The crystal structure of the PTK domain of FGF receptor 1 has been determined. The activation loop of the FGF receptor kinase domain contains two tyrosine autophosphorylation sites, Tyr[653] and Tyr[654], corresponding to Tyr[1162] and Tyr[1163] in the insulin receptor. The conformation of the unphosphorylated FGF RTK activation loop as seen in the crystal structure is significantly different from that found in insulin RTK (Figure 4.10). In the FGF RTK structure, neither of the activation-loop tyrosines is bound in the active site. Rather, the tyrosine-kinase-invariant proline at the end of the activation loop and nearby residues is positioned to interfere with the binding of a substrate

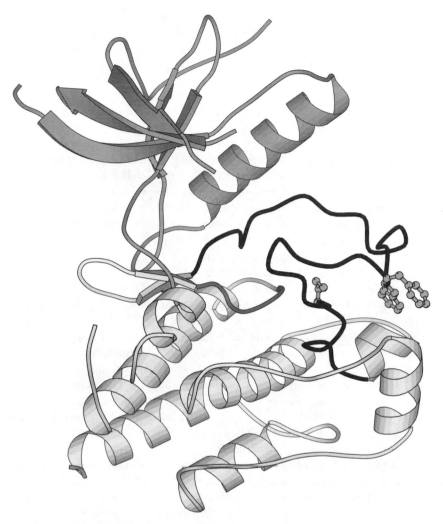

FIGURE 4.10 Structure of the PTK domain of the FGF receptor 1. The N-terminal kinase lobe is composed of one α helix and five β sheets that are shown in medium gray. The C-terminal lobe is composed of α helices and β sheets that are shown in light gray with the catalytic loop in medium gray. The activation loop is in dark gray with Tyr[653], Tyr[654] and Pro[663] in medium gray. PDB id: 1FGK. (Mohammadi, M. et al., *Cell*, 86, 577, 1996.)

tyrosine. Furthermore, in contrast to insulin RTK, the beginning of the activation loop does not obstruct the ATP binding site in FGF RTK.

The crystal structure of the PTK domain of the VEGF receptor 2 KDR reveals similarities and differences with insulin and FGF RTKs. The VEGF receptors (KDR and Flt-1), like the PDGF receptors, possess a large kinase insert between helices D and E in the carboxyl-terminal lobe. The kinase insert contains several tyrosine autophosphorylation sites that serve as docking sites for SH2 domain proteins. Attempts to crystallize VEGF RTK with the insert failed, but crystals of a protein lacking 50 residues of the insert were obtained. VEGF RTK has two tyrosine autophosphorylation sites in the activation loop, Tyr[1054] and Tyr[1059], which correspond to Tyr[1158] and Tyr[1163] in the insulin receptor. However, a tyrosine residue corresponding to the autoinhibitory Tyr[1162] in the insulin receptor is not present in the VEGF receptor. The crystal structure, determined in an unligated, phosphorylated state, reveals an overall fold and catalytic residue positions similar to those observed in other tyrosine kinase structures. The kinase activation loop, autophosphorylated on Tyr[1059] prior to crystallization, is mostly disordered. However, a portion of the activation loop in the vicinity of conserved Pro[1168] adopts the same inhibitory conformation as that seen in the structure of unphosphorylated FGR RTK: this region occupies a position inhibitory to substrate binding. The ends of the kinase insert form a β-like structure, not observed in other known tyrosine kinase structures, that packs near to the kinase C terminus. The unique structure may also occur in other PDGF receptor family members and may serve to properly orient the kinase insert for autophosphorylation of tyrosine residues and binding of adaptor proteins.

Tie2 (also known as Tek) is an endothelium-specific RTK involved in both angiogenesis and vasculature maintenance. The crystal structure of the RTK domain of Tie2 contains the catalytic core, the kinase insert domain, and the C-terminal tail. The overall fold of Tie2 is similar to that observed in other serine/threonine and tyrosine kinase structures. However, several features distinguish the Tie2 structure from those of other kinases. The Tie2 nucleotide binding loop is in an inhibitory conformation, which is not seen in other kinase structures, while its activation loop adopts an "activated-like" conformation in the absence of phosphorylation. Tyr[897], located in the N-terminal domain, may negatively regulate the activity of Tie2 by preventing dimerization of the kinase domains or by recruiting phosphatases when it is phosphorylated. Activation of the RTK activity of Tie2 is a complex process that requires conformational changes in the nucleotide binding loop, activation loop, C helix, and the carboxyl-terminal tail for ATP and substrate binding.

The crystal structure of the entire catalytic domain of EphB2 and the latter half of the juxtamembrane region, including two tyrosine phosphorylation sites Tyr[604] and Tyr[610] mutated to phenylalanines, has been solved. The structure of the catalytic domain conforms to that generally observed for protein kinases, consisting of two lobes, a smaller N-terminal lobe and a larger C-terminal lobe. The autoinhibited EphB2 catalytic domain adopts a closed conformation that superficially resembles an active state (Figure 4.11). The EphB2 juxtamembrane region preceding the catalytic domain is highly ordered, consisting of an extended strand segment Ex1, a single-turn 3/10 helix αA′, and a four-turn helix αB′. These elements associate intimately with helix αC of the N-terminal catalytic lobe and also interact in a limited way with the C-terminal lobe. The juxtamembrane segments adopt a helical conformation that distorts the small N-terminal lobe of the kinase domain by imposing a significant curvature on helix αC. This distortion couples to local distortions in other N-terminal lobe elements, most critically the glycine-rich loop and the invariant lysine–glutamate salt bridge. Together, the N-terminal distortions appear to impinge on catalytic function by adversely affecting the coordination of the sugar and phosphate groups of the bound nucleotide. With limited contacts to the lower lobe of the catalytic domain, the juxtamembrane segment also sterically impedes the activation segment from adopting the productive conformation that typifies the active state of PTK. Together, the effects on nucleotide coordination and the activation segment form the basis for autoinhibition of EphB2 RTK by the juxtamembrane segment. In EphB2, and most likely Eph RTKs in general, the switch to an active state is coordinated by phosphorylation at highly conserved sites within both the juxtamembrane region and the catalytic domain. Phosphorylation of EphB2 at Tyr[788] likely promotes the ordering of the activation segment to a catalytically competent conformation. In contrast, the phosphorylation at Tyr[604] and Tyr[610] may serve to destabilize the juxtamembrane structure and cause it to dissociate from the catalytic domain. This would allow for a return of the N-terminal lobe to an undistorted active conformation.

4.5.3 STRUCTURE OF ACTIVATED RECEPTOR TYROSINE KINASES

The crystal structure of the phosphorylated, activated form of the insulin RTK in complex with a peptide substrate and an ATP analog has been determined. The activation loop undergoes a major conformational change upon autophosphorylation of Tyr[1158], Tyr[1162], and Tyr[1163] within the loop, resulting in unrestricted access of ATP and protein substrates to the kinase active site (Figure 4.12). Phosphorylated Tyr[1163] (pTyr[1163]) is the key phosphotyrosine in stabilizing the conformation of the

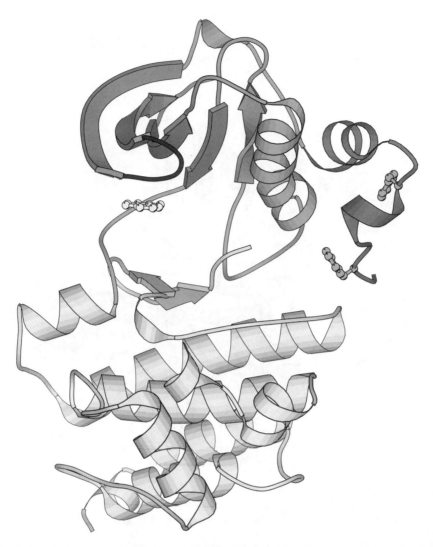

FIGURE 4.11 Structure of the autoinhibited EphB2 PTK domain. The juxtamembrane region is composed of two α helices that are shown in dark gray with Tyr[604] and Tyr[610] in medium gray. The N-terminal kinase lobe is composed of one α helix and five β sheets that are shown in medium gray with the nucleotide-binding loop in dark gray. The adenine moiety of AMP-PNP is in light gray. The C terminal kinase lobe is composed of α helices and β sheets that are shown in light gray. PDB id: 1JPA. (Wybenga-Groot, L. E. et al., *Cell,* 106, 745, 2001.)

tris-phosphorylated activation loop, whereas pTyr[1158] is completely solvent exposed, suggesting availability for interaction with downstream signaling proteins. The YMXM-containing peptide substrate binds as a short antiparallel β strand to the C-terminal end of the activation loop, with the methionine side-chains occupying two hydrophobic pockets on the C-terminal lobe of the kinase. The structure reveals the molecular basis for insulin receptor activation via autophosphorylation, and provides insights into RTK substrate specificity and the mechanism of phosphotransfer.

The insulin-like growth factor I receptor is closely related to the insulin receptor. The RTK activity of the IGF-I receptor is regulated by intermolecular autophosphorylation at three sites within the activation loop. The crystal structure of the trisphosphorylated form of IGF-I RTK domain with an ATP analog and a specific peptide substrate showed that autophosphorylation stabilizes the activation loop in a conformation that facilitates catalysis. Furthermore, the structure revealed how

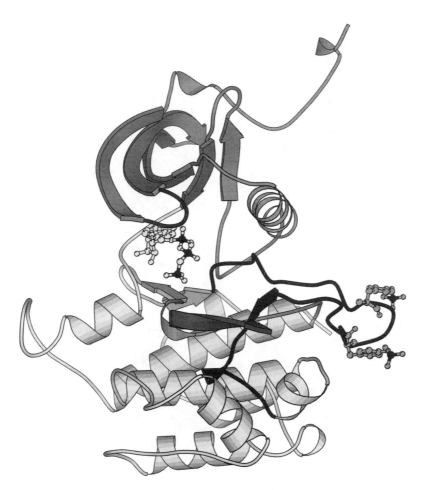

FIGURE 4.12 Structure of the tris-phosphorylated insulin receptor. The N-terminal kinase lobe is composed of one α helix and five β sheets that are shown in medium gray with the nucleotide-binding loop in dark gray. AMP-PNP is in light gray with the three phosphate residues in dark gray. The C-terminal kinase lobe is composed of α helices and β sheets that are shown in light gray with the catalytic loop in medium gray and the peptide substrate in dark gray. (Hubbard, S. R., *EMBO J.*, 16, 5572, 1997.)

the RTK recognizes tyrosine-containing peptides with hydrophobic residues at the P+1 and P+3 positions. Overall, the activated IGF-I RTK structure is similar to the activated insulin RTK structure, although sequence differences could potentially be exploited for anticancer drug design.

Another group solved the crystal structure of the IGF-I RTK domain phosphorylated at two tyrosine residues within the activation loop and bound to an ATP analog. The ligand is not in a conformation compatible with phosphoryl transfer, and the activation loop is partially disordered. IGF-I RTK is trapped in a half-closed, previously unobserved conformation. This conformation may be intermediary between the open, inactive conformation and closed, active conformation of insulin and IGF-I RTKs.

4.5.4 RECEPTOR TYROSINE KINASE INHIBITORS

Receptor tyrosine kinases are critical components of signaling pathways that control cell proliferation and differentiation. Enhanced RTK activity due to activating mutations or overexpression has been implicated in human cancers. Thus, selective inhibitors of RTKs have considerable value. Although a number of compounds have been identified as effective inhibitors of RTKs, the precise molecular mechanisms by which these agents inhibit RTK activity have not been elucidated. Two studies have reported the crystal structure of RTK inhibitors in complex with the tyrosine kinase domain of FGF receptor 1. One class of RTK inhibitors is based on an oxindole core (indolinones). Two compounds of this class inhibited the kinase activity of FGF receptor 1 and showed differential specificity toward other RTKs. The structure of the complex revealed that the oxindole occupies the site in which the adenine of ATP binds, whereas the moieties that extend from the oxindole contact residues in the hinge region between the two lobes of the kinase. The more specific inhibitor of FGF receptor 1 induces a conformational change in the nucleotide-binding loop. Another class of RTK inhibitors includes a synthetic compound of the pyrido-2,3-d-pyrimidine class that selectively inhibits the PTK activity of FGF and VEGF receptors. The structure of the complex of the compound and the kinase domain of FGF receptor 1 shows a high degree of surface complementarity between the pyrimidine analog and the hydrophobic ATP-binding pocket of FGF receptor 1. These inhibitors are promising candidates for therapeutic angiogenesis inhibitors and antiproliferative drugs to be used to be used in the treatment of cancer and other growth disorders.

4.6 FURTHER READING

de Vos, A. M., Ultsch, M., and Kossiakoff, A. A., Human growth hormone and extracellular domain of its receptor: crystal structure of the complex, *Science*, 255, 306–312, 1992.

Favelyukis, S., Till, J. H., Hubbard, S. R., and Miller, W. T., Structure and autoregulation of the insulin-like growth factor 1 receptor kinase, *Nat. Struct. Biol.*, 8, 1058–1063, 2001.

Gammeltoft, S., Insulin receptors: binding kinetics and structure-function relationship of insulin, *Physiol. Rev.*, 64, 1321–1378, 1984.

Gronborg, M., Wulff, B. S., Rasmussen, J. S., Kjeldsen, T., and Gammeltoft, S., Structure–function relationship of the insulin-like growth factor-I receptor tyrosine kinase, *J. Biol. Chem.*, 268, 23435–13440, 1993.

Heldin, C. H., Dimerization of cell surface receptors in signal transduction, *Cell*, 80, 213–223, 1995.

Hubbard, S. R., Crystal structure of the activated insulin receptor tyrosine kinase in complex with peptide substrate and ATP analog, *EMBO J.*, 16, 5572–5581, 1997.

Hubbard, S. R. and Till, J. H., Protein tyrosine kinase structure and function, *Annu. Rev. Biochem.*, 69, 373–398, 2000.

Hubbard, S. R., Wei, L., Ellis, L., and Hendrickson, W. A., Crystal structure of the tyrosine kinase domain of the human insulin receptor, *Nature*, 372, 746–754, 1994.

Hubbard, S. R., Mohammadi, M., and Schlessinger, J., Autoregulatory mechanisms in protein-tyrosine kinases, *J. Biol. Chem.*, 273, 11987–11990, 1998.

Hunter, T., The Croonian Lecture 1997. The phosphorylation of proteins on tyrosine: its role in cell growth and disease, *Philos. Trans. Roy. Soc. London B (Biol. Sci.)*, 353, 583–605, 1998.

Jiang, G. and Hunter, T., Receptor signaling: when dimerization is not enough, *Curr. Biol.*, 9, R568–R571, 1999.

Kossiakoff, A. A. and De Vos, A. M., Structural basis for cytokine hormone-receptor recognition and receptor activation, *Adv. Protein Chem.*, 52, 67–108, 1998.

Kuriyan, J. and Cowburn, D., Modular peptide recognition domains in eukaryotic signaling, *Annu. Rev. Biophys. Biomol. Struct.*, 26, 259–288, 1997.

Livnah, O. et al., Functional mimicry of a protein hormone by a peptide agonist: the EPO receptor complex at 2.8 Å, *Science*, 273, 464–471, 1996.

Mohammadi, M., Schlessinger, J., and Hubbard, S. R., Structure of the FGF receptor tyrosine kinase domain reveals a novel autoinhibitory mechanism, *Cell*, 86, 577–578, 1996.

Pawson, T. and Scott, J. D., Signaling through scaffold, anchoring, and adaptor proteins, *Science*, 278, 2075–2080, 1997.

Plotnikov, A. N., Schlessinger, J., Hubbard, S. R., and Mohammadi, M., Structural basis for FGF receptor dimerization and activation, *Cell*, 98, 641–650, 1999.

Schlessinger, J., Cell signaling by receptor tyrosine kinases, *Cell*, 103, 211–225, 2000.

Schlessinger, J. et al., Crystal structure of a ternary FGF–FGFR–heparin complex reveals a dual role for heparin in FGFR binding and dimerization, *Mol. Cell.,* 6, 743–750, 2000.

Wiesmann, C. et al., Crystal structure at 1.7 Å resolution of VEGF in complex with domain 2 of the Flt-1 receptor, *Cell,* 91, 695–704, 1997.

Wiesmann, C., Ultsch, M. H., Bass, S. H., and de Vos, A. M., Crystal structure of nerve growth factor in complex with the ligand-binding domain of the TrkA receptor, *Nature*, 401, 184–188, 1999.

Wybenga-Groot, L. E. et al., Structural basis for autoinhibition of the EphB2 receptor tyrosine kinase by the unphosphorylated juxtamembrane region, *Cell,* 106, 745–757, 2001.

Section III

Ligand-Binding Studies of Receptors

5 Direct Measurement of Drug Binding to Receptors

Dennis G. Haylett

CONTENTS

0-8493-1029-6/03/$0.00+$1.50
© 2003 by CRC Press LLC

5.1   INTRODUCTION

In this chapter, we look at ways in which the binding of ligands to macromolecules can be directly investigated. Although most interest centers on the interaction of drugs and hormones with receptors, the approach taken here can be applied to any similar process — for example, the combination of drugs with ion channels or membrane transport systems. The binding of ligands, including drugs, to plasma proteins has been studied for more than 50 years, but the study of binding to the much smaller amounts of protein (e.g., receptors) in cell membranes is more recent, having become feasible only when suitable radioactively labeled ligands became available. The first rigorous study of drug binding to receptors was that of Paton and Rang (1965), who investigated ^{3}H-atropine binding to muscarinic receptors in smooth muscle. The use of radiolabeled drugs in radioligand-binding studies is now common and for many pharmaceutical manufacturers forms an essential part of the screening process, providing a rapid means of determining the affinity of new drugs for a wide range of receptors. Labeling of drugs with radioisotopes is attractive because very small quantities, often as low as 1 fmol, can be readily and accurately measured. Receptor pharmacologists are also interested in the measurement of ligand concentration by fluorescence, but this, of course, requires the availability or novel synthesis of ligands with suitable fluorescent moieties, and currently this method requires substantially higher ligand concentrations. Fluorescent probes do, however, have a particular utility in kinetic experiments, where the changes in fluorescence that occur on binding are immediate, allowing the binding to be continuously monitored.

5.1.1   Objectives of Radioligand Binding Studies

These include:

- *Measurement of dissociation equilibrium constants*, which is of particular value in receptor classification and in the study of structure/activity relationships, where the effects of changes in chemical structure on affinity (and efficacy) are explored.
- *Measurement of association and dissociation rate constants.*
- *Measurement of receptor density,* including changes in receptor density occurring under different physiological or pathological conditions. Examples include the reduction in β-adrenoreceptor density that occurs with the use of β-agonists in the treatment of asthma (down-regulation) and the increase in β-adrenoreceptor numbers in cardiac muscle in response to thyroxin. The densities of receptors may be measured either directly in tissue samples or in intact tissues by quantitative autoradiography. Autoradiography, in which a picture of the distribution of the radiolabel in a section of tissue is obtained by placing a photographic film in contact with the tissue, has provided valuable information on the distribution of many receptors in the brain. Positron emission tomography (PET) and single-photon-emission computerized tomography (SPECT) utilizing ligands labeled with either positron emitters (e.g., ^{11}C) or gamma emitters are increasingly used to investigate receptor densities or occupancy of receptors by drugs *in vivo*.
- *Recognition and quantification of receptor subtypes*, which may be possible if subtype-selective ligands are available.
- *Use of radioligands in the chemical purification of receptors.* Here, the bound radioligand allows the receptors to be tracked through the various purification steps — for example, in the fractions eluting from separation columns. In such experiments, it is important for the radioligand to be irreversibly bound to the receptor.

- Finally, it may be possible to obtain some limited information on the *mechanisms of action of agonists* from the shapes of binding curves. For example, as discussed later, the binding of some agonists is affected by guanosine triphosphate (GTP), immediately suggesting the involvement of G-proteins in the transduction mechanism.

5.1.2 NOMENCLATURE

Compared with the conventions adopted for discussing the relationship between drug concentration and response (Chapter 1), a rather different terminology has evolved for ligand-binding studies.

R: Binding site, most often a true receptor (but quite commonly the term *receptor* is applied indiscriminately to any binding site)

L: Radiolabeled ligand whose binding is directly measured; L can be an agonist or antagonist or even a channel blocker, etc.

I: An inhibitor of the binding of L; I can be an agonist or an antagonist

B: Often used to denote the amount of radioligand bound, B_{max}, the maximum binding capacity

K_L, K_I: Dissociation equilibrium constants for binding of L and I (reciprocals of affinity constants)

K_d: Used more generally for the dissociation equilibrium constant of any ligand

5.1.3 SPECIFICITY OF BINDING

An all-important consideration in binding studies is the extent to which the measured binding of a radioligand represents association with the receptor or other site of interest. (In functional studies, this is not difficult, as the response can only be elicited by the binding of an agonist to the receptor and, for competitive antagonism, at least, it is likely that the antagonist also binds to the receptor.) Invariably in binding studies, uptake of the radioligand by other tissue components occurs (unless, of course, binding to a purified, soluble protein is under investigation). The binding to the receptor is normally termed *specific binding*, whereas the binding to non-receptor tissue components is referred to as *nonspecific binding*. Nonspecific binding may be attributable to:

1. Ligand bound to other sites in the tissue (e.g., other receptors, enzymes or membrane transporters). For example, some muscarinic antagonists will also bind to histamine receptors, and some adrenoreceptor ligands will also bind to the neuronal and extraneuronal uptake mechanisms for noradrenaline. Such uptake might be properly considered "specific," but it is not the binding of primary interest to the investigator. Unlike other sources of nonspecific binding, this binding will be saturable, though it may be hoped that it will be of lower affinity and so will increase in an approximately linear fashion over the concentration range of ligand used. If the characteristics of nonspecific binding of this sort are well established, it may be possible to eliminate it by the use of selective blockers (e.g., by the use of specific inhibitors of the uptake-1 process for noradrenaline).
2. Distribution of ligand into lipid components of the preparation (e.g., cell membranes) or uptake into intact cells or membrane vesicles
3. Free ligand that is not separated from bound ligand during the separation phase of the experiment, including ligand bound to a filter or trapped in the membrane or cell pellet during centrifugation

Unlike category 1 above, nonspecific binding arising from categories 2 and 3 will be nonsaturable and will increase linearly with radioligand concentration. Nonspecific binding of types 1 and 2 and radioligand trapped in pellets should increase in proportion to the amount of tissue used in the binding reaction; binding to filters and to the walls of centrifuge tubes should not. If the investigator is fortunate, in that nonspecific binding in category 1 is linear over the range of radioligand concentrations used, then the types of binding for all three categories simply combine to constitute a single, nonspecific component. Nonspecific binding is usually estimated by measuring the binding of the radioligand in the presence of an agent that is believed to bind selectively to the receptor, at a concentration calculated to prevent virtually all specific binding without appreciable modification of nonspecific binding (further details are provided in Section 5.3.5).

5.2 TYPES OF RADIOLIGAND-BINDING EXPERIMENTS

Four kinds of ligand-binding studies will be discussed: (1) saturation, (2) kinetic, (3) competition, and (4) retardation.

5.2.1 SATURATION EXPERIMENTS

These experiments examine the binding of the radioligand at equilibrium directly and can provide estimates of K_L and B_{max}. Initially, we consider the simple reaction:

$$R + L \rightleftharpoons RL \tag{5.1}$$

This represents binding in isolation and would be applicable to the binding of a competitive antagonist (or a channel blocker) that produces insignificant structural change in the receptor. (The case for an agonist that must produce such a change, often an isomerization, to generate the active state is considered later). The binding at equilibrium is given by the following equation (equivalent to Eq. (1.2)):

$$[RL] = R_{TOT} \frac{[L]}{K_L + [L]} \tag{5.2}$$

Alternatively,

$$B = B_{max} \frac{[L]}{K_L + [L]} \tag{5.3}$$

Typical units for B are pmol.mg protein^{-1}, pmol.mg dry tissue^{-1}, etc. A curve of B vs. [L] has the form of a rectangular hyperbola, exactly equivalent to the curve describing receptor occupancy presented in Chapter 1, Figure 1.1.

It is convenient at this point to consider nonspecific binding. Ideally, nonspecific binding should be entirely independent of specific binding, so that the total uptake of radioligand by the tissue should be the simple sum of the two. If we can assume that the nonspecific binding is a linear function of the ligand concentration, then the observed binding will be given by:

$$B = B_{max} \frac{[L]}{K_L + [L]} + c \cdot [L] \tag{5.4}$$

where c is a constant. The relationship among total, specific, and nonspecific binding is indicated in Figure 5.1.

In practice, total and nonspecific binding are measured over a range of concentrations of L that will allow specific binding to approach saturation. The analysis of saturation experiments to obtain estimates of K_L and B_{max} is described later.

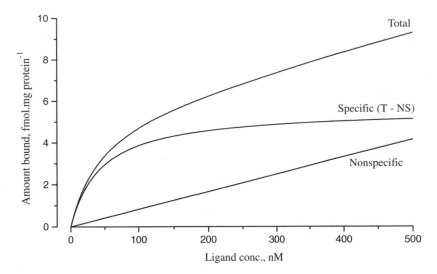

FIGURE 5.1 The binding of a radioligand to a receptor preparation normally involves a nonspecific component in addition to the specific, receptor binding. In principle, at least, specific binding can be estimated from the total binding (T) by subtracting nonspecific binding (NS). (Curves are theoretical, with B_{max} = 5.6 fmol.mg protein^{-1}, K_L = 45 nM, and c = 0.0083 fmol.nM^{-1}.)

It is useful now to recall the Hill coefficient, which has been discussed in detail in Chapter 1. In binding studies, the Hill coefficient, n_H, is generally a convenient means of describing the steepness of the plot of specific binding against the log of the ligand concentration, generally without any attempt to define the underlying mechanism. In the simplest case, a plot of specific binding against [L] is analyzed to provide a fit of the following equation (equivalent to Eq. (1.6)):

$$B = B_{max} \frac{[L]^{n_H}}{K_L^{n_H} + [L]^{n_H}}$$ (5.5)

For a simple bimolecular reaction following the law of mass action, n_H would be unity. If n_H is greater than 1, the plot of specific binding against log [L] will be steep; if less than 1, it will be shallow. Under these circumstances, a Hill plot (see Chapter 1) would have slopes either greater or less than unity.

5.2.1.1 Multiple Binding Sites

It is, of course, quite possible that more than one kind of specific binding site exists for the radioligand. For example, receptor subtypes may be present (subtypes of 5HT receptors, adreno-receptors, etc.) or the binding sites might be functionally quite different. Also, some receptor ligands may also be channel blockers (e.g., tubocurarine) or inhibitors of transmitter uptake (e.g., phenoxybenzamine). The question then arises as to whether or not the sites are interacting or noninteracting. In the case of only two sites that do not interact, an additional term can simply be added to the binding equation. For total binding,

$$B = B_{max_1} \frac{[L]}{K_{L1} + [L]} + B_{max_2} \frac{[L]}{K_{L2} + [L]} + c \cdot [L]$$ (5.6)

where subscripts 1 and 2 specify the two sites (further terms can be added for additional components).

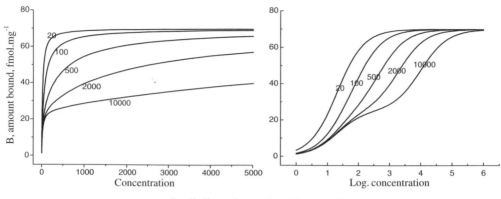

Radioligand concentration (nM)

FIGURE 5.2 Theoretical curves for the specific binding of a radioligand to a preparation containing two classes of binding site. A high-affinity component with a B_{max} of 25 fmol.mg^{-1} has a fixed K_L of 20 nM. The second component, with a B_{max} of 45 fmol.mg^{-1} is given K_L values varying between 20 and 10,000 nM, as indicated. The K_L values for the two sites must differ considerably before the existence of two components becomes obvious. (Data are displayed using both linear and logarithmic concentration scales.)

The curve for specific binding will no longer be a simple rectangular hyperbola, though whether distinct components can be distinguished by eye will depend on the difference in the K_L values and on the number of observations and their accuracy. Theoretical curves are shown in Figure 5.2. For relatively small differences in the K_L values of the two sites, the curve appears to have a single component, but analysis would show it to have a low Hill coefficient. The separate components are revealed more clearly when a logarithmic scale is used for the radioligand concentration. Thus, two components are very apparent in the right-hand panel of Figure 5.2.

5.2.1.2 Interacting Sites

In some instances (for example, the nicotinic acetylcholine receptor), the binding site is duplicated on identical subunits incorporated into a multimeric protein, which allows for the possibility that binding to one site may influence binding to the other. The two sites could in principle behave in an identical fashion, but it is more likely that incorporation of the subunits into the assymetrical multimer (a heteropentamer for the nicotinic receptor) introduces constraints that lead to different affinities for ligands. Of particular importance is the likelihood that occupation of one site by the ligand will increase or decrease the affinity for binding to the other (i.e., show positive or negative cooperativity). The following provides the simplest representation of this two-binding-site model:

$$R + L \overset{K_1}{\rightleftharpoons} RL + L \overset{K_2}{\rightleftharpoons} RL_2 (\overset{E}{\rightleftharpoons} RL_2^*) \tag{5.7}$$

This scheme is also discussed in Chapter 1 (at Appendix 1.2C) and in Chapter 6. In this scheme, the two binding sites are considered identical. RL_2^* is the active state produced when L is an agonist. The shape of the binding curve depends on the relative magnitudes of K_1 and K_2. When $K_1 > K_2$, positive cooperativity will occur (i.e., binding to the first site will increase affinity for the second); when $K_1 < K_2$, negative cooperativity will occur. Figure 5.3 illustrates the shapes of the binding curves predicted by Eq. (1.14) for various ratios of K_1 to K_2.

In competition experiments, it is possible that the binding of the radioligand is inhibited not by competition at a common site, but by the inhibitor affecting the binding remotely through interaction with a different part of the receptor molecule (i.e., by an allosteric action).

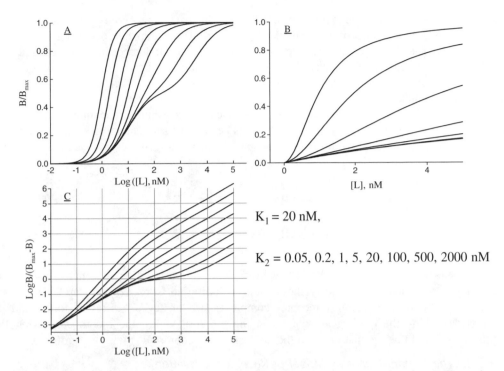

FIGURE 5.3 Binding of a radioligand to a receptor containing two identical binding sites (scheme shown in Eq. (5.7) but ignoring isomerization). Binding of the first ligand molecule is given a K_1 of 20 nM. The K_2 value for binding of a second ligand molecule is given a range of values to represent varying degrees of cooperativity, from strongly positive (0.05 nM) to strongly negative (2000 nM). As illustrated in A, for a logarithmic concentration scale, positive cooperativity steepens the curve, whereas negative cooperativity makes it shallower. Two components become quite evident for the larger values of K_2. In panel B, the linear concentration scale has been expanded to show the S-shaped foot of the binding curve, indicative of positive cooperativity. The Hill plot, C, shows that with a large degree of positive cooperativity n_H approaches 2 for intermediate concentrations of radioligand, becoming unity at either very high or very low concentrations (see Eq. (1.15)).

5.2.1.3 Agonists

The foregoing discussion of saturation experiments considered the binding step in isolation; however, for agonists to produce a tissue response, there must be some change in the receptor (isomerization) — for example, a conformational change to open an integral ion channel or to promote association with a G-protein. The complications arising with agonists will now be discussed.

5.2.1.3.1 The del Castillo–Katz Model of Receptor Activation

This model, represented below, has been discussed in Chapter 1, Sections 1.4.4 to 1.4.5.

$$A + R \overset{K_A}{\rightleftharpoons} AR \overset{E}{\rightleftharpoons} AR * \tag{5.8}$$

In a ligand-binding study, the measured binding includes AR^* as well as AR. The relevant equation then is:

$$B_{(AR+AR^*)} = B_{max} \frac{[A]}{\left(\dfrac{K_A}{1+E}\right) + [A]} \tag{5.9}$$

In this equation, A has been used in preference to L to emphasize that an *agonist* is being considered. The equation retains the form of a rectangular hyperbola, 50% occupancy occurring when [A] = $K_A/(1 + E)$. $K_A/(1 + E)$ is thus an effective equilibrium constant and accordingly is referred to as K_{eff}. The important point to note is that binding measurements do not give an estimate of K_A alone. K_{eff} is smaller than K_A, so the isomerization step increases affinity (in effect, dragging the receptor into the occupied state).

Another complication is receptor desensitization. Desensitization of the nicotinic acetylcholine receptor is attributed to the receptor, especially in its activated form, changing spontaneously to a desensitized, inactive state. The following is a scheme incorporating all possible desensitized states of the receptor:

$$A+R \rightleftharpoons AR+A \rightleftharpoons A_2R \rightleftharpoons A_2R^*$$
$$\updownarrow \qquad \updownarrow \qquad \quad \updownarrow \qquad \quad \updownarrow$$
$$A+R_D \rightleftharpoons AR_D+A \rightleftharpoons A_2R_D \rightleftharpoons A_2R_D{}^*$$

(This scheme is based on the Katz–Thesleff cyclic model of desensitization, modified to incorporate the binding of two molecules of acetylcholine and including an isomerization step.) It is evident from this scheme that the agonist–receptor complexes are of several different forms and the equations describing the binding are correspondingly complex. For the nicotinic acetylcholine receptor, it is found that agonist binds to the desensitized receptor (R_D) with high affinity.

5.2.1.3.2 The Ternary Complex Model of Receptor Activation

The following model has already been introduced in Chapter 1 (Section 1.4.6):

$$A + R \rightleftharpoons AR + X \rightleftharpoons ARX \qquad\qquad (5.10)$$

ARX, three reacting species, is the ternary complex. This scheme is often used to describe G-protein-mediated responses, when X is replaced by G, but it clearly is an oversimplification. For example, it does not include the additional states introduced by the binding of GTP or guanosine diphosphate (GDP). From the point of view of ligand-binding studies, we need to note that measured binding will include both AR and ARX. The equation that gives the bound concentration (AR + ARX) at equilibrium is complex (and in the case of G-protein coupled responses must also take into account the concentrations of receptors and G-protein, as discussed in Chapter 1, and of GTP and GDP). A particular feature of the binding of agonists to receptors that couple to G-proteins is that the concentration of GTP will affect the binding curve. The binding of agonists often exhibits components with high and low affinities, and GTP is found to increase the proportion in the low-affinity state. This will be considered further when discussing competition experiments.

5.2.2 KINETIC STUDIES

Both the onset of binding, when the radioligand is first applied, and offset, when dissociation is promoted, can be studied directly. The relevant kinetic equations relating to the simple bimolecular interaction of ligand with receptor are presented in Chapter 1, Section 1.3.

5.2.2.1 Measurement of the Dissociation Rate Constant, k_{-1}

To measure the dissociation rate constant, all that is necessary, in principle, is first to secure a satisfactory occupancy of the receptors by the radioligand and then to prevent further association, either by adding a competing agent in sufficient concentration or by lowering [L] substantially by dilution. The amount of drug bound to the receptors is measured at selected times after initiating net dissociation and, for the simple model considered in Sections 1.2 and 1.3 of Chapter 1, will show an exponential decline.

$$RL \xrightarrow{k_{-1}} R + L \tag{5.11}$$

$$B_t = B_0 e^{-k_{-1}t} \tag{5.12}$$

$$\log_e B_t = \log_e B_0 - k_{-1}t \tag{5.13}$$

B_0 and B_t are the amounts bound initially (at $t = 0$) and at specific times (t) after initiating dissociation. A plot of $\log_e B_t$ against t is linear with a slope of $-k_{-1}$; k_{-1} may thus be estimated directly from the slope of this plot or may be obtained by nonlinear least-squares curve fitting to Eq. (5.12). It is always desirable to plot $\log_e B_t$ against t to detect any nonlinearity that might reflect either the presence of multiple binding sites or the existence of more than one occupied state of the receptor.

5.2.2.2 Measurement of the Association Rate Constant, k_{+1}

For the simple bimolecular reaction involving a single class of binding site, the onset of binding should also contain an exponential term. Thus,

$$B_t = B_\infty (1 - e^{-k_{on}t}) \tag{5.14}$$

where B_t is the binding at time t, B_∞ is the binding at equilibrium, and k_{on} is the observed onset rate constant. However, as shown in Chapter 1, k_{on} is not a simple measure of k_{+1}; rather:

$$k_{on} = k_{-1} + k_{+1}[L] \tag{5.15}$$

Equation (5.15) can be converted into a linear form:

$$\log_e \left(\frac{B_\infty - B_t}{B_\infty} \right) = -k_{on}t \tag{5.16}$$

and k_{on} can be obtained from the slope of the plot of the left-hand side of the equation against t.

Once k_{on} is known, k_{+1} can be estimated in at least three different ways. First, an independent estimate of k_{-1} can be obtained from dissociation studies as described above, where, from Eq. (5.15), $k_{+1} = (k_{on} - k_{-1})/[L]$. Second, k_{on} can be measured at several different concentrations of L and a plot of k_{on} against [L] constructed in which, according to Eq. (5.15), k_{+1} is given directly by the slope. This plot will also provide an estimate of k_{-1} (intercept). Third, it is possible to perform a simultaneous nonlinear least-squares fit of a family of onset curves (obtained by using different concentrations of L), the fitting routine providing estimates of k_{+1}, k_{-1}, and B_{max} (Problem 5.2 provides an opportunity to calculate binding rate constants).

In the case of multiple binding sites or if the ligand–receptor complex isomerizes, the onset and offset curves will be multiexponential. It is generally assumed that nonspecific binding will occur rapidly, and this should certainly be so for simple entrapment in a membrane or cell pellet. If, however, specific binding is very rapid or nonspecific binding particularly slow (possibly

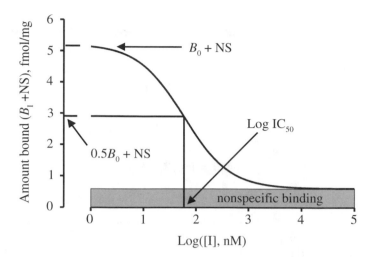

FIGURE 5.4 In this illustration of a competition experiment, a fixed concentration of radioligand, in the absence of inhibitor, produces specific binding of B_0. The specific binding in the presence of a competitive inhibitor is denoted by B_I. A constant amount of nonspecific binding is assumed to be present. The concentration of inhibitor that reduces specific binding by 50% is referred to as the IC_{50}.

reflecting uptake of the ligand by cells), then the time course of nonspecific binding also must be determined to allow an accurate assessment of the onset of specific binding. Note, too, that the onset of ligand binding will be slowed in the presence of an inhibitor, a phenomenon that is employed in *retardation* experiments (discussed in Section 5.2.4).

5.2.3 COMPETITION EXPERIMENTS

Of course, saturation experiments are only possible when a radiolabeled form of the ligand of interest is available. Competition experiments, on the other hand, are particularly useful in allowing the determination of dissociation constants for unlabeled drugs which compete for the binding sites with a ligand that is available in a labeled form. This approach has been widely adopted by the pharmaceutical industry as a rapid means of determining the affinity of novel compounds for a particular receptor for which a well-characterized radioligand is available.

In competition experiments, a fixed amount of radioligand, generally at a concentration below K_L, is equilibrated with the receptor preparation in the presence of a range of concentrations of the unlabeled inhibitor I. In these studies, the amount of radioligand bound is usually plotted against log[I]. Figure 5.4 provides an example for the simple case where the radioligand and inhibitor compete reversibly for a single class of site. In this illustration, the constant level of nonspecific binding has not been subtracted, whereas in most published studies it would be. The amount of nonspecific binding could, of course, be defined by applying high concentrations of the inhibitor itself; but if the competing agent is expensive or in short supply, it is possible to employ another well-characterized inhibitor for the same purpose. The two main features of this curve are its position along the concentration axis and its slope. The position along the concentration axis is conventionally indicated by the IC_{50}, the concentration of inhibitor that reduces the specific binding by 50%. The predicted relationship (see also Eq. (1.48)) between the amount of specific binding in the presence of I (B_I) and [I] is given by:

$$B_I = B_{max} \frac{[L]}{K_L\left(1 + \dfrac{[I]}{K_I}\right) + [L]} \tag{5.17}$$

Provided that a value for K_L is available, it is possible to use this equation to obtain a value for K_I, the dissociation equilibrium constant for the inhibitor, by nonlinear least-squares analysis of the displacement curve. Alternatively, K_I can be calculated from the IC_{50}, which may be obtained by simple interpolation by eye from a Hill plot or by fitting a curve to an equation of the type:

$$B_I = B_0 \frac{IC_{50}}{IC_{50} + [I]}$$

(5.18)

where B_0 is the specific binding observed in the absence of competing ligand.

5.2.3.1 Relationship between K_I and IC_{50}

B_0 is given by Eq. (5.3):

$$B_0 = B_{max} \frac{[L]}{K_L + [L]}$$

and, by definition, when $[I] = IC_{50}$, $B_I = 0.5 B_0$; therefore, from Eq. (5.17):

$$B_{IC_{50}} = B_{max} \frac{[L]}{K_L \left(1 + \dfrac{IC_{50}}{K_I}\right) + [L]}$$

(5.19)

$$= 0.5 B_{max} \frac{[L]}{K_L + [L]}$$

by cancellation and rearrangement:

$$K_I = IC_{50} \frac{K_L}{K_L + [L]} = \frac{IC_{50}}{\left(1 + \dfrac{[L]}{K_L}\right)}$$

(5.20)

The term $1 + ([L]/K_L)$ is often referred to as the Cheng–Prusoff correction. It is clear from this analysis that the IC_{50} does not give a direct estimate of K_I unless $[L]$ is very low, when IC_{50} tends to K_I. Just as with saturation experiments, the situation will be complicated by the presence of different classes of binding sites (e.g., receptor subtypes) and by the involvement of G-proteins in agonist binding.

5.2.3.2 Multiple Binding Sites

The effect of multiple binding sites on displacement curves will be determined by the relative affinities of the radioligand and displacing agent for the various sites. Considering the simple situation where the radioligand exhibits the same affinity for each of two sites (e.g., propranolol for β-adrenoreceptors), the displacement curve for an inhibitor will show two components only if the K_I values for the binding of the inhibitor to the two sites are sufficiently different and if the measurements of displacement are accurate and made over an adequate range of concentrations of I (see also Figure 5.2 and Section 5.4.4).

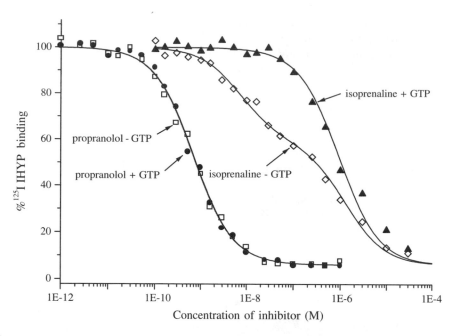

FIGURE 5.5 Effect of GTP on the competition binding curves of isoprenaline and propranolol. Membranes prepared from L6 myoblasts were incubated with ^{125}I-iodopindolol (50 pM) in the presence of either (–)-isoprenaline or (–)-propranolol with or without 100 μM GTP for 90 min at 25°C. GTP has no effect on the binding of the antagonist but shifts the curve for displacement by the agonist to the right (by abolishing the high-affinity component of binding). (Redrawn using data of Wolfe, B. B. and Molinoff, P. B., in *Handbook of Experimental Pharmacology,* Trendelenburg, U. and Weiner, N., Eds., Springer–Verlag, Berlin, 1988, chap. 7.)

5.2.3.3 G-Protein-Linked Receptors

As already mentioned, GTP affects binding of agonists to G-protein-coupled receptors, which has been much studied because of the light it can throw on the mechanism of action of such receptors. These receptors often exhibit two states that bind agonists with different affinities. The interactions of G-proteins with receptors are discussed in Chapter 7, and here it is only necessary to note that the high-affinity form of the receptor is coupled to the G-protein. In the simplest model, when GTP replaces GDP on the α subunit, the G-protein splits to release the α-GTP and βγ subunits, which mediate the cellular effects of the agonist. The receptor then dissociates, reverting to the low-affinity state. Hence, in the absence of GTP, a significant proportion of the receptors will be in the high-affinity state, but in its presence most will adopt the low-affinity state. The resulting "GTP shift" is illustrated in Figure 5.5. Note that it applies only to the binding of agonists, as antagonists do not promote coupling of the receptors to the G-protein. If there is a relatively low concentration of G-protein so that it is depleted by association with the receptor, then the competition curve for an agonist in the absence of GTP may exhibit two components, as in the figure.

5.2.4 RETARDATION EXPERIMENTS

It is useful to consider a particular variant of competitive binding experiment which has been used especially to investigate the nicotinic acetylcholine receptor. In essence, it is possible to determine the dissociation equilibrium constant for a reversible competitive inhibitor by the reduction it produces in the rate of binding of an irreversible radioligand (e.g., α-bungarotoxin). In practice, the time-course of binding of the irreversible ligand is studied in the absence and presence of the inhibitor. The expected outcome is shown in Figure 5.6.

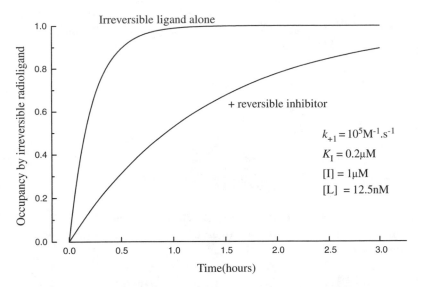

FIGURE 5.6 Retardation experiment. A reversible inhibitor will slow down the rate of association of an irreversible ligand with its receptor. These curves have been constructed according to Eq. (5.26) using the numerical values indicated in the figure. These have been chosen to illustrate the effect of an antagonist, such as tubocurarine, on the binding of α-bungarotoxin to the nicotinic receptor of skeletal muscle.

When the irreversible ligand is applied by itself, the change in the proportion of sites occupied, p_{LR}, with time will be given by:

$$\frac{dp_{LR}(t)}{dt} = k_{+1}[L]\{1 - p_{LR}(t)\} \tag{5.21}$$

where $1 - p_{LR}(t)$ is the proportion of receptors remaining free and available to bind with L. If p_{LR} = 0 at t = 0, the solution is :

$$p_{LR}(t) = 1 - e^{-k_{+1}[L]t} \tag{5.22}$$

This equation is the application of Eq. (1.22) to an irreversible ligand (i.e., k_{-1} = 0), and in the long run all of the receptors will be occupied so that $p_{LR}(\infty)$ is unity. The rate constant for equilibration is thus given by $k_{+1}[L]$. For the case where binding is studied in the presence of an inhibitor, Eq. (5.21) becomes:

$$\frac{dp_{LR}(t)}{dt} = k_{+1}[L]\{1 - p_{LR}(t) - p_{IR}(t)\} \tag{5.23}$$

where p_{IR} is the proportion of receptor sites occupied by the inhibitor. The rate of association is slowed because the free concentration of binding sites has been reduced through occupation by I. If we assume that I equilibrates rapidly with the available sites:

$$p_{IR}(t) = \{1 - p_{LR}(t)\}\frac{[I]}{K_I + [I]} \tag{5.24}$$

Substituting in Eq. (5.23):

$$\frac{dp_{LR}(t)}{dt} = k_{+1}[L]\left\{1 - p_{LR}(t) - (1 - p_{LR}(t)) \cdot \frac{[I]}{K_I + [I]}\right\}$$

$$= k_{+1}[L](1 - p_{LR}(t))\left(1 - \frac{[I]}{K_I + [I]}\right)$$

(5.25)

The solution for $p_{LR} = 0$ at $t = 0$ is:

$$p_{LR}(t) = 1 - e^{-k_{+1}[L]\left(1 - \frac{[I]}{K_I + [I]}\right)t}$$

(5.26)

The onset rate constant (see Eq. (5.22)) is reduced by the factor $1 - [I]/(K_I + [I])$. If the rate constants for binding of the irreversible ligand are determined in the absence and presence of the inhibitor and denoted k_0 and k_I, respectively, then:

$$\frac{k_0}{k_I} = \frac{k_{+1}[L]}{k_{+1}[L]\left(1 - \frac{[I]}{K_I + [I]}\right)} = \frac{[I]}{K_I} + 1$$

(5.27)

Thus, for a given concentration of I an estimate of its equilibrium constant can be determined.

5.3 PRACTICAL ASPECTS OF RADIOLIGAND-BINDING STUDIES

The majority of binding studies estimate the amount of binding by the separation of bound from free ligand, using either centrifugation or filtration, followed by measurement of the quantity bound. The separation stage, however, can be avoided in scintillation proximity assays (SPAs). These assays are applicable to ligands containing radioisotopes (e.g., tritium) that produce low-energy β-particles that travel only a very short distance (less than 10 μm) in aqueous solution. In one form of SPA, the receptor preparation is immobilized on microbeads containing scintillant molecules. The scintillant molecules are able to detect β-radiation emanating from radioligand bound to receptors located on the bead surface (and thus in close proximity) but will not respond to radiation from the relatively remote radioligand molecules free in the aqueous solution. For this technique to work, it must be possible to couple the receptor preparation to the bead in a way that does not interfere with the binding of the ligand. Provided this can be done, scintillation proximity counting provides a simple method of detecting binding and can, furthermore, be used to follow the time-course of binding while the reaction mixture remains in the scintillation counter. Techniques employing fluorescently labeled ligands (e.g., fluorescence polarization and fluorescence resonance energy transfer methods) are being developed and can also avoid the need to separate bound from free ligand. These techniques have the additional advantage of avoiding the hazards associated with the use and disposal of radioisotopes.

5.3.1 RECEPTOR PREPARATIONS

Most receptors (a notable exception being the steroid receptors that influence DNA transcription) are located on the cell surface, and purified cell membranes are thus an obvious choice of preparation. When a tissue is homogenized, however, any membrane fraction isolated may well contain membranes from intracellular organelles in addition to cell membranes from all the cell types present in the tissue. Thus, brain membranes will contain membranes not only from neurons but also from glia, as well as the smooth muscle and endothelial cells of blood vessels. It may, however, be possible to prepare membranes from pure cell preparations (e.g., cell lines in culture or cells obtained by disaggregation of the tissue with enzymes and subsequently subjected to purification by differential centrifugation). Increasingly, binding studies are performed on membranes from cell lines transfected with cloned human receptor genes, and a wide range of such cloned receptors is now available for routine drug screening.

A feature of cell disruption is that it may expose receptors that were not originally on the cell surface. Some of the receptors will have been in the process of insertion while others may have been endocytosed. This would lead to an overestimate of the cell-surface receptor density. On the other hand, cell membranes may form vesicles that can have either an outside-out or inside-out orientation. Cell-surface receptors in inside-out vesicles will not bind the ligand unless it can penetrate the vesicle. It is usually necessary to wash membrane preparations several times to remove endogenous material that might affect the binding (e.g., proteolytic enzymes, endogenous ligands). One important advantage of cell membranes is that often the preparation can be stored deep-frozen for many weeks without any change in binding properties.

The use of cell membranes can be criticized on the grounds that the receptors have been removed from their natural environment and will no longer be subject to cellular control mechanisms; for example, the phosphorylation of intracellular domains may be modified. These problems can be avoided by using intact cells for binding studies. Tissue slices (e.g., brain, heart) are used, as are cells isolated from dissected tissue by collagenase or trypsin digestion. Permanent cell lines in culture can also be used. However, the possibility that application of proteolytic enzymes to aid the disaggregation of tissues might modify the receptors is of some concern. When using intact cells, it is also possible that some ligands will be transported into the cells, leading to a higher nonspecific binding. Furthermore, some cells may contain enzymes that metabolize the radioligand. On the other hand, because cells must be maintained under physiological conditions to remain viable, binding results are, perhaps, more likely to reflect the true *in vivo* situation. Studies on purified, soluble receptors are much less common and subject to the uncertainty that removal from the lipid environment of the cell membrane may modify binding.

5.3.2 THE RADIOLIGAND

Although nonlinear least-squares methods allow complex binding curves to be analyzed, single-component curves will yield more precise estimates of the binding parameters. If, however, it is not possible to avoid multiple components, the curves will be more satisfactorily analyzed if the individual components of binding exhibit substantially different dissociation equilibrium constants. There is thus an obvious advantage in using *selective* radioligands that have greater affinity for one type of binding site. A *high affinity* is also desirable, as it allows the binding to be studied at a low concentration, which, other things being equal, will reduce nonspecific binding. A high ratio of specific to nonspecific binding will reduce the errors in the estimated parameters. A high affinity, however, also has consequences for the rate at which the binding reaches equilibrium. The association rate constant, k_{+1}, has an upper limit, determined by collision theory, of about 10^8 $M^{-1}sec^{-1}$, from which it follows that ligands with high affinities must have very low k_{-1} values. From Eqs. (5.12) and (5.15), it is seen that this will lead to both a slow onset (at the low concentrations of L being used) and a slow offset of binding. A slow rate of offset is advantageous in the separation of bound from free ligand by filtration, where it is important to ensure that the washing steps do not cause significant dissociation.

The radioligand should also have a *high specific activity* so that very small quantities of bound ligand can be accurately measured. The specific activity, simply defined as the amount of radioactivity, expressed in becquerels (Bq) or curies (Ci) per mole of ligand, is dependent on the half-life of the isotope used and on the number of radioactive atoms incorporated into the ligand molecule. A radioisotope with a short half-life decays rapidly so that many disintegrations occur in unit time, resulting in a high specific activity. The isotopes used most frequently for labeling are ^{125}I and ^3H, with half-lives of 60 days and 12.3 years, respectively (labeling with ^{14}C, with a half-life of 5760 years, would result in a low specific activity). Ligands labeled with single atoms of either ^{125}I or ^3H will have maximum specific activities of 2200 and 29 Ci per mmol, respectively. A basic difference exists between labeling with ^3H and with ^{125}I. With ^3H, the radioisotope can replace hydrogen atoms in the molecule with only insignificant changes in the chemical properties; indeed, it would be possible to replace several H by ^3H without a significant change in chemical properties but with a useful gain in specific activity. In contrast, most natural ligands and nearly all drugs do not contain an iodine atom that can be replaced by ^{125}I. Instead, it is necessary to produce an iodinated derivative that *will* have different chemical properties and quite likely a different affinity for the receptor. (For this reason, it is usual to incorporate only one atom of ^{125}I in each ligand molecule.) It is, therefore, necessary to check that the radioiodinated derivative retains the desired properties of the parent compound. With radioiodine, it is possible to achieve 100% isotopic labeling, as it is possible to obtain pure ^{125}I and to separate the labeled ligand from both unincorporated $^{125}I-$ and noniodinated parent compound. It is obviously important to ensure that the label is associated only with the intended ligand. Potential problems include the possibilities that contaminating substances might also have been labeled and that the radioligand may have suffered chemical modification during storage. Highly radioactive ligands can suffer radiation damage, and the presence of radioactive impurities will almost certainly lead to a reduction in the ratio of specific to nonspecific binding.

For many receptors, both hydrophilic and hydrophobic radioligands are available. In some cases, the hydrophobic ligands have been found to give higher estimates of B_{max}, suggesting that they have access to receptors within the cell that are denied to hydrophilic ligands. This is exemplified by the greater B_{max} values observed (in neuroblastoma membranes) for the muscarinic receptor ligand ^3H-scopolamine (tertiary amine) compared with ^3H-N-methylscopolamine (quaternary ammonium). These differences in access to receptors can actually be exploited to study receptor internalization.

5.3.3 INCUBATION CONDITIONS

5.3.3.1 Incubation Medium

Binding to intact cells must of necessity be performed in a physiological solution, and the results obtained are hence quite likely to correlate with functional studies. It would be wise to avoid the inclusion of protein (e.g., albumin), as protein may well bind the radioligand to a significant extent which would not be detected by measurement of the radioactivity of the supernatant obtained by centrifugation. Binding to membranes, by contrast, is quite often performed in a simple buffer solution (for example, 20- or 50-mM Tris or HEPES buffers). It is clear, however, that the affinity of some ligands for receptors is increased in solutions of low ionic strength. This effect has been clearly demonstrated for muscarinic cholinergic receptors. In principle, it could be avoided by including sufficient NaCl to make the incubation medium isotonic with the appropriate physiological solution. Particular ions have been shown to have effects on certain receptor systems. Mg^{2+}, for example, commonly affects binding to G-protein-coupled receptors, which is in keeping with its known effects on G-protein activation. The ionization of weakly acidic or basic groups in both receptor and ligand will be affected by pH and is likely to modify binding. Accordingly, binding studies should be done at physiological pH, if at all possible.

5.3.3.2 Temperature

Temperature has effects on both the rates of reaction and dissociation equilibrium constants. A rise in temperature will increase the rates of both association and dissociation, as shown in Table 5.1

TABLE 5.1
Effect of Temperature on the Kinetics of [³H]-Flunitrazepam Binding to Rat Brain Homogenates

Temperature (°C)	k_{+1} (M^{-1}sec^{-1})	k_{-1} (sec^{-1})	K_D (nM)
0	7.3×10^5	7.3×10^{-4}	1.0
22	4.6×10^6	1.0×10^{-2}	2.2
35	1.1×10^7	5.9×10^{-2}	5.3

Source: From Speth, R.C. et al., *Life Sci.*, 24, 351, 1979. With permission.

---

for the binding of ³H-flunitrazepam to rat brain membranes. The effect on the dissociation equilibrium constant is less because the changes in k_{+1} and k_{-1} are in the same direction. It has been found for some receptors that the effect of temperature on affinity is greater for agonists than for antagonists. Table 5.2 illustrates the results for binding to β-adrenoreceptors obtained by Weiland et al. (1979). It was suggested that the difference in the effect of temperature on agonist as compared with antagonist binding reflected the structural changes in the receptor (isomerization) that occurs with agonists but not antagonists. More recent investigations of this issue have not, however, confirmed the generality of this conclusion.

In the light of these results, it might seem best to measure binding only at the relevant physiological temperature; however, conducting the incubation at low temperature has some advantages. For example, proteolytic damage to the receptor and breakdown of the ligand, if it is chemically unstable, will be reduced during very long incubations (though this advantage may be offset by the longer incubation time required for equilibration).

TABLE 5.2
K_I Values for Inhibition of ¹²⁵I-Iodohydroxybenzylpindolol Binding to β-Adrenoreceptors in Turkey Erythrocyte Membranes at 1°C and 37°C

	K_I (nM) 37°C	K_I (nM) 1°C	$K_I(37°C)/K_I(1°C)$
Agonists:			
Isoprenaline	254	11	23.3
Noradrenaline	2680	48	55.5
Adrenaline	5230	326	16
Antagonists:			
Propranolol	1.6	0.59	2.6
Pindolol	4.5	1.5	2.95
Atenolol	5300	2530	2.09

Note: The binding curves for both agonists and antagonists were unaffected by GTP.

Source: Data from Weiland et al., *Nature*, 281, 114, 1979.

5.3.3.3 Duration of Incubation

Equilibrium studies clearly require an incubation period that is long enough to allow equilibration to be achieved. As discussed above, the time required will be longer at lower temperatures. It is critically dependent on the affinity of the ligand for the receptor. As outlined earlier, the rate constant for the onset of binding is given by $k_{-1} + k_{+1}[L]$. If k_{+1} is given a value of 10^7 $M^{-1}sec^{-1}$, it can be estimated that to achieve 97% of equilibrium for a ligand with a K_L of 100 pM, at relevant concentrations, would require about 1 hour at 37°C and as much as 58 hours at 0°C. The effect of a competing drug is to slow the rate of equilibration. These considerations demonstrate the desirability of conducting pilot kinetic studies before any detailed equilibrium measurements are made.

5.3.3.4 Amount of Tissue

The aim should be to employ sufficient material to give a good ratio of specific to nonspecific binding without causing significant *depletion* of the radioligand. Nonspecific binding associated with binding to a filter is likely to be a fixed amount at any given ligand concentration, so increasing the amount of receptor present should increase the signal-to-noise ratio. A large concentration of receptor may, however, bind a substantial fraction of the radioligand present and so reduce the free concentration. Such depletion is an important consideration. If the free ligand concentration can be measured directly, this should be done, and the concentration so obtained is applicable to the equations presented in this chapter. An alternative, if [L] cannot be measured, is to derive equations that allow for depletion arising from both specific and nonspecific binding. Such equations have been presented by Hulme and Birdsall (1992), but some of the assumptions made are necessarily oversimplifications. It is preferable to try to design the study so that depletion is kept to an insignificant level (say, <5%) and so can be ignored.

5.3.4 Methods of Separating Bound from Free Ligand

For particulate receptor preparations (intact cells or membranes), it is usual to separate bound from free ligand by either centrifugation or filtration. (For soluble receptor preparations, equilibrium dialysis, using a semipermeable membrane, or gel filtration can be employed.)

5.3.4.1 Filtration

At the appropriate time, the reaction mixture is either tipped or drawn by suction onto the filter and the supernatant immediately filtered under vacuum. The filter, often made of glass fiber, must retain all of the receptor preparation, while at the same time allowing a rapid separation. It is also necessary to check for binding of ligand to the filter. Several examples of "specific," saturable binding of radioligand to filters can be found in the literature. The receptor preparation retained by the filter is normally washed two or three times with a small volume of incubation buffer that does not contain the radioligand in order to remove superficial radiolabel. It is essential to minimize any dissociation of bound ligand during these washes. This can be achieved by using only a few, rapid washes and by washing with buffer at a low temperature. Commercially available filtration systems now allow many samples to be handled simultaneously. Commonly used filtration equipment does not, however, allow the supernatant to be collected for the determination of the free ligand concentration.

5.3.4.2 Centrifugation

Incubation is often performed in small plastic tubes, which can be centrifuged directly to form, within seconds, a cell or membrane pellet. The supernatant can then be either tipped off or removed by suction. The radioactivity of the supernatant can be measured to determine the free ligand concentration. Any supernatant remaining on the surface of the pellet or tube can be reduced by washing, again using cold buffer. Most receptors will be within the pellet and will not be exposed to the wash solution, so dissociation should be limited. It is obviously important that washing does not disturb the pellet, causing loss of receptors. In some experiments using intact cells, separation has been achieved by conducting the incubation over a layer of oil of appropriate density. At the desired time, the cells are centrifuged through the oil layer, with virtually all of the supernatant remaining on top. Supernatant and oil are then removed by suction and no washing step is needed. If plastic tubes are used, the tip of the tube containing the pellet can be cut off, so reducing further any counts due to radioligand attached to the tube wall. Finally, the bound radioligand (on the filter or in the pellet) is quantified using standard methods for measuring radioactivity (usually scintillation counting).

5.3.5 DETERMINATION OF NONSPECIFIC BINDING

Nonspecific binding is estimated by setting up additional incubation mixtures which, in addition to the radioligand, also include enough of a displacing agent to virtually eliminate the specific receptor binding. Because most of the displacing agents employed to define nonspecific binding act competitively, it is necessary to use a concentration that is 100 to 1000 times larger than its K_d to ensure that higher concentrations of the radioligand do not overcome the inhibition. It is also important to check that the displacing agent does not reduce nonspecific binding. This is likely to be more of a problem if a nonlabeled form of the radioligand itself is used; therefore, preference should be given to a chemically distinct displacing agent. Extra reassurance can be obtained if similar values for nonspecific binding are estimated using more than one displacing agent. This is often the case in competition experiments where several competing drugs produce an identical maximal inhibition of binding, thus providing a reliable estimate of the residual nonspecific binding.

5.4 ANALYSIS OF BINDING DATA

The analysis of binding experiments essentially has two steps:

1. Preliminary inspection and analysis of the data to try to establish a model that adequately describes the binding. For example, multiple components or cooperativity may be identified.
2. Estimation of the model parameters (e.g., B_{max}, K_L) with some indication of the errors associated with the estimates.

It is always desirable to plot the data in terms of the amount of radioligand bound as a function either of the radioligand concentration (saturation experiments) or inhibitor concentration (competition experiments). A logarithmic concentration scale usually provides a clearer picture of the relationship, with deviations from a simple monotonic curve being more obvious. It is also common to use linearizing transformations of the binding curves, both to reveal binding complexities and to provide initial estimates of binding parameters. Various linear transformations have been used to analyze saturation experiments, as will now be outlined.

5.4.1 SCATCHARD PLOT

Equation (5.3) can be rearranged to give:

$$\frac{B}{[L]} = \frac{B_{max}}{K_L} - \frac{B}{K_L} \tag{5.28}$$

The Scatchard plot is bound free ($B/[L]$, y-axis) vs. bound (B, x-axis) (the Eadie–Hofstee plot is bound vs. bound/free). If this equation is applicable (i.e., the binding represents a simple bimolecular interaction), the data points will fall on a straight line, the slope will be $-K_L^{-1}$, and the intercept on the x-axis (when $B/[L] = 0$) will give B_{max}. (See Figure 5.10 for a Scatchard plot of the data provided in Problem 5.1.) Curved Scatchard plots can indicate positive or negative cooperativity or the presence of sites (e.g., receptor subtypes) with different affinities for the ligand. The Scatchard plot, in the past, has been the primary means of obtaining estimates of K_L and B_{max}, but it is only reliable if the data are very good and a straight line is obtained. It should be noted that simple linear regression should not be applied to the Scatchard plot, as B with its associated error occurs in both x and y values. Linear regression of Scatchard plots systematically overestimates K_d and B_{max}. Because nonlinear Scatchard plots are even more difficult to handle, there is often a strong temptation to fit straight lines to plots that clearly are not straight. Nonlinear least-square methods (see below) are much to be preferred for the estimation of parameters with their confidence limits.

5.4.2 LINEWEAVER–BURK PLOT

This double-reciprocal plot is based on another rearrangement of Eq. (5.3):

$$\frac{1}{B} = \frac{K_L}{B_{max}} \cdot \frac{1}{[L]} + \frac{1}{B_{max}} \tag{5.29}$$

A plot of $1/B$ vs. $1/[L]$ will give a straight line providing that Eq. (5.3) applies; when $1/B = 0$, then $1/[L] = -1/K_L$, and when $1/[L] = 0$, then $1/B = 1/B_{max}$. A Lineweaver–Burk plot is shown in Figure 5.10, where it may be compared with the Scatchard plot of the same data. The double-reciprocal plot spreads the data very poorly and is inferior to the Scatchard plot.

5.4.3 HILL PLOT

This plot has already been discussed in detail in Chapter 1 and earlier in this chapter. Yet another rearrangement of Eq. (5.3) gives:

$$\frac{B}{B_{max} - B} = \frac{[L]}{K_L}$$

$$\log\left(\frac{B}{B_{max} - B}\right) = \log[L] - \log K_L \tag{5.30}$$

The Hill plot is $\log (B/(B_{max} - B))$ vs. $\log [L]$. As noted earlier, the slope of the Hill plot (the Hill coefficient, n_H) is of particular utility. If the equation holds, a straight line of slope = 1 should be obtained. A value greater than 1 may indicate positive cooperativity, and a slope less than 1 either negative cooperativity or commonly the presence of sites with different affinities. The data of Problem 5.1 are also presented as a Hill plot in Figure 5.10.

5.4.4 ANALYSIS OF COMPETITION EXPERIMENTS

Equation (5.18), which describes competitive binding, can also be transformed into the form of a Hill plot:

$$\log\left(\frac{B_I}{B_0 - B_I}\right) = \log IC_{50} - \log[I] \tag{5.31}$$

For simple competitive interaction at a single class of site, a plot of $\log (B_I/(B_0 - B_I))$ vs. $\log[I]$ will be linear with a slope of -1 and intercept on the x-axis of $\log (IC_{50})$. This estimate of IC_{50} can be

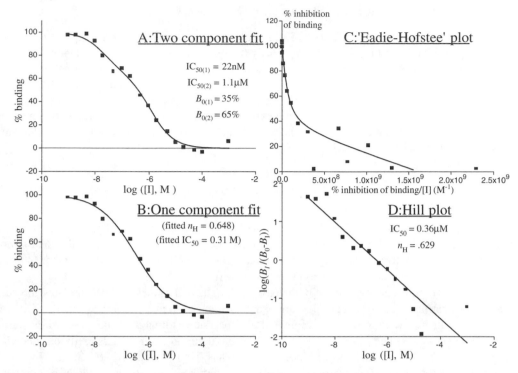

FIGURE 5.7 Analysis of a competition experiment in which the binding of a radiolabeled β-adrenoreceptor antagonist (^{125}I-iodopindolol) is inhibited by a β_1-β_2 selective antagonist. The four panels indicate various ways in which the data can be analyzed (see text). (The data for the figure have been extracted from Fig. 4, Chapter 7, of Wolfe, B. B. and Molinoff, P. B., in *Handbook, of Experimental Pharmacology*, Trendelenburg, U. and Weiner, N., Eds., Springer-Verlag, Berlin, 1988.)

used to derive a value for K_I as discussed earlier. A different plot, equivalent to the Eadie–Hofstee plot for saturation experiments, has also been used to reveal more complex binding characteristics in competition experiments. Figure 5.7 provides an example of the analysis of a competition study in which two sites are indicated.

A plot of B vs. log[I] (Figures 5.7A and B) might initially suggest two components, but the scatter of the observations would counsel caution. The Hill plot (Figure 5.7D) reveals a slope (by linear regression) of –0.629 (significantly different from –1), which is not consistent with simple 1:1 competition at a single binding site but is instead suggestive of multiple binding sites or negative cooperativity. An Eadie–Hofstee plot (Figure 5.7C) is clearly nonlinear. Nonlinear least-squares analysis of the data (see next section) is shown in Figures 5.7A and B. In B, a single component is fitted using Eq. (5.18), but with the terms raised to the power n_H. The fit is quite reasonable and yields an n_H of –0.648, close to the value from the Hill plot. A closer fit (Figure 5.7A) (predictably) is obtained with a two-component model (in which n_H is constrained to one) according to:

$$B_I = B_{0(1)}\left(\frac{IC_{50(1)}}{IC_{50(1)} + [I]}\right) + B_{0(2)}\left(\frac{IC_{50(2)}}{IC_{50(2)} + [I]}\right) \qquad (5.32)$$

The conversion of each IC_{50} into K_I for the two sites will depend on a knowledge of the affinity of the radioligand for the sites. Note also that the ratio of $B_{0(1)}$ to $B_{0(2)}$ will only give the relative proportions of the two sites in the tissue if the sites have identical affinities for the radioligand.

5.4.5 Nonlinear Least-Squares Methods of Data Analysis

As already noted, with the advent of powerful microcomputers and software incorporating appropriate fitting routines, binding data can be readily analyzed by means of nonlinear least-squares fitting procedures. It is beyond the scope of these notes to give a full description of this method. In essence, however, the procedure first requires the selection of an expression that is believed to represent the system being investigated. Initial guesses are then made of the unknown parameters (e.g., K_L, B_{max}), and by using these guesses the expected binding is calculated corresponding to the ligand concentration at each datum point. The deviations of the observed points from the calculated points are squared and added together. Thus,

$$\text{Sum of squares} = \sum w(B_{obs} - B_{calc})^2 \qquad (5.33)$$

where B_{obs} is the measured binding, B_{calc} is the binding calculated using the guesses, and w is a weighting factor. This allows the investigator to give more or less weight to particular data points according to their perceived reliability. Where each datum point has an associated standard error, it is quite common, for example, to weight inversely with the variance.

The program then makes systematic changes to the guessed values and recalculates the sum of squares, repeating this process until the sum of squares reaches a minimum (i.e., the least-squares estimate is obtained). Many of the programs will also produce estimates of the standard deviation of the estimated values. The process is described in more detail in Colquhoun's textbook, *Lectures on Biostatistics,* and its application to binding studies has been considered specifically by Wells (see Further Reading section). *Sigmaplot* (Jandel) and *Origin* (Microcal) are examples of commercially available graphing and curve-fitting programs. Programs designed specifically for the analysis of ligand binding experiments are *Ligand* (Biosoft) and *Prism* (GraphPad Software).

Closer least-squares fits can obviously be obtained by adopting more complicated models involving extra parameters. The use of more complicated models can, of course, be more readily justified if there is independent supporting evidence available (e.g., knowledge of multiple binding sites from functional studies).

5.5 RELEVANCE OF RESULTS FROM BINDING STUDIES

Binding studies are done independently of any biological response, and it is obviously desirable to have some check to ensure that the binding is occurring at a relevant or identifiable site. Thus, wherever possible, the binding results should be compared with results from functional studies. This can be achieved most easily for competitive antagonists. In this case, Schild plots (see Chapter 1) can provide an estimate of affinity from the shift of concentration–response curves that should correspond to the K_d obtained in binding studies. Hulme and Birdsall (1992) provide an excellent illustration of such a correlation for muscarinic receptors, and a further example is provided in Figure 5.8, which compares functional and binding studies of potassium channel blockers. It will clearly be more difficult to establish such relationships when there are subtypes of a receptor in a tissue. In these circumstances, the availability of agents that exhibit selectivity for subtypes will assist the interpretation.

5.6 PROBLEMS

These problems are provided to afford an opportunity for the reader to analyze binding data of different sorts. The problems do not require nonlinear least squares analysis, but this would be recommended to those with access to appropriate facilities. It must be emphasized that, while linearizing transformations allow binding data to be clearly visualized, parameter estimation should

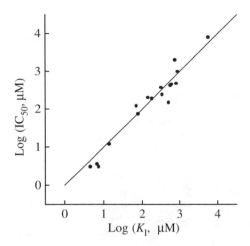

FIGURE 5.8 Correlation between the abilities of various compounds to inhibit ^{125}I-monoiodoapamin binding to guinea-pig hepatocytes (K_I values, abscissa) and their abilities to inhibit the K^+ permeability increase induced by angiotensin II in these cells (IC_{50} values, ordinate). The straight line is that expected for direct equivalence. The measurements are highly correlated, suggesting that the compounds do indeed produce their effects by binding to the apamin-sensitive K^+ channels. (Data from Cook, N. S. and Haylett, D. G., *J. Physiol.*, 358, 373, 1985. With permission.)

utilize nonlinear least squares fits of the untransformed data. The analysis of each set of data is discussed in detail in Section 5.8.

Problem 5.1: Saturation Binding

The data in Table 5.3 are from an experiment measuring ^{125}I-monoiodoapamin binding to guinea-pig hepatocytes. Conditions were such that depletion of radioligand was negligible over the entire concentration range studied.

TABLE 5.3
Data for Problem 5.1

Radioligand Concentration [L] (pM)	Amount Bound (fmol · mg dry tissue⁻¹)	
	Total	Noninhibitable
20	0.110	0.018
50	0.224	0.046
100	0.351	0.071
150	0.495	0.143
200	0.557	0.180
300	0.708	0.275
500	0.942	0.462
1000	1.530	0.900
1500	1.920	1.310

1. Plot specific (inhibitable) binding against [L]. Make initial estimates of K_L and B_{max} from this graph.
2. Construct a Scatchard plot of the data and derive new estimates of K_L and B_{max}.

3. Construct a Hill plot ($\log(B/(B_{max} - B))$) vs. $\log [L]$). What can be concluded from the slope of this plot?

TABLE 5.4
Data for Problem 5.2

Time (sec)	Specific Binding (fmol/mg dry tissue)		
	[L] = 30 pM	[L] = 100 pM	[L] = 300 pM
5	.025	.071	.165
10	.029	.112	.294
15	.041	.135	.340
20	.063	.166	.392
30	.063	.218	.460
50	.098	.257	.481
100	.102	.260	.503
200	.112	.270	.488

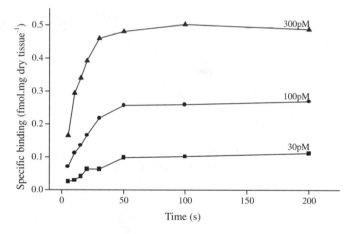

FIGURE 5.9 Plot of the data for Problem 5.2.

Problem 5.2: Kinetics

The onset of binding of radiolabeled apamin to guinea-pig hepatocytes was studied for three concentrations of the ligand over a 200-sec period and provided the results provided in Table 5.4. These data are plotted in Figure 5.9 and indicate how the rate constant for onset of binding increases with the ligand concentration. For each set of results the expected binding is given by:

$$B_t = B_\infty (1 - e^{-(k_{-1} + k_{+1}[L])t})$$ (5.34)

Estimate k_{+1} and k_{-1} from the data (see Section 5.2.2.2).

Problem 5.3: Competition Experiment

The binding of three concentrations of ^{125}I-labeled iodohydroxybenzylpindolol (IHYP) to membranes from turkey erythrocytes was studied in the absence and presence of a range of sotalol concentrations. Table 5.5 presents the results. Plot the total amount of IHYP bound against log [sotalol] and draw smooth curves by eye through each set of points. Estimate the IC_{50} for each

TABLE 5.5
Data for Problem 5.3

[Sotalol] (M)	Total Binding (fmol/mg protein)		
	[IHYP] = 30 pM	[IHYP] = 100 pM	[IHYP] = 300 pM
0.0	34.0	56.2	75.1
1.0×10^{-8}	33.8	57.0	74.0
3.2×10^{-8}	32.5	55.3	74.6
1.0×10^{-7}	31.0	55.0	73.8
3.2×10^{-7}	26.2	51.8	69.6
1.0×10^{-6}	20.0	42.6	67.0
3.2×10^{-6}	9.7	26.3	50.6
1.0×10^{-5}	4.2	13.0	35.0
3.2×10^{-5}	3.0	7.9	22.5
1.0×10^{-4}	1.9	5.0	12.5
3.2×10^{-4}	1.4	3.8	11.9
1.0×10^{-3}	1.2	3.5	10.0

curve. Given that the K_L for IHYP is 37 pM, calculate K_I from each IC_{50} (see Eq. (5.20)). Tabulate the specific binding for each set of data, and construct Hill plots (Eq. (5.31)). Are the results consistent with a single population of receptors? Compare each IC_{50} from these plots with your previous estimates.

5.7 FURTHER READING

First rigorous study of radioligand binding

Paton, W. D. M. and Rang, H. P., The uptake of atropine and related drugs by intestinal smooth muscle of the guinea-pig in relation to acetylcholine receptors, *Proc. Roy. Soc. London Ser. B*, 163, 1, 1965.

Scintillation proximity method

Udenfriend, S., Gerber, L., and Nelson, N., Scintillation proximity assay: a sensitive and continuous isotopic method for monitoring ligand/receptor and antigen/antibody interactions, *Anal. Biochem.*, 161, 494, 1987.

Effect of ionic strength on ligand binding

Birdsall, N. J. M., Burgen, A. S. V., Hulme, E. C., and Wells, J. W., The effects of ions on the binding of agonists and antagonists to muscarinic receptors, *Br. J. Pharmacol.*, 67, 371, 1979.

Comprehensive treatment of theoretical and practical aspects of radioligand experiments

Hulme, E. C. and Birdsall, N. J. M., Strategy and tactics in receptor binding studies, in *Receptor–Ligand Interactions: A Practical Approach*, Hulme, E. C., Ed., IRL Press, Oxford, 1992, chap. 4.

Parameter estimation including nonlinear least-squares methods

Colquhoun, D., *Lectures on Biostatistics*, Clarendon Press, Oxford, 1971.
Wells, J. W., Analysis and interpretation of binding at equilibrium, in *Receptor–Ligand Interactions: A Practical Approach*, Hulme, E. C., Ed., IRL Press, Oxford, 1992, chap. 11.

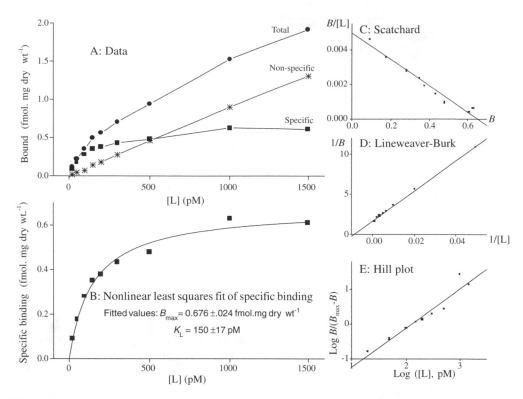

FIGURE 5.10 Analysis of the saturation data provided for Problem 5.1 (see accompanying text).

5.8 SOLUTIONS TO PROBLEMS

Problem 5.1: Saturation Data

The raw data are plotted in Figure 5.10A. The top two points of the specific data might suggest that B_{max} has been reached by about 1000 pM, with a value between measured values at 1000 and 1500 pM, say 0.62 fmol/mg dry wt. An estimate of K_L can be obtained by reading from the graph the ligand concentration that produces binding of 0.5 B_{max} (i.e., 0.31 fmol/mg dry wt.; see Eq. (5.3)). This estimate will depend on how the curve has been drawn but is likely to be around 120 pM.

A Scatchard plot of the data is shown in Figure 5.10C. For convenience, the fitted line is the regression of B/F on B (though, as noted earlier, this is statistically unsound) and provides an estimate for B_{max} (x-intercept) of 0.654 fmol/mg dry wt. and an estimate for K_L (–1/slope) of 132 pM. A Lineweaver–Burk (double-reciprocal) plot is provided for comparison in Figure 5.10D. Linear regression gives another estimate for B_{max} (1/y-intercept; see Eq. (5.29)) of 0.610 fmol/mg dry wt. The estimate of K_L from this plot (slope $\times B_{max}$) is 114 pM.

To construct the Hill plot (Figure 5.10E), it was assumed that B_{max} was 0.654 fmol/mg dry wt., the Scatchard value. The slope of the plot is 1.138 with a standard deviation of 0.12, so it would not be unreasonable to suppose n_H was indeed 1 and so consistent with a simple bimolecular interaction. Figure 5.10B shows a nonlinear least-squares fit of Eq. (5.3) to the specific binding data (giving all points equal weight). The least-squares estimates are 0.676 fmol/mg dry wt. for B_{max} and 150 pM for K_L. (Estimates of the standard errors of these values are noted in the figure.) A nonlinear least-squares fit of the *total* binding data to Eq. (5.4) gave B_{max} = 0.686 fmol/mg dry wt. and K_L = 151 pM. The data for Problem 5.1 was in fact generated by setting the points randomly about a curve with B_{max} = 0.68 fmol/mg dry wt. and K_L = 150 pM. Both the Scatchard and double-reciprocal plots, in this case, underestimate both parameters, the latter plot being particularly inaccurate.

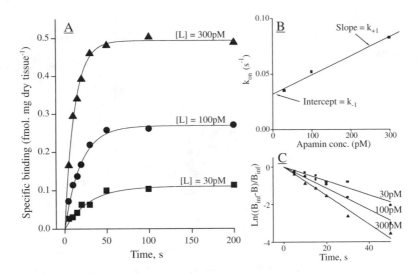

FIGURE 5.11 Analysis of the kinetic data provided for Problem 5.2 (see accompanying text).

Problem 5.2: Kinetic Data

A graphical analysis, which allows the determination of k_{+1} and k_{-1} from the given data, is described in Section 5.2.2.2. For each set of data, it is necessary to determine k_{on}. These values can be obtained from the semilogarithmic plots of $\ln((B_\infty - Bt)/B_\infty)$ vs. t. But, what value should be taken for B_∞? Estimates can be made by eye from the data, and for Figure 5.11C the B_∞ for 30 and 100 pM have been taken as the highest recorded values and for 300 pM as the mean of the values at 100 and 200 sec.

In plotting Figure 5.11C, the points beyond 50 sec have been ignored because the errors in $(B_\infty - B_t)$ become proportionately very large. Linear regressions have been fitted to the three lines, giving k_{on} estimates of 0.0377 sec^{-1} (30 pM), 0.0572 sec^{-1} (100 pM), and 0.0765 sec^{-1} (300 pM). Nonlinear least-squares fits, using Eq. (5.14), were also made of each set of data (using *Origin*), and the fitted curves are shown in Figure 5.11A. The fitted values for B_∞ were 0.110 ± 0.005, 0.269 ± 0.006, and 0.494 ± 0.006 fmol.mg dry wt.$^{-1}$ and for k_{on} 0.0351 ± 0.004, 0.0518 ± 0.003, and 0.0828 ± 0.003 sec^{-1}. These latter values have been plotted against [L] in Figure 5.11B, and linear regression gives a slope ($\equiv k_{+1}$) of 1.72×10^{-4} pM^{-1} sec^{-1} ($= 1.7 \times 10^{8}$ M^{-1} sec^{-1}) and intercept ($\equiv k_{-1}$) of 0.032 sec^{-1}. (All three curves were also fitted simultaneously to Eqs. (5.14) and (5.15) using a nonlinear least-squares program (D. Colquhoun, unpublished) and provided values for k_{+1} and k_{-1} directly: $k_{+1} = 1.63 \times 10^{-4}$ pM^{-1} sec^{-1}, $k_{-1} = 0.034$ sec^{-1}.)

Problem 5.3: Competition Data

The individual plots of the data will produce curves equivalent to that in Figure 5.4, the nonspecific binding, of course, increasing with radioligand concentration. The IC$_{50}$ can be read from the curves directly (taking account of nonspecific binding) or can be obtained from Hill plots for specific binding (see Eq. (5.31)). Hill plots of the data are presented in Figure 5.12, the points for concentrations outside 3×10^{-8} to 3×10^{-4} M being excluded because of the large errors associated with them. The lines are seen to be straight, and linear regression indicates slopes not significantly different from −1. The fitted lines have therefore been constrained to have a slope of −1. The x-intercepts corresponding to the IC$_{50}$ are 1.43 μM, 2.48 μM, and 5.74 μM. (Compare these with estimates obtained by direct interpolation on the plots of the raw data.) Nonlinear least-squares fits of each set of data to Eq. (5.18) provided IC$_{50}$ estimates of 1.20 ± 0.07 μM, 2.51 ± 0.13 μM, and

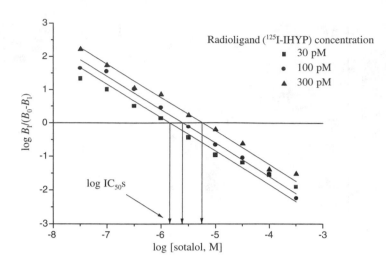

FIGURE 5.12 Hill plots of the results of the competition experiment used for Problem 5.3. The fitted lines have been constrained to have a slope of –1. IC_{50} values are given by the x-intercepts and can be used to determine K_I for the binding of sotalol (see accompanying text). The IC_{50} values, as expected from Eq. (5.20), increase with radioligand concentration.

6.17 ± 0.45 μM. The K_I can be obtained from the IC_{50} using Eq. (5.20). Taking K_L as 37 pM gives K_I values of 0.66, 0.68, and 0.68 μM, respectively, which as expected are very similar. The data for this problem were actually generated using a starting value for K_I of 0.68 μM.

Section IV

Transduction of the Receptor Signal

6 Receptors Linked to Ion Channels: Mechanisms of Activation and Block

Alasdair J. Gibb

CONTENTS

6.1 INTRODUCTION

Many measurements in pharmacology rely on a chain of events following receptor activation to produce a measurable response — for example, contraction of the smooth muscle of a piece of guinea-pig ileum in response to muscarinic receptor activation by acetylcholine. This means that the relationship between receptor occupancy and response is likely to be complex, and mechanisms of drug action in such systems are often difficult to define.

In contrast to this, agonist responses at ligand-gated ion channels and drug effects at ion channels are often more amenable to mechanistic investigation because the response (ionic current through open ion channels when measured with voltage or patch-clamp techniques) is directly proportional to receptor activation. This is a great advantage and has allowed electrophysiological techniques to be used to study ion-channel activation and drug block of ion-channel receptors in great detail.

This chapter deals mainly with information that can be obtained from equilibrium, or at least steady-state, recordings of ion-channel receptor activity. However, a great deal of information has also been obtained from kinetic studies of ion channels where the aim has been to determine values for the rate constants in a receptor mechanism. In general, only equilibrium constants can be determined from equilibrium studies.

6.1.1 THE RESPONSE TO RECEPTOR ACTIVATION

Activation of a ligand-gated ion-channel receptor causes opening of the ion channel, which forms a central pore through the receptor structure. Ions such as Na^+ and K^+, and often also Ca^{2+} (depending on the ionic selectivity of the channel), flow through cationic channels formed by nicotinic acetylcholine receptors (nAChRs), ionotropic glutamate receptors, $5HT_3$ receptors, or P2X adenosine triphosphate (ATP) receptors. These ionic currents are generally excitatory and lead to depolarization of the cell. Chloride ions, with some contribution from HCO_{3-} ions, are the main charge carriers through γ-aminobutyric acid ($GABA_A$) and glycine receptor channels, and these currents are generally, but not always, inhibitory.

The ligand-gated ion-channel receptors mediate fast synaptic transmission at the neuromuscular junction and throughout the central and peripheral nervous system. These receptors are also located presynaptically on nerve terminals at many synapses where they affect transmitter release. In addition, where the receptor channels are permeable to Ca^{2+}, they are involved in the control of the intracellular Ca^{2+} concentration and hence feed into many of the transduction mechanisms that involve Ca^{2+} as a second messenger. Ca^{2+} influx through glutamate receptors of the N-methyl-D-aspartate (NMDA) subtype (Ascher and Nowak, 1988) is of particular importance in the processes of synaptogenesis and control of the strength of synaptic connections in the brain, while excess Ca^{2+} influx through NMDA receptor channels is thought to be the main cause of neuronal cell death during hypoxia or ischemia in the brain.

Over the past 50 years, the development of electrophysiological techniques has allowed the effects of agonists and antagonists at the ligand-gated ion-channel receptors to be studied with great precision. This has been particularly useful in studies of the mechanism of action of drugs because the result of receptor activation (current through the ion channel) can be measured directly, and channel opening is directly linked to receptor activation. Thus, it should be no surprise that the first physically plausible mechanism for receptor activation was the result of electrophysiological studies of AChR activation. Those experiments were performed by Katz and co-workers in the Biophysics Department at University College, London, more than 40 years ago.

6.2 AGONIST MECHANISMS

The simplest agonist mechanism that can be used to describe activation of the ligand-gated ion-channel receptors is that first suggested by del Castillo and Katz (1957) for activation of nAChRs at the neuromuscular junction:

$$A + R \underset{k_{-1}}{\overset{k_{+1}}{\rightleftharpoons}} AR \underset{\alpha}{\overset{\beta}{\rightleftharpoons}} AR* \tag{6.1}$$

This mechanism makes the vital point that receptor activation must represent a distinct step (most likely several steps) subsequent to agonist binding (see also Chapter 1). However, this mechanism does not allow for the fact that considerable functional, biochemical, and structural evidence now suggests that there are two ACh binding sites on nicotinic acetylcholine receptors of muscle and electric organs (Unwin, 1996), and it is probably the case that other four-transmembrane (4TM)-domain subunit receptors (see Chapter 3) such as the glycine and GABA receptors also require binding of two agonist molecules for efficient activation of the receptor. At present, the mechanism most commonly (e.g., Colquhoun and Sakmann, 1981) used to describe AChR activation is as follows:

$$A + R \underset{k_{-1}}{\overset{2k_{+1}}{\rightleftharpoons}} AR + A \underset{2k_{-2}}{\overset{k_{+2}}{\rightleftharpoons}} A_2R \underset{\alpha}{\overset{\beta}{\rightleftharpoons}} A_2R* \tag{6.2}$$

Here, the microscopic association and dissociation rate constants for each step in the receptor activation mechanism are given, where k_{+1} and k_{+2} refer to agonist binding, k_{-1} and k_{-2} refer to agonist dissociation, and β and α are the rate constants for channel opening and closing, respectively. The factor of 2 before k_{+1} and k_{-2} occurs because the mechanism assumes that either of the two agonist binding sites can be occupied or vacated first. In addition, note that the two sites are assumed to be equivalent before agonist binding.

6.2.1 EVIDENCE FOR NONIDENTICAL AGONIST BINDING SITES

The agonist binding sites on the receptor are some distance from the ion channel and outside the membrane. They are in pockets formed within each α-subunit (Unwin, 1996). The environment of the two binding sites cannot, in principle, be identical because of the nonidentical adjacent subunits and the fact that the receptor is a pentamer. However, functional evidence demonstrating nonequivalance of the two binding sites has not been consistent between species.

The best evidence that the binding sites are different comes from studies of the *Torpedo* AChR, for which both binding studies of native receptors and patch-clamp studies of cloned receptors expressed in fibroblasts suggest that there is on the order of a 100-fold difference in affinity for ACh between the two sites (Lingle et al., 1992). Similar experiments on the BC3H1 cell line also suggest heterogeneity of the agonist binding sites on this embryonic mouse muscle AChR. In contrast, some experiments have found no evidence for a large difference between ACh binding at the two sites on frog endplate AChRs (Colquhoun and Ogden, 1988).

At present, this issue has not been resolved, and further functional and structural work continues to address this question. However, it should be noted that the presence on a receptor of two agonist/antagonist binding sites, which may be different, adds considerably to the complexity of the results expected from binding studies or dose-ratio experiments such as the Schild method, as described later in this chapter. It can also be noted here that homomeric receptors (such as the neuronal nicotinic α_7 receptor or homomeric AMPA receptor; see Chapter 3) will have equivalent agonist binding sites before agonist binding. A further interesting point is that if the glutamate receptor subunit stoichiometry is tetrameric, then heteromeric non-NMDA receptors composed of, for example, two GluR1 and two GluR2 subunits will, in principle, have nonidentical binding sites on the equivalent subunits if the subunits are adjacent to each other in the molecule, but they will have equivalent binding sites when the GluR1 and GluR2 subunits alternate in position around the central ion channel. These are very good examples of how information on receptor structure can be indispensable in interpreting the results of functional studies of drug action.

6.2.2 APPLICATION OF THE TWO-BINDING-SITE MECHANISM

Equation (6.2) has proved to be a good description of AChR activity in a wide range of experimental situations (reviewed by Edmonds et al., 1995) and more recently has been used as a starting point in developing mechanisms to describe the activation of other ligand-gated ion channels such as glutamate receptors, $5HT_3$ receptors, and GABA receptors.

Expressions relating the equilibrium occupancy of any state in this mechanism to agonist concentration can be derived as described in Chapter 1. If we define the equilibrium constants for agonist binding as $K_1 = k_{-1}/k_{+1}$ and $K_2 = k_{-2}/k_{+2}$ and a constant E describing the efficiency of channel opening (equivalent to *efficacy*) as $E = \beta/\alpha$, then the equilibrium occupancy of the open state (A_2R^*) will be:

$$p_{A_2R^*} = \frac{[A]}{[A] + \dfrac{1}{E}\left\{[A] + K_2\left(2 + \dfrac{K_1}{[A]}\right)\right\}} \tag{6.3}$$

It is instructive to write this equation in the form analogous to that for a single agonist binding site mechanism,

$$p_{A_2R^*} = \frac{[A]^2}{\dfrac{K_1K_2}{E} + [A]\left\{[A] + \dfrac{[A]}{E} + \dfrac{2K_2}{E}\right\}} \tag{6.4}$$

as this form illustrates the low-concentration dependence of $p_{A_2R^*}$ on the square of the agonist concentration, which steepens the dose–response curve.

The equilibrium occupancy of the open state of an ion channel is usually referred to as the p_{open} and is the fraction of time that a single channel is open or, equally, the fraction of a population of channels that are open at equilibrium. For a two-binding site agonist mechanism, the relationship between the p_{open} and the agonist concentration (p_{open} curve) has the familiar sigmoid shape (when the agonist concentration is plotted on a logarithmic scale) of a dose–response curve but is steeper than for a single binding site mechanism.

6.2.3 HILL COEFFICIENTS AND COOPERATIVITY

In Chapter 1 (Section 1.2.4.3), the Hill equation and the Hill coefficient, n_H, are described. Hill coefficients greater than or less than unity are often interpreted as indicating positive or negative cooperativity, respectively, in the relationship between receptor occupancy and response. For example, positive cooperativity could arise due to amplification in a transduction mechanism mediated by G-proteins and changes in cell calcium concentration.

If the receptor has two agonist binding sites, the question arises as to whether binding of agonist at one site can influence the binding of the agonist at the other site, referred to as *cooperativity between agonist binding sites*. *Negative cooperativity* occurs when binding at one site reduces the affinity at the second site, while *positive cooperativity* occurs if binding at one site increases the affinity at the second site. Note that there may be cooperativity between agonist binding sites even though the unoccupied sites have the same affinity for the agonist. However, it is also possible that the two agonist binding sites are different before agonist binding occurs (on average, one site is then more likely to be occupied before the other), and in this case it is still possible for the binding of agonist at one site to influence binding at the other site.

The slope of the p_{open} curve for Eq. (6.2) is more complex than for a single agonist binding site; Eq. (6.4) does not have the same form as the Hill–Langmuir equation, and the Hill plot is not

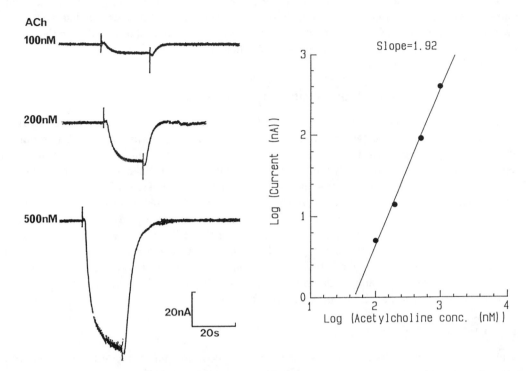

FIGURE 6.1 Macroscopic AChR responses and the Hill slope for AChR activation. (Left) Current through AChR ion channels in response to increasing concentrations of ACh was recorded from *Xenopus* oocytes which had been injected 3 days previously with cRNA (courtesy of Prof. S. F. Heinemann, Salk Institute) for the α, β, γ, and δ subunits of the mouse muscle AChR. An inward current through the AChR ion channels is shown as a downward deflection of the trace. Small artifacts on the trace indicate the time when the solution flowing into the bath was changed from control to the indicated ACh concentrations and then back to control. Currents were recorded with two-microelectrode voltage clamp. The membrane potential was –60 mV and the recordings were made at room temperature. (Right) The response (in nA) to increasing concentrations of ACh is plotted against ACh concentration (in nM) on log–log scales. The slope of the line (1.92) is an approximation to the Hill coefficient (when receptor occupancy is small) and suggests that two agonist molecules must bind to the receptor to produce efficient receptor activation.

a straight line (as mentioned in Chapter 1, Section 1.2.4.3). This is because for the two-agonist binding site mechanism the Hill coefficient n_H depends on the agonist concentration:

$$n = 2\left(\frac{1+[A]/K_1}{1+2[A]/K_1}\right) \tag{6.5}$$

When $[A] \ll K_1$, then $n_H = 2$ but falls to $n_H = 1$ when $[A] \gg K_1$. In a study of AChR activation at the frog endplate, estimates were made of $EC_{50} = 15$ μM, $K_1 = K_2 = 77$ μM, and $n_H = 1.6$ at the half-maximal response, EC_{50}, concentration.

An approximation to the Hill plot is often used with agonist-response data for ligand-gated ion channels to suggest a lower limit for the number of agonist binding sites on the receptor. It turns out that, for many (but not all) mechanisms, if $[A] \ll K_A$, then the slope of a plot of log (response) vs. log $[A]$ approaches the number of agonist binding reactions required for receptor activation. Figure 6.1 illustrates this using data recorded from a *Xenopus* oocyte expressing embryonic mouse muscle AChR receptors. In this example, the response being measured is the summed current flowing through many thousands of open receptor channels in the oocyte membrane. At these low agonist concentrations ($[A] \ll K_A$), the slope of the plot (in this case, 1.92) suggests that the binding of two ACh molecules is necessary for receptor activation, and this correlates well with the known subunit stoichiometry of muscle AChRs of $\alpha_2\beta\gamma\delta$, where the ACh binding sites are known to be formed by the α subunits.

6.2.4 HILL COEFFICIENT FOR HOMOMERIC RECEPTOR CHANNELS

Several functional receptors have been described in expression systems where the receptor is expressed from a single receptor subunit. Receptor subunits that form functional homomeric channels include the neuronal nicotinic α_7 subunit, the $5HT_3$ receptor subunit, some non-NMDA receptor subunits, the embryonic glycine receptor α subunit, and the P2X ATP receptor subunits. Based on analogy with the known structure of *Torpedo* AChRs, it is assumed that AChRs, $5HT_3$ receptors, and glycine receptors have a pentameric structure of five subunits surrounding a central ion channel pore. Such a structure suggests that there will be five agonist binding sites on a homomeric receptor. What, then, should we expect the Hill coefficient to be for these receptors? Hill coefficients for these receptors are generally found to be in the range from 1 to 3. Such measurements are complicated by receptor desensitization (see below). However, these results can be interpreted as indicating that, in situations with five agonist binding sites on the receptor, perhaps only any two must be occupied for full receptor activation.

6.2.5 RECEPTOR DESENSITIZATION

Desensitization can be defined as the tendency of a response to wane, despite the presence of a stimulus of constant intensity (e.g., constant agonist concentration). In the case of the nicotinic ACh receptor, good evidence suggests that desensitization results from a change in receptor conformation to an inactive refractory state (Rang and Ritter, 1970). To describe this in terms of the AChR activation mechanism, we could add a desensitized state to the scheme shown in Eq. (6.2) to give:

$$\mathrm{A + R} \underset{k_{-1}}{\overset{2k_{+1}}{\rightleftharpoons}} \mathrm{AR + A} \underset{2k_{-2}}{\overset{k_{+2}}{\rightleftharpoons}} \mathrm{A_2R} \underset{\alpha}{\overset{\beta}{\rightleftharpoons}} \mathrm{A_2R^*} \underset{2k_{-D}}{\overset{k_{+D}}{\rightleftharpoons}} \mathrm{A_2R_D} \tag{6.6}$$

Here, k_{+D} and k_{-D} are the rate constants for entry into and exit from the desensitized state A_2R_D. Investigation of the applicability of a range of mechanisms like the linear scheme in Eq. (6.6) to AChR desensitization (Katz and Thesleff, 1957; Rang and Ritter, 1970) provided good evidence that linear schemes could not adequately account for AChR desensitization. In particular, it was noted that onset was often slower than the offset of desensitization at agonist concentrations producing around 50% steady-state desensitization, and, while the rate of onset was dependent on the nature of the agonist, offset was independent of the agonist. These results are not expected from linear schemes like Eq. (6.6). It was concluded that a cyclic scheme such as the following was necessary:

$$
\begin{array}{ccc}
\mathrm{A + R} \underset{}{\overset{K_A}{\rightleftharpoons}} \mathrm{AR} \underset{\alpha}{\overset{\beta}{\rightleftharpoons}} \mathrm{A_2R^*} \\
\big\updownarrow K'_D \qquad\quad \big\updownarrow K_D \\
\mathrm{A + R_D} \overset{K'_A}{\rightleftharpoons} \mathrm{AR_D}
\end{array}
\tag{6.7}
$$

Here, the equilibrium constants for each reaction are given and only a single agonist binding step is shown for simplicity.

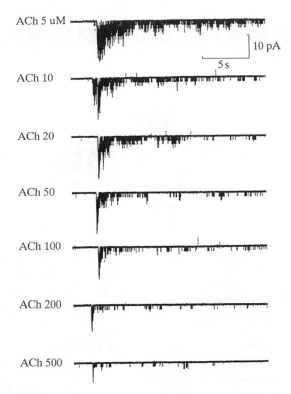

FIGURE 6.2 Activation of single AChR channels in an outside-out membrane patch and responses to increasing concentrations of ACh of a membrane patch containing several AChRs. A small artifact near the beginning of each trace indicates the time when the solution flowing into the recording chamber was changed to solution containing the indicated concentration of ACh. With increasing ACh concentration, it can be seen that the channels are activated more rapidly, and that receptor desensitization becomes increasingly more rapid such that the peak response is reduced at the higher ACh concentrations. Once the response to agonist has reached a steady state, probably more than 90% of the receptors in the patch are desensitized. It is then possible to see individual clusters of channel openings, which reflect periods when single AChRs briefly exit from a desensitized state and undergo repeated activation by the agonist ACh, before reentering the desensitized state again. Identification of these clusters provides a means of directly observing and measuring the p_{open} for the receptor at high agonist concentrations, as illustrated in Figure 6.3.

The desensitized state of the receptor has very high affinity for the agonist ($K_A' \ll K_A$) and receptors are more likely to desensitize when occupied by agonist ($K_D \ll K_D'$). These observations have important consequences for radioligand-binding studies utilizing ligand-gated ion-channel receptor agonists. Generally, because desensitization is fast relative to the time scale of a binding experiment, what is measured will be dominated by the equilibrium constant for binding of the agonist to the desensitized state of the receptor, and this may be of higher affinity by several orders of magnitude than the affinity of the agonist for the resting, nondesensitized receptor. This is simply another case of the results developed in Chapter 1 showing that, in general, the *apparent* affinity of agonists estimated by methods such as radioligand binding will be a function of all the equilibrium constants in the receptor mechanism.

Desensitization is probably a quite general receptor phenomenon, although it varies widely in extent and rate of onset and offset. The scale and time course of AChR desensitization is illustrated in Figure (6.2), which shows responses of a patch of cell membrane containing several AChRs to increasing concentrations of ACh. Two things are obvious: first, during each ACh application, the response rises rapidly to a peak and then wanes to a level where the trace can be seen stepping

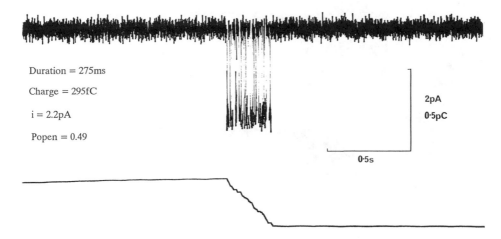

Duration = 275ms

Charge = 295fC

i = 2.2pA

Popen = 0.49

2pA

0·5pC

0·5s

FIGURE 6.3 Measurement of receptor p_{open} during clusters of AChR channel openings in an outside-out patch expressing mouse muscle AChR as described for Figure 6.1. The upper trace shows a single cluster of AChR channel openings activated by 10 μM ACh. The lower trace shows a trace of the output from an analog integrator circuit. The duration of the cluster is 275 msec, and the charge passed was 295 fC. The average single-channel current was 2.2 pA, giving a p_{open} for this cluster of 0.49.

between single-channel current levels. Second, it can be seen that with increasing ACh concentration the peak response does not simply become greater; instead, it first increases and then decreases due to the increasing rate of onset of desensitization.

6.2.6 Determination of the P_{OPEN} Curve

Due to the occurrence of desensitization, the shape of the full relationship between agonist concentration and response cannot be determined from experiments like that illustrated in Figure 6.1A. In practice, the most accurately determined part of the macroscopic dose–response curve is often at the low concentration limit, where the effects of desensitization on the dose–response curve are small.

Single-channel recording provides a way around the problem of desensitization because periods when all the receptors in the membrane patch are desensitized are obvious at high agonist concentrations as long stretches of recording where no channel openings occur; therefore, desensitization has been used to provide a means of obtaining groups of successive openings, all due to the activity of a single AChR, referred to as *clusters*. The desensitized periods are simply discarded, and the channel p_{open} is measured during the clusters of activity between desensitized periods.

In each trace in Figure 6.2, after several seconds of exposure to ACh it becomes possible to identify individual clusters of AChR channel openings. Analysis of these clusters of channel openings, as illustrated in Figure 6.3, allows the relationship between ACh concentration and p_{open} to be determined.

Figure 6.3 shows an example of a cluster of AChR channel openings recorded from an outside-out membrane patch in the presence of 10 μM ACh. The p_{open} during the cluster is, in principle, simple to calculate; the fraction of time the channel is open is the total time spent in the open state divided by the duration of the cluster. However, the limited bandwidth of any recording system means that some short openings will be too short to be measured. It is, therefore, preferable to measure the charge passed during the cluster (because charge is not lost with filtering) and use the accumulated charge (the integral of the current during the cluster) to calculate the p_{open}:

$$p_{open} = \frac{\text{charge passed during cluster (pC)}}{\text{single channel current (pA)} \times \text{cluster duration (secs)}} \qquad (6.8)$$

a

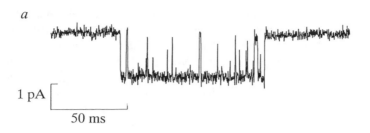

1 pA

50 ms

b

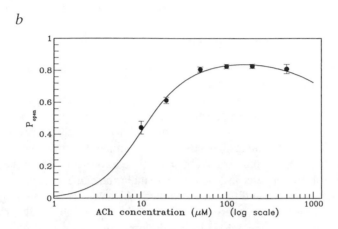

FIGURE 6.4 The p_{open} curve for mouse muscle AChR expressed in *Xenopus* oocytes. (a) A cluster of AChR channel openings activated in response to 200 µM ACh is shown; the cluster p_{open} = 0.87. (b) The relationship between cluster p_{open} and ACh concentration is shown. The data points show the mean ± S.E. (n = 8–82 clusters) at each ACh concentration. The solid line shows the fit of the data to the reaction mechanism given in Eq. (6.24), where the agonist can both activate the receptor and block the open ion channel. The equilibrium constants for agonist binding to the two binding sites on the receptor were assumed to be equal (K_A) and were estimated to be 22 µM, the ratio of channel opening to closing rate constants (β/α) was 7.9, and the equilibrium constant for open channel block (K_B) was 4.9 mM. (Adapted from Gibb et al., *Proc. Roy. Soc. London Ser. B*, **242**, 108–112, 1990.)

Using the method of integrating the charge passed during each cluster of channel activity, it is possible to accurately determine the p_{open} curve at high agonist concentrations. However, notice that this method depends on identification of clusters of channel openings where each cluster can be assigned unambiguously as resulting from the activity of a single receptor channel: at low p_{open}, it is possible for two channels to be active during a cluster without giving any clear double openings but, of course, giving about double the true p_{open} for a single receptor. Therefore, the lower part of the p_{open} curve cannot be determined in this type of experiment. Ideally, the entire p_{open} curve should be determined from experiments where there is only one receptor present in the patch of membrane being recorded. In practice, this is extremely difficult to achieve because the density of receptors is too high in most cell membranes and it is not possible to determine how many receptors are in the patch.

Figure 6.4 shows an example of a cluster of AChR channel openings and the p_{open} curve obtained from the same patch. It was possible to identify clusters clearly when the p_{open} was greater than about 0.4. The results are complicated by the presence of open channel block of the AChR channel by the agonist, ACh (see Section 6.3.3 and Eq. (6.24)). This causes the p_{open} to gradually decrease at high agonist concentrations, particularly above 1 mM. The maximum p_{open} for the patch illustrated in Figure 6.4a was 0.83 ± 0.01 (n = 45 clusters) and occurred at 200 µM ACh (Figure 6.4b). How should these results be interpreted? The p_{open} curve in Figure 6.4b was fitted with the relationship between p_{open} and the ACh concentration predicted for the two-agonist binding site mechanism extended to allow for block of the open ion channel by ACh (Eq. (6.34)). This fitting allows estimates to be made for each of the equilibrium constants in the reaction mechanism.

There is, however, one difficulty with interpreting the results of fitting the p_{open} curve. The difficulty is that when the maximum p_{open} approaches unity, increasing β/α or decreasing K_A has a very similar effect on the p_{open} curve, both changes simply shifting it to the left. Thus, β/α and K_A cannot be estimated independently ($E = \beta/\alpha$ and K_A are correlated) when the maximum p_{open} is high. One solution to this is to estimate β/α separately and then fix this value when fitting the p_{open} curve to estimate K_A. Fortunately, estimates of β and α can be obtained from the analysis of bursts of single-channel openings recorded at low agonist concentrations as detailed below.

6.2.7 ANALYSIS OF SINGLE-CHANNEL RECORDINGS

Development of the single-channel recording technique was an enormous advance for studies of ion-channel receptor function (Neher and Sakmann, 1976). For the first time it became possible to ask detailed questions about the mechanism of activation and block of the ligand-gated ion-channel receptors. It became possible to measure directly the duration of ion-channel openings and closings and so avoid some of the most limiting assumptions that had been necessary when interpreting macroscopic current records. An interesting point is that, although single-channel recordings are generally made at equilibrium, it is possible to obtain detailed information about the rates of channel opening and closing. This is because, in a sense, any single molecule is never at equilibrium but spends randomly distributed times in different conformational states. The mean length of time spent in any individual states is equal to the inverse of the sum of the rates of all possible routes for leaving that state, so measurement of channel open times and closed times provides information about the rate constants for transitions in a reaction mechanism. A complete description of the interpretation of single-channel data is beyond the scope of this chapter (see Further Reading section).

6.2.8 ANALYSIS OF BURSTS OF ION-CHANNEL OPENINGS

Equation (6.2) predicts that channel openings will occur in groups or *bursts*. Bursts of openings occur because each time the receptor reaches state A_2R the channel may open or an agonist molecule can dissociate from the receptor. When the agonist dissociation rate k_{-2} is similar to the channel opening rate β, the channel may open and close several times before agonist dissociation occurs, generating a burst of openings. The burst of openings and closings is also referred to as an *activation*, which can be defined as everything that occurs from the first opening following agonist binding until the end of the last opening before all agonist molecules dissociate from the receptor (obviously, occasions where the agonist binds and then dissociates without channel opening are invisible). It was predicted that ligand-gated ion-channel receptor activation would result in bursts of channel openings given what was known about fast synaptic transmission (reviewed by Edmonds et al., 1995), and this idea has been used to interpret data from single-channel recordings of AChR channel openings at the frog neuromuscular junction (Colquhoun and Sakmann, 1985).

From Eq. (6.2), the mean open time is predicted to be the reciprocal of the rate constant for channel closing ($\tau_{open} = 1/\alpha$). For bursts recorded at very low agonist concentrations, the mean closed time within bursts, τ_g, is equal to $1/(\beta + 2k_{-2})$, and the mean number of gaps per burst, N_g, is equal to $\beta/2k_{-2}$. Using these two simultaneous equations, it is then possible to calculate β and k_{-2}.

From recordings of bursts of recombinant embryonic mouse muscle AChR channel openings at low concentrations of ACh (less than 1 μM), the duration of openings and closings and the number of closings per burst was measured. On average $\tau_{open} = 3.0$ msec, $\tau_g = 94$ μsec, and $N_g = 0.86$, giving $\alpha = 333$ sec^{-1}, $\beta = 4919$ sec^{-1}, and $k_{-2} = 2860$ sec^{-1}. If we assume $k_{+2} = 2 \times 10^8$ M^{-1}sec^{-1}, then $K_A = 14$ μM. Thus, $\beta/\alpha = 15$ and the maximum $p_{open} = \beta/(\alpha + \beta) = 0.94$. These values are consistent with those obtained from fitting the p_{open} curve in Figure 6.4. The ratio $\beta/(\alpha + \beta)$ indicates that ACh is a high-efficacy agonist, while the large value for β indicates that a high [ACh] will very rapidly (within a few hundred microseconds) activate the channel, as is observed during neuromuscular transmission (Edmonds et al., 1995).

6.3 ANTAGONISM OF ION-CHANNEL RECEPTORS

The use of the Schild method for estimation of the dissociation equilibrium constant of a competitive antagonist is described in detail in Chapter 1. The great advantage of the Schild method lies in the fact that it is a null method: agonist *occupancy* in the absence or presence of antagonist is assumed to be equal when *responses* in the absence or presence of the antagonist are equal. Even when the relationship between occupancy and response is complex, the Schild method has been found to work well.

6.3.1 COMPETITIVE ANTAGONISM AND THE SCHILD EQUATION

Using the procedures outlined in Chapter 1, it is straightforward to show that the Schild equation is also obtained for competitive antagonism of ion-channel receptors in the case of a single agonist binding site. However, when considering two agonist binding sites, the situation is more complicated as several new questions about the mechanism must be answered:

- Is the antagonist affinity for both binding sites equal? It is quite possible that even if the agonist has the same affinity for both sites, an antagonist will not.
- Can two antagonist molecules occupy the receptor at the same time?
- Does binding of the antagonist at one site influence the affinity of the other site for either agonist or antagonist?

The situation can be simplified by assuming:

- Agonist affinity at each site is the same.
- Antagonist affinity at each site is the same.
- Occupancy of one site by either agonist or antagonist does not influence the affinity of the second site for either agonist or antagonist.

Even with these simplifying assumptions, a mechanism to describe the simultaneous action of both agonist and antagonist at a two-binding-site receptor is complex:

$$
\begin{array}{ccccccc}
 & & 2k_{+A} & & k_{+A} & & \beta \\
B + R + A & \rightleftharpoons & B + AR + A & \rightleftharpoons & A_2R & \rightleftharpoons & A_2R^* \\
 & k_{-A} & & 2k_{-A} & & \alpha & \\
k_{-B} \updownarrow 2k_{+B} & & k_{-B} \updownarrow k_{+B} & & & & \\
 & 2k_{-B} & & k_{+A} & & & \\
B_2R & \rightleftharpoons & B + BR + A & \rightleftharpoons & BRA & & \\
 & k_{+B} & & k_{-A} & & &
\end{array}
\tag{6.9}
$$

An expression for the equilibrium occupancy of $p_{A_2R^*}$ can again be obtained using the methods outlined in Chapter 1. A potential complication is that this mechanism contains a cycle, so the product of the reaction rates in both clockwise and counterclockwise directions should be equal in order to ensure the principle of microscopic reversibility is maintained. In this case, microscopic reversibility is maintained. Thus,

$$
2k_{+A} \cdot k_{+B} \cdot k_{-A} \cdot k_{-B} = 2k_{+B} \cdot k_{+A} \cdot k_{-B} \cdot k_{-A}
\tag{6.10}
$$

In the presence of both agonist A and antagonist B, p_{A_2R*} depends on both the agonist and antagonist concentration in quite a complicated fashion; however, the relationship is essentially an extension of Eq. (6.3) and is arrived at as follows:

1. The proportions of all forms of the receptor must add up to one:

$$p_{B_2R} + p_{BR} + p_{BRA} + p_R + p_{AR} + p_{A_2R} + p_{A_2R*} = 1 \tag{6.11}$$

2. When the system is at equilibrium, each individual reaction step in Eq. (6.9) can be used to write expressions for each form of the receptor in terms of the active form of the receptor, A_2R*:

$$p_{A_2R} = \frac{1}{E} p_{A_2R*}, \quad p_{AR} = \frac{2K_A}{[A]E} p_{A_2R*}, \quad p_R = \frac{K_A^2}{[A]^2 E} p_{A_2R*} \tag{6.12}$$

$$p_{BAR} = \frac{2[B]K_A}{K_B[A]E} p_{A_2R*}, \quad p_{BR} = \frac{[B]K_A^2}{2K_B[A]^2 E} p_{A_2R*}, \quad p_{B_2R} = \frac{[B]^2 K_A^2}{K_B^2[A]^2 E} p_{A_2R*} \tag{6.13}$$

The relationship between p_{A_2R*} and both agonist and antagonist concentration can then be written as:

$$p_{A_2R*} = \frac{[A]}{[A] + \dfrac{1}{E}\left\{[A] + K_A\left[2 + \dfrac{2[B]}{K_B} + \dfrac{K_A}{[A]}\left(1 + \dfrac{[B]}{K_B}\right)^2\right]\right\}} \tag{6.14}$$

It is clear from comparison of Eq. (6.14) with Eq. (6.3), reproduced below as Eq. (6.15) with $K_A = K_1 = K_2$,

$$p_{A_2R*} = \frac{[A]}{[A] + \dfrac{1}{E}\left\{[A] + K_A\left(2 + \dfrac{K_A}{[A]}\right)\right\}} \tag{6.15}$$

that there is now no simple expression relating dose ratio to antagonist concentration. After equating occupancies in the absence and presence of the blocker and multiplying the agonist concentration in Eq. (6.14) by the dose ratio, r can be found from the expression:

$$\left(2 + \frac{K_A}{[A]}\right) = \frac{1}{r}\left[2 + \frac{2[B]}{K_B} + \frac{K_A}{r[A]}\left(1 + \frac{[B]}{K_B}\right)^2\right] \tag{6.16}$$

This expression can be rearranged to give a quadratic equation in r:

$$\frac{2[A]}{K_A} + 1 = \frac{1}{r}\left(\frac{2[A]}{K_A} + \frac{2[A][B]}{K_A K_B}\right) + \frac{1}{r^2}\left(1 + \frac{[B]}{K_B}\right)^2 \tag{6.17}$$

and this can be rearranged to have the standard form:

$$r^2(a) + r(b) + (c) = 0 \tag{6.18}$$

whose two solutions are found from the equation:

$$r_1, r_2 = \frac{-b \pm \sqrt{b^2 - 4ac}}{2a} \tag{6.19}$$

One solution is negative and the other is (perhaps surprisingly!) the familiar Schild equation:

$$r = \frac{[B]}{K_B} + 1 \tag{6.20}$$

More directly, it may be seen by inspection of Eqs. (6.14) and (6.15) that:

$$\left(2 + \frac{K_A}{[A]}\right) = 2\left(\frac{1 + [B]/K_B}{r}\right) + \frac{K_A}{[A]}\left(\frac{1 + [B]/K_B}{r}\right)^2 \tag{6.21}$$

so for the right and left sides of this equation to be equal,

$$\frac{1 + [B]/K_B}{r} = 1 \tag{6.22}$$

and the Schild equation applies.

Thus, if we assume that the two binding sites are identical and independent, then the Schild equation holds for the two-binding-site mechanism. If however, the antagonist binds with different affinity to each site, then the dose ratio becomes a complex function of both agonist and antagonist concentrations and equilibrium constants (Colquhoun, 1986). It is, therefore, not surprising that a parallel shift of the p_{open} curve with increasing concentration of antagonist is predicted not to be observed when the binding sites are different, so the dose ratio will depend on the response level at which it is measured. However, some simplifying assumptions can still be made. If the p_{open} is small ([A] << K_A), then an approximately parallel shift of the dose–response curve occurs and the dose ratio is:

$$r \approx \sqrt{\left(1 + \frac{[B]}{K_{B1}}\right)\left(1 + \frac{[B]}{K_{B2}}\right)} \tag{6.23}$$

Here, K_{B1} and K_{B2} are the equilibrium constants for the blocker at the two sites. In this situation, the Schild plot is not linear; it has a slope of less than unity at antagonist concentrations around K_B (where $K_B = (K_{B1}K_{B2})^{1/2}$) and tends to unity at high or at low antagonist concentrations (Colquhoun, 1986).

An example of the use of the Schild plot in examining the action of the antagonist tubocurarine on AChRs at the frog neuromuscular junction (Colquhoun et al., 1979) is shown in Figure 6.5. This figure illustrates an experiment where the net inward current measured in response to different concentrations of carbachol is plotted first in the absence (control) and then in the presence of increasing concentrations of tubocurarine. Recordings were made at two different membrane potentials and the Schild plot for each membrane potential constructed. The results illustrate that, at –70 mV, the Schild plot is linear and has a slope close to unity, suggesting competitive antagonism

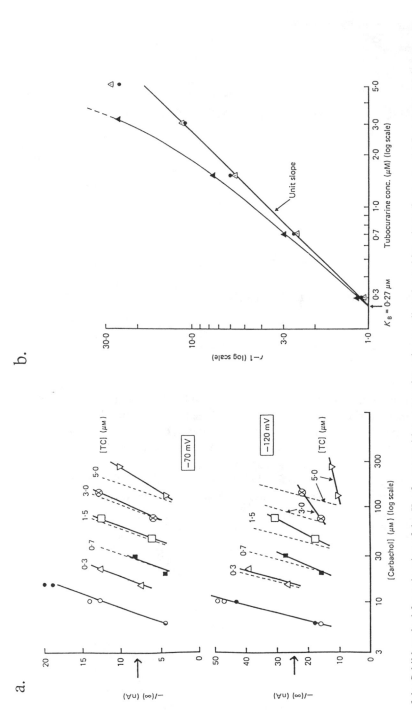

FIGURE 6.5 Use of the Schild method for estimation of the K_B of a competitive antagonist acting at a ligand-gated ion-channel receptor. (a) Log concentration–response curves for the equilibrium net inward current ($-I_\infty$) evoked by carbachol in the presence of increasing concentrations of tubocurarine (TC) at a membrane potential of –70 mV (upper panel) and at a membrane potential of –120 mV (lower panel). It can be seen that, except for the highest concentration of TC (5 μM), at –70 mV this antagonist produces an approximately parallel shift of the carbachol dose–response curve as expected for competitive antagonism. However, in the same experiment at a membrane potential of –120 mV, the shift of the dose–response curves is far from parallel. This is because the positively charged tubocurarine molecule is being attracted into the AChR channel when the inside of the cell is made more negative. The dashed lines in the upper and lower panels show the responses predicted for pure competitive antagonism with K_B = 0.27 μM. Dose ratios were calculated at a response level of –8 nA at –70 mV and –24 nA at –120 mV. (b) Schild plot of log (r – 1) against log (tubocurarine concentration). The filled circles show equilibrium dose ratios at –70 mV, filled triangles show equilibrium dose ratios at –120 mV, and open triangles show the peak response at –120 mV. Because open channel block by tubocurarine is relatively slow to develop, when the peak response is measured mainly competitive antagonism is seen and the Schild slope is close to unity. The fact that both curves coincide at low antagonist concentrations (small dose ratios) suggests that the K_B for competitive binding to the receptor is independent of the membrane potential, as might be expected if the agonist binding site is outside the membrane potential field. (Adapted from Colquhoun, D. et al., *J. Physiol.*, 293, 247–284, 1979.)

(without any distinction between binding sites for the antagonist). However, at a membrane potential of -120 mV, the Schild plot is nonlinear and has a slope steeper than unity. This occurs because tubocurarine also blocks the open ion channel of the endplate AChR, and, when the membrane potential is made more negative, the positively charged tubocurarine molecule is attracted into the ion channel, resulting in a noncompetitive block of the receptor, as discussed in the next section.

6.3.2 ION-CHANNEL BLOCK

The ion-channel blocking mechanism has been widely tested and found to be important in both pharmacology and physiology. Examples are the block of nerve and cardiac sodium channels by local anesthetics, or block of NMDA receptor channels by Mg^{2+} and the anesthetic ketamine. The channel-block mechanism was first used quantitatively to describe block of the squid axon K^+ current by tetraethylammonium (TEA) ions. The effects of channel blockers on synaptic potentials and synaptic currents were investigated, particularly at the neuromuscular junction, and the development of the single-channel recording technique allowed channel blockages to be observed directly for the first time.

6.3.3 A MECHANISM FOR CHANNEL BLOCK

The idea that drugs could act by directly blocking the flow of ions through ion channels probably started, like any hypothesis, as some sort of abstract idea without any physical basis. It is easy to draw a scheme that includes something like the plug in a sink, blocking the flow of water down the drain (ion channel); however, to progress, it is necessary to convert the drawing into a mechanism that is physically plausible (i.e., does not contravene any of the accepted laws of physics) and provides quantitative predictions that can be tested experimentally.

Ideally, the aim would be to estimate the association and dissociation rate constants for the channel-blocking drug. This would then give the dissociation equilibrium constant (K_B) for drug binding. Just as in the use of the Schild method to quantify competitive antagonism, a quantitative estimate of the K_B for channel block allows comparison of various drugs and a pharmacological classification of the ion channels to which they bind.

In other words, we could say that when an ion channel is open, the drug binding site is exposed. If a drug binds to that site, flow of ions through the channel is blocked. We might further suppose that the drug has to unblock before the channel can close normally. A standard mechanism used to describe channel block of ligand-gated ion-channel receptors is then:

$$A + R \underset{k_{-1}}{\overset{2k_{+1}}{\rightleftharpoons}} AR + A \underset{2k_{-2}}{\overset{k_{+2}}{\rightleftharpoons}} A_2R \underset{\alpha}{\overset{\beta}{\rightleftharpoons}} A_2R* + B \underset{k_{-B}}{\overset{[B]k_{+B}}{\rightleftharpoons}} A_2RB \qquad (6.24)$$

where β and α are the channel opening and closing rates, and k_{+B} and k_{-B} are the microscopic association and dissociation rate constants for blocking the channel by the drug B. Here, [B] is indicated on the transition into the blocked state to remind the reader that the rate of this reaction depends on [B]. Notice that this mechanism does not take into account the possibility that a drug could bind to the channel in the closed (occupied or unoccupied) conformation.

With mechanisms such as these, it is often possible to simplify the analysis of the action of a channel blocker by assuming that agonist binding is much faster than channel opening and closing and then combining several closed states together so that the mechanism approximates a three-state system:

$$A_2R \underset{\alpha}{\overset{\beta'}{\rightleftharpoons}} A_2R* + B \underset{k_{-B}}{\overset{[B]k_{+B}}{\rightleftharpoons}} A_2RB \qquad (6.25)$$

Notice that the channel opening rate is now denoted β'. Because the channel can only open from the A_2R state, the effective opening rate, β', is obtained by multiplying the real opening rate β by the equilibrium occupancy of A_2R:

$$\beta' = p_{A_2R}\beta \tag{6.26}$$

6.3.4 MACROSCOPIC KINETICS: RELAXATIONS (SUCH AS SYNAPTIC CURRENTS) AND NOISE

Changes in the occupancy of the open-channel state of the receptor as a function of time ($p_{A_2R*}(t)$) in response to a perturbation of the receptor equilibrium can be used to obtain information about the rates of channel gating and the interaction of drugs with ion-channel receptors. The system is said to *relax* towards a new equilibrium. The time course of the relaxation is used to measure rates from the average behavior of many ion channels in a recording, while noise analysis uses the frequency of the moment-to-moment fluctuations in occupancy of the open-channel state at equilibrium to provide information about the rates in the receptor mechanism.

For k states, a relaxation (or noise spectrum) will contain k_{-1} exponential (or Lorentzian) components. Thus, the mechanism in Eq. (6.25) above will have two states in the absence of blocker and so give rise to relaxations (or noise spectra) that can be fitted with single exponential (or Lorentzian) functions. Addition of the blocker creates an extra state (the blocked state), giving $k = 3$. For $k = 3$, the occupancy of the open state as a function of time will be described by two exponentials:

$$p_{A_2R*}(t) = p_{A_2R*}(\infty) + w_1 \exp\left(-\frac{t}{\tau_1}\right) + w_2 \exp\left(-\frac{t}{\tau_2}\right) \tag{6.27}$$

The reciprocals of the time constants, τ_1 and τ_2, are the rate constants λ_1 and λ_2. The weights of the exponentials (w_1 and w_2) are complicated functions of the transition rates in Eq. (6.25). However, the rate constants are eigenvalues found by solving the system of differential equations that describe the above mechanism. λ_1 and λ_2 are the two solutions of the quadratic equation:

$$\lambda^2 + b\lambda + c = 0 \tag{6.28}$$

where

$$-b = \lambda_1 + \lambda_2 = \alpha + \beta' + [B]k_{+B} + k_{-B} \tag{6.29}$$

and

$$c = \lambda_1\lambda_2 = \alpha k_{-B}\left[1 + \frac{\beta'}{\alpha}\left(1 + \frac{[B]}{k_{-B} / k_{+B}}\right)\right] \tag{6.30}$$

Notice that when β' is small (i.e., when the occupancy of A_2R is very small, as it will be if the agonist concentration is low), then

$$\lambda_1 + \lambda_2 = \alpha + [B]k_{+B} + k_{-B} \tag{6.31}$$

and

$$\lambda_1 \lambda_2 = \alpha k_{-B} \tag{6.32}$$

With the simplifying assumption of a small β', the sum and the product of the rate constants measured in an experiment can be used to calculate k_{-B} and k_{+B} if α is known from experiments in the absence of the blocker. This is simply done by plotting the sum or the product of the measured rate constants against blocker concentration. From Eq. (6.32) above, the product of the rate constants should be independent of blocker concentration with a value equal to αk_{-B}, while the sum of the rate constants (Eq. (6.31)) will give a straight line with slope equal to k_{+B} and intercept of $\alpha + k_{-B}$. If the experimental data is consistent with these predictions, then the data points plotted in this way should lie on a straight line, and this is good evidence that the mechanism of action of the drug is to block the open ion channel.

The assumption that β' is very small has been used when studying the effects of channel blockers on synaptic currents, as the transmitter concentration (and hence p_{A_2R}) is probably small during the decay phase of the current. During noise analysis experiments, a low agonist concentration is used so that, again, under these conditions β' should be small.

6.3.5 CHANNEL BLOCK AT EQUILIBRIUM

The relationship between p_{open} ($p_{control}$) and agonist concentration for the two-agonist binding site mechanism is given in Eq. (6.4) and reproduced below in a slightly different form:

$$p_{control} = \cfrac{1}{1 + \cfrac{1}{E} + \cfrac{2K_2}{[A]E} + \cfrac{K_1 K_2}{[A]^2 E}} \tag{6.33}$$

When an open channel blocker is added, the p_{open} in the presence of the blocker ($p_{blocker}$) given below is a function of both agonist (A) and blocker (B) concentration:

$$p_{blocker} = \cfrac{1}{1 + \cfrac{1}{E} + \cfrac{2K_2}{[A]E} + \cfrac{K_1 K_2}{[A]^2 E} + \cfrac{[B]}{K_B}} \tag{6.34}$$

Taking the ratio of $p_{control}/p_{blocker}$ gives this simple result:

$$\frac{p_{control}}{p_{blocker}} = 1 + \frac{p_{control}}{K_B} \cdot [B] \tag{6.35}$$

Because the current recorded in a voltage clamp experiment is directly proportional to the channel p_{open}, the ratio of current in the absence of blocker to current in the presence of increasing concentrations of blocker can be used to calculate K_B. The experimental design is intended to obtain a fairly large response to agonist alone and then calculate the ratio of this control response to responses to the same concentration of agonist in the presence of increasing concentrations of channel blocker. The ratio $p_{control}/p_{blocker}$ when plotted against [B] will be a straight line that intercepts the y-axis at 1 and has a slope of $p_{control}/K_B$. If $p_{control} = 1$, then the slope $= 1/K_B$. If $p_{control}$ is known for a particular agonist concentration, then obviously K_B can still be estimated. If we assume $p_{control} = 1$, then the calculated K_B will be greater than the true K_B: for example, by a factor of 2 if $p_{control} = 0.5$ and by a factor of 10 if $p_{control} = 0.1$.

6.3.6 SINGLE-CHANNEL ANALYSIS OF CHANNEL BLOCK

Below is an outline of some of the information that can be obtained from single-channel data using fairly simple measurements such as the mean open time and mean shut time. This analysis is illustrated in Figure 6.6 for the block of NMDA receptor channels by Mg^{2+} ions.

6.3.6.1 Open Times

Channel blockers will produce a reduction of the mean open time from:

$$\tau_o = \frac{1}{\alpha} \tag{6.36}$$

in the control to:

$$\tau_o = \frac{1}{\alpha + k_{+B}[B]} \tag{6.37}$$

in the presence of blocker, calculated from the rule that the mean lifetime of any state is equal to the reciprocal of the sum of the rates for leaving that state (Colquhoun and Hawkes, 1982). A plot of $1/\tau$ against [B] should, therefore, give a straight line of slope k_{+B}. This is illustrated in Figure 6.6C, where for a range of membrane potentials and Mg^{2+} concentrations the inverse NMDA channel mean open time follows this linear relationship, giving k_{+B} values in the range 6.6×10^6 $M^{-1}sec^{-1}$ at –40 mV to 8.4×10^7 $M^{-1}sec^{-1}$ at –80 mV.

6.3.6.2 Closed Times

Closed periods due to channel blockages have, from the same rule, a mean lifetime of:

$$\tau_g = \frac{1}{k_{-B}} \tag{6.38}$$

Note that the duration of channel blockages is predicted to be independent of the blocker concentration, as illustrated in Figure 6.6D, where the blockage duration shows no clear dependence on Mg^{2+} concentration.

6.3.6.3 Blockage Frequency

The frequency of blockages, per second of open time, is $k_{+B}[B]$, so the mean *number* of blockages in each channel opening is simply the blockage frequency multiplied by the mean open time:

$$N_g = \frac{k_{+B}[B]}{\alpha} \tag{6.39}$$

6.3.6.4 Bursts of Openings

Where the channel blocker converts single openings into obvious bursts (e.g., local anesthetic block of nicotinic channels), the mean number of openings per burst is one more than the mean number of gaps (blockages):

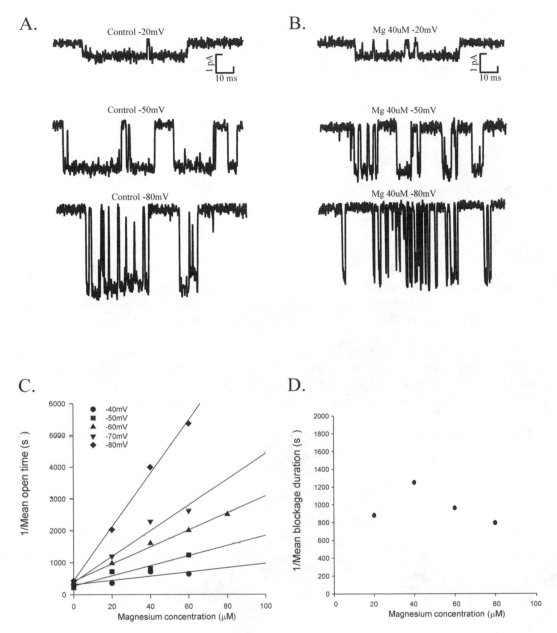

FIGURE 6.6 Single-channel analysis of ion-channel block. Representative recordings of single-channel currents through NMDA receptor channels recorded are illustrated at membrane potentials of –20 mV, –50 mV, and –80 mV in control recordings (A) and in the presence of 40-μM magnesium (B). The rapid blocking and unblocking of the channel are particularly evident at more negative voltages. The inverse mean open time and inverse mean duration of the additional channel closings caused by Mg^{2+} are plotted against Mg^{2+} concentration in (C) and (D). These results confirm the linear relationship between Mg^{2+} concentration and inverse mean open time and the lack of Mg^{2+} concentration dependence of the channel predicted by the simple open-channel block mechanism. The solid lines in (C) illustrate linear regression of the data recorded at each membrane potential. The slopes of these lines give estimates of the value of k_{+B} of 6.6, 15.7, 26.6, 40.4, and 84.0×10^6 M^{-1} sec^{-1} at –40-, –50-, –60-, –70-, and –80-mV membrane potential.

$$N_o = 1 + \frac{k_{+B}[B]}{\alpha} \tag{6.40}$$

Notice that the mean total open time per burst will be:

$$N_o \tau_o = \left(1 + \frac{k_{+B}[B]}{\alpha}\right) \frac{1}{\alpha + k_{+B}[B]} \tag{6.41}$$

$$N_o \tau_o = \left(\frac{\alpha + k_{+B}[B]}{\alpha}\right) \frac{1}{\alpha + k_{+B}[B]} \tag{6.42}$$

$$N_o \tau_o = \frac{1}{\alpha} \tag{6.43}$$

This is an important result. The simple open-channel block mechanism predicts that the total open time per burst is the same as the mean open time in the absence of blocker (Neher, 1983), even though openings are now chopped up by channel blockages. In fact, for channels that give bursts of openings in control recordings, the total open time per burst is constant in the presence or absence of blocker.

This result is also of importance because it shows that simple open-channel blockers do not reduce the charge passed by the channel during each activation so they will not reduce the charge injected at a synapse by a synaptic current. Instead, they prolong the time over which the charge is injected, which can have quite dramatic effects on synaptic transmission.

6.3.6.5 Burst Length

The mean burst length is found as shown below:

$$\tau_b = \frac{1}{\alpha} + N_g \cdot \tau_g \tag{6.44}$$

$$\tau_b = \frac{1}{\alpha} + \frac{1}{k_{-B}} \cdot \frac{k_{+B}[B]}{\alpha} \tag{6.45}$$

$$\tau_b = \frac{1}{\alpha}\left(1 + \frac{[B]}{K_B}\right) \tag{6.46}$$

$$\tau_b = \frac{1}{\alpha} + \frac{1}{\alpha K_B} \cdot [B] \tag{6.47}$$

Thus a plot of the mean burst length vs. [B] will give a straight line of intercept $1/\alpha$ and slope $1/(\alpha K_B)$.

6.3.7 THE TIME SCALE OF CHANNEL BLOCK

Channel blockers are often classified as slow, intermediate, or fast blockers, based on the very wide range of values that have been found for the microscopic dissociation rate constant of different channel blockers. Nearly all channel blockers have been found to have microscopic association rate constants (k_{+B}) in the range around 10^7 $M^{-1}sec^{-1}$. In contrast, microscopic dissociation rate constants (k_{-B}) range over several orders of magnitude from around 10^5 sec^{-1} (e.g., block of nicotinic receptor channels by ACh) to 0.01 sec^{-1} for MK-801 (dizocilpine) block of NMDA channels. The mean lengths of the blockage gaps can therefore range from 10 μsec up to 100 sec. It is only when the blockages are in the intermediate range, on the order of 1 msec in duration, that the gaps are easily detected in single-channel recordings. If the blocker is a slow blocker with very long blockage gaps, the data record looks as though the frequency of channel openings has decreased. If the blocker is fast, the single-channel amplitude appears decreased because the blocking and unblocking are too fast to be resolved.

6.3.8 Use Dependence of Channel Blockers

It follows from the fact that the blocker is assumed to bind only to the activated state of the channel that the degree of block will be not only concentration dependent but also use dependent; in other words, the more the channels are activated, the more they become blocked.

It follows from the above discussion on the time scales of channel block that the degree of use dependence will be critically dependent on the microscopic dissociation rate constant. Slow blockers show extreme use dependence, which is augmented with blockers displaying the *trapping* phenomenon. Trapping occurs when the channel can close and the agonist dissociate with the blocker still bound in the channel. The blocker is then trapped in the channel until the next time the receptor is activated. Important examples of trapping block include the action of hexamethonium at autonomic ganglia and the block of the NMDA receptor channel by MK801 or the anesthetic ketamine.

6.3.9 Voltage Dependence of Channel Block

One of the interesting results arising from early voltage-clamp experiments with channel-blocking drugs was that the potency of the blocker was dependent on the membrane voltage. In contrast, this was found not to be the case for competitive antagonism at endplate nicotinic receptors (Figure 6.5). These results were interpreted as indicating that the acetylcholine binding site on the receptor (and therefore competitive block at that site by tubocurarine) is not influenced by the potential difference across the membrane; whereas, if binding is affected by the membrane potential, then the binding site must be at a region of the protein that is part of the way across the electric field of the membrane.

Binding of a charged drug at a site within an electric field will be influenced by chemical interactions (such as hydrogen bonding, common to all drug–receptor interactions) and by the electric field and charge on the drug.

The microscopic rate constants for association and dissociation at a site within an electric field (for block by charged drugs) are exponential functions of the membrane voltage:

$$k_{+B}(V) = k_{+B}(0)\exp\left(\frac{-\delta zFV}{RT}\right) \tag{6.48}$$

$$k_{-B}(V) = k_{-B}(0)\exp\left(\frac{\delta zFV}{RT}\right) \tag{6.49}$$

Here, δ refers to the fraction of the membrane voltage that the blocking drug senses at the binding site, and the sign on the δ is determined by whether the blocking drug approaches the binding site from the inside or outside of the membrane. As expressed here, these equations describe the rate constants for block from the outside. The valence of the blocking drug is given as z, and F, R, and

T are the Faraday constant (9.65×10^4 C mol^{-1}), the gas constant (8.32 J K^{-1} mol^{-1}), and the absolute temperature (293 K at room temperature), respectively. The voltage dependence of the dissociation equilibrium constant is given by:

$$\frac{k_{-B}(V)}{k_{+B}(V)} = k_B(V) = K_B(0)\exp\left(\frac{\delta z F V}{RT}\right) \qquad (6.50)$$

From this relationship it can be seen that a semilogarithmic plot of $\ln K(V)$ vs. membrane potential will give a straight line with slope of $\delta z F/RT$ and intercept of $\ln K(0)$. The inverse of the slope gives the change in membrane voltage required to give an e-fold change in the equilibrium constant. It can be seen that the maximum slope will be obtained when $\delta = 1$. For a blocker with a single charge, this will give a maximum slope of 25 mV for an e-fold change while for a divalent ion, the maximum slope will be 13 mV for an e-fold change. This analysis is illustrated in Figure 6.7 for the block of NMDA receptor channels by Mg^{2+} ions.

Figure 6.7A shows that a plot of log k_{+B} against membrane potential gives a linear relation with the slope corresponding to $\delta = 0.76$, while a plot of log k_{-B} against membrane potential (Figure 6.7B) is also linear but not as steeply voltage dependent with $\delta = 0.21$. How should these results be interpreted? They may either mean that the energy barriers for Mg^{2+} approaching its binding site and dissociating from its binding site back to the extracellular solution are not symmetrical, or that a proportion of Mg^{2+} ions leave their binding site by permeating through the channel to the inside of the cell membrane. The voltage dependence of the equilibrium constant, K_{+B}, shows that the affinity of Mg^{2+} for the channel is steeply voltage dependent with $\delta = 0.97$, implying that Mg^{2+} ions sense almost 100% of the membrane electric field at their binding site (Ascher and Nowak, 1998).

Given that channel blocking drugs, by definition, act within the permeation path of the channel, it is not unexpected to discover that interaction between the channel-blocking drug and the normal permeant ions may affect the behavior of a channel blocker. This is the case for NMDA receptors, where occupation of permeant ion binding sites has a significant effect on the observed voltage dependence of Mg^{2+} block. Antonov and Johnson (1999) have demonstrated that taking this effect into account places the Mg^{2+} ion binding site at a much shallower position ($\delta = 0.47$) in the membrane electric field, which is consistent with the predicted position of two asparagine residues near the apex of the M2 loop of the NMDA receptor subunits, which have been identified from structural modification of the NMDA receptor as being crucial for Mg^{2+} block of the channel.

The steep voltage dependence of channel block underlies the crucial role that Mg^{2+} block of NMDA channels plays in giving NMDA receptors the property of being "coincidence detectors" in the nervous system. This property may underlie the Hebbian behavior of excitatory synapses in the brain and can, in principle, allow networks of neurons to adapt their behavior according to experience; hence, in effect, this property allows the nervous system to learn from experience. A simulation of the effect of Mg^{2+} block on the steady-state current through NMDA receptor channels is illustrated in Figure 6.7D. It can be seen that the linear relationship between membrane potential and NMDA receptor current becomes steeply voltage dependent with increasing Mg^{2+} concentration. At physiological levels of Mg^{2+} (1 mM), the current through the channels increases between –80 mV and –20 mV as the Mg^{2+} block is relieved by depolarization. It is important to appreciate that this type of effect will also happen to a greater or lesser extent with any drug that acts to block ion channels and makes predicting the action of channel-blocking drugs, particularly on the nervous system, extremely complicated.

Figure 6.8 shows a diagrammatic representation of the energy barriers that a channel-blocking drug might be supposed to overcome to reach its binding site within the channel. This diagram allows for the possibility that the blocking drug could actually permeate the channel after binding rather than returning after dissociation to the same side it had originally come from. This generalized mechanism can be used to describe channel block from either side of the membrane, access to the

A. Blocking rate (M⁻¹s⁻¹)

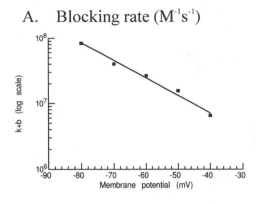

B. Unblocking rate (s⁻¹)

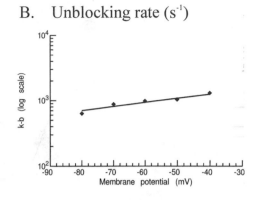

C. Equilibrium Constant (µM)

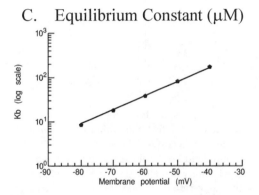

D. Current-voltage relation

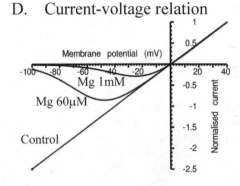

FIGURE 6.7 Analysis of the voltage-dependence of the block of NMDA receptor channels by Mg^{2+}. (A) Channel-blocking rate, k_{+B}, estimated from the slope of the lines fitted to the data in Fig 4A, is plotted against membrane potential. The solid line shows the fit of Eq. (6.48) to the data with $\delta = 0.76$ (reflecting an e-fold increase in blocking rate for every 16.6 mV hyperpolarization of the membrane potential) and a blocking rate of 2.66×10^7 M^{-1} sec^{-1} at –60 mV. (B) Channel unblocking rate, k_{-B}, estimated as the mean of the values at each Mg^{2+} concentration, shows a shallower voltage dependence than that of the channel blocking rate. The solid line shows the fit to the data of Eq. (6.49) with $\delta = 0.21$ (reflecting an e-fold increase in blocking rate for every 61 mV hyperpolarization of the membrane potential) and a blocking rate of 2.66×10^7 M^{-1} sec^{-1} at –60 mV. (C) Voltage dependence of the equilibrium constant, K_B, for channel block, calculated from the ratio of k_{-B}/k_{+B}. The solid line shows the fit of the data to Eq. (6.50) with $\delta = 0.97$ and illustrates the steep voltage dependence of K_B which increases e-fold for every 13 mV depolarization. (D) Simulation of the current–voltage relationship in the presence of a steeply voltage-dependent channel block. The control current is a linear function of the membrane voltage; however, in the presence of a low concentration (60 µM) or a physiological concentration (1 mM) of Mg^{2+}, the current through the channel rectifies steeply at negative potentials, reflecting the steep voltage dependence of the equilibrium constant, K_B.

binding site being dependent on the height of the energy barriers that the drug molecule has to cross. More generally, Figure 6.8 helps to illustrate the idea that the difference between permeation of an ion through the channel and block of the channel may be one of degree and not necessarily a reflection of any fundamental difference in the way a permeant ion or blocker interacts with the channel protein.

6.4 CONCLUDING REMARKS

The material in this chapter has centered around the effects of drugs at receptors in the ligand-gated ion channel class. In particular, the aim has been to emphasize that a quantitative treatment

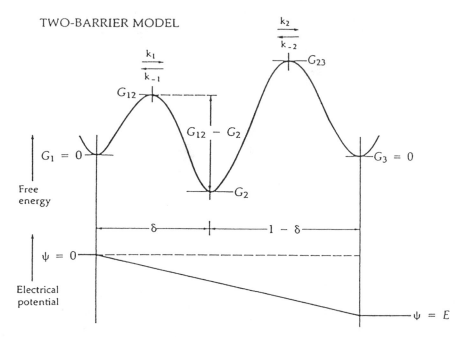

FIGURE 6.8 Shown is a representation of a two-energy-barrier model that can be used to describe the energy barriers a channel-blocking drug might have to overcome to reach its binding site within the channel. The barriers are shown as symmetrical in this case, although they need not necessarily be so, in which case the δ value for access to the binding site would not be equal in magnitude to the δ value for unbinding and return to the same side of the membrane. This diagram allows for the possibility that the blocking drug could actually permeate the channel after binding rather than returning to the same side of the membrane it had originally come from. This generalized mechanism can be used to describe channel block from either side of the membrane, access to the binding site being dependent on the height of the energy barriers that the drug must cross. The free energy, G, is shown relative to that outside the membrane. The transition rates k_1, k_{-1}, k_2, and k_{-2} will depend on both the height of the energy barrier and the membrane potential and can be calculated as described in Hille (1992). (Adapted from Hille, B., *Ionic Channels of Excitable Membranes*, 2nd ed., Sinauer, Sunderland, MD, 1992, fig. 5, chap. 14.)

of some simple mechanisms can allow experimentally testable predictions to be made for the effects of a drug and estimates of the affinity of a drug for its binding site/sites on the receptor. Because quantifying the interactions of drugs with their receptors is at the heart of advances in the development of selective drugs and the classification of receptors, this approach is likely to continue to be an essential part of pharmacology. This is particularly so for studies of the central nervous system, where a bewildering array of receptor subtypes await the development of subtype-selective drugs so the functional and therapeutic significance of this receptor diversity can be determined.

6.5   PROBLEMS

Problem 6.1

An experiment in which single AChR ion-channel currents were recorded at a membrane potential of –60 mV showed that the duration of individual channel openings followed a single exponential distribution. The mean open time was 5.0 msec. When the experiment was repeated in the presence of an antagonist, drug B, in a concentration of 10 µM, it was found that the mean open time was reduced to 2.5 msec and that the channel openings were interrupted by brief shut periods with a mean duration of 1.0 msec such that openings were grouped into bursts. When the experiment was repeated at a membrane potential of –120 mV, the mean open time was 10 msec in the absence of drug B but only 2 msec in its presence; the interruptions of the channel openings had become longer, lasting 2 msec on average at –120 mV. These results are consistent with drug B being an open channel blocker.

a. Calculate the microscopic association and dissociation rate constants and equilibrium constant for the action of drug B.
b. What can you say about the probable site of action of drug B given that the drug has a single positive charge?

Hint: The reciprocal of the mean lifetime of an individual state is the sum of the rates (in sec⁻¹) for leaving that state.

Problem 6.2

With endplate nicotinic receptors it has been found that, as well as activating the receptor, acetylcholine (ACh) blocks the ion channel. A possible mechanism to describe this situation (assuming for simplicity only a single agonist binding is required to activate the receptor) might therefore be:

$$A + R \underset{k_{-1}}{\overset{k_{+1}}{\rightleftharpoons}} \underset{\text{closed}}{AR} \underset{k_{-2}}{\overset{k_{+2}}{\rightleftharpoons}} \underset{\text{open}}{AR^*} + A \underset{k_{-3}}{\overset{k_{+3}}{\rightleftharpoons}} \underset{\text{blocked}}{ARA} \qquad (6.51)$$

$$\underset{\text{closed}}{}$$

a. Stating any assumptions you need to make, derive an expression for the equilibrium occupancy of the AR* state (p_{AR*}) in Eq. (6.51).
b. Write down expressions for the mean open time (τ_o) and mean duration of the blocked state (τ_b). (*Hint:* The mean lifetime of any state is equal to the reciprocal of the sum of the rates for leaving that state.) In experiments designed to test the mechanism in scheme (6.51), two high concentrations of ACh (300 and 800 µM) were tested in single-channel recording experiments, and τ_o, τ_b, and the channel open probability (p_{open}) were measured. The results were as follows:

[ACh] (µM)	τ_o (msec)	τ_b (msec)	p_{open}
300	0.2	0.04	0.5
800	0.1	0.04	0.4

c. Using a plot of $1/\tau_o$ vs. [ACh], calculate k_{-2} and k_{+3}. In addition, calculate k_{-3} from the duration of the blockages (τ_b) and then calculate the equilibrium constant (K_3) for block of the channel by ACh. In other experiments, values of 10^7 M⁻¹ sec⁻¹, 10^4 sec⁻¹, and 10^4 sec⁻¹ were found for k_{+1}, k_{-1}, and k_{+2}.
d. Using the expression you derived in (a), calculate the p_{AR*} you would expect at 300 and 800 µM ACh. How does this compare with the experimentally observed p_{open} given in the table above? Suggest reasons why the calculated and observed p_{open} might be different.

Problem 6.3

A simple mechanism for competitive antagonism of a ligand-gated ion-channel receptor would be as follows:

$$BR \underset{k_{+B}}{\overset{k_{-B}}{\rightleftharpoons}} B + R + A \underset{k_{-A}}{\overset{k_{+A}}{\rightleftharpoons}} AR \qquad (6.52)$$

a. Derive an expression for the equilibrium occupancy of state AR given the concentration of antagonist [B] and agonist [A] and their microscopic rate constants for association and dissociation with the receptor. In an experiment designed to measure k_{-B} and k_{+B}, the agonist was applied at a concentration of 100 μM (the equilibrium constant for the agonist is known to be 11 μM). Then, a step change in the antagonist concentration was made from zero to [B] and back to zero again. On application of the antagonist, the response was observed to decline (relax) exponentially toward a steady-state level of block with time constant τ_{on}. If it is assumed that equilibration with the agonist is much faster than equilibration with the antagonist, then the relaxation time constant τ_{on} can be shown for scheme (6.52) to be described by the equation:

$$\tau_{on} = \frac{1}{p_{free} k_{+B}[B] + k_{-B}} \tag{6.53}$$

where p_{free} is the fraction of receptors in state R before the antagonist is applied. The antagonist was tested at three concentrations and the results were as follows:

[B] (μM)	τ_{on} (sec)	Percent Block at Equilibrium (%)
7.5	0.4	62
20	0.2	83
45	0.1	95

b. Calculate the microscopic rate constants k_{+B} and k_{-B} and the equilibrium constant K_B. Using these and the equation you derived in part (a), calculate the percent block expected at equilibrium for each of the antagonist concentrations used. How well do these calculated values agree with those observed experimentally? Suggest possible reasons why the calculated equilibrium block might not agree with that observed experimentally. Describe what a single-channel recording of the receptor activity would look like at equilibrium in the presence of the agonist alone and in the presence of agonist plus antagonist.

6.6 FURTHER READING

Textbooks with relevant material

Hille, B., *Ionic Channels of Excitable Membranes*, 2nd ed., Sinauer, Sunderland, MD, 1992 (see chap. 7, Endplate channels and kinetics; chap. 15, Channel-block mechanisms).

Ogden, D. C., *Microelectrode Techniques: The Plymouth Workshop Handbook*, 2nd ed., The Company of Biologists, Ltd., Cambridge, U.K., 1994 (excellent discussion of both methods and principles).

Sakmann, B. and Neher, E., *Single Channel Recording*, 2nd ed., Plenum Press, New York, 1995 (many good articles that discuss methods and principles).

Original papers

Antonov S. M. and Johnson J. W., Permeant ion regulation of *N*-methyl-D-aspartate receptor channel block by Mg(2+). *Proc. Natl. Acad. Sci.*, 96, 14571–14576, 1999.

Ascher P. and Nowak L., The role of divalent cations in the *N*-methyl-D-aspartate responses of mouse central neurones in culture, *J. Physiol.*, 399, 247–266, 1988.

Colquhoun, D., On the principles of postsynaptic action of neuromuscular blocking agents, in *New Neuro-muscular Blocking Agents*, Kharkevich, D. A., Ed., Springer–Verlag, Berlin/New York, 1986.

Colquhoun, D. and Ogden, D. C., Activation of ion channels in the frog end-plate by high concentrations of acetylcholine, *J. Physiol.*, 395, 131–159, 1988.

Colquhoun, D. and Sakmann, B., Fluctuations in the microsecond time range of the current through single acetylcholine receptor ion channels, *Nature,* 294, 464–466, 1981. (The full version of this paper can be found in *J. Physiol.,* 369, 501–557, 1985.)

Colquhoun, D., Dreyer, F., and Sheridan, R. E., The actions of tubocurarine at the frog neuromuscular junction, *J. Physiol.*, 293, 247–284, 1979.

del Castillo, J. and Katz, B., Interaction at endplate receptors between different choline derivatives, *Proc. Roy. Soc. London Ser. B*, 146, 369–381, 1957.

Edmonds, B., Gibb, A. J., and Colquhoun, D., Mechanisms of activation of muscle nicotinic acetylcholine receptors and the time course of endplate currents, *Annu. Rev. Physiol.*, 57, 469–493, 1995.

Katz, B. and Thesleff, S., A study of the 'desensitization' produced by acetylcholine at the motor end-plate, *J. Physiol.,* 138, 63–80, 1957.

Lingle, C. L., Maconochie, D., and Steinbach, J. H., Activation of skeletal muscle nicotinic acetylcholine receptors, *J. Memb. Biol.*, 126, 195–217, 1992 (excellent review of much of the evidence concerning the mechanism of receptor activation).

MacDonald, J. F. and Nowak, L. M., Mechanisms of blockade of excitatory amino acid receptor channels, *TIPS,* 11(4), 167–172, 1990.

Neher, E., The charge carried by single-channel currents of rat cultured muscle cells in the presence of local anaesthetics. *J. Physiol.*, 339, 663–678, 1983.

Rang, H. P. and Ritter, J. M., On the mechanism of desensitization at cholinergic receptors, *Mol. Pharmacol.*, 6, 357–382, 1970.

Triggle, D. J., Desensitization, *Trends Pharmacol. Sci.,* 14, 395–398, 1980.

Unwin, N., Neurotransmitter action: opening of ligand-gated ion channels, *Neuron*, 10(Suppl. 1), 31–41, 1993.

Unwin, N., Projection structure of the nicotinic acetylcholine receptor: distinct conformations of the alpha subunits, *J. Mol. Biol.*, 257, 586–596, 1996.

6.7 SOLUTIONS TO PROBLEMS

Problem 6.1

Notice that the problem states that the distribution of open times is a single exponential. This tells you that a mechanism containing a single open state of the receptor can describe the data. Using the above hint, the channel closing rate (call this α) is therefore the reciprocal of the mean open time. Thus, at –60 mV, $\alpha = 1/5$ msec, or 200 sec^{-1}; at –120 mV, $\alpha = 1/10$ msec, or 100 sec^{-1}. This indicates that the channel closing conformational change is affected by the electric field across the membrane.

In the presence of drug B, the mean duration of the blockages (assuming a single blocked state) will be the reciprocal of the rate for leaving the blocked state (say, k_{-B}). Thus, at –60 mV, $k_{-B} = 1/1.0$ msec, or 1000 sec^{-1}; at –120 mV, $k_{-B} = 1/2.0$ msec, or 500 sec^{-1}. Apparently, the rate of dissociation of drug B from the channel is slowed when the membrane potential is made more negative. For a positively charged drug, this is a common finding and suggests the drug is binding within the membrane electric field. However, it could also be that the change in membrane potential has altered the receptor protein conformation and thus affected the binding of the drug to the receptor.

To calculate the microscopic association rate for drug B, use the hint above to show that the mean open time in the presence of drug B will be equal to $1/(\alpha + [B]k_{+B})$. Thus, the reciprocal of the mean open time in the presence of drug B will be equal to $(\alpha + [B]k_{+B})$, so $(\alpha + [B]k_{+B}) = 400$ sec^{-1} at –60 mV and 500 sec^{-1} at –120 mV. α was 200 sec^{-1} at –60 mV and 100 sec^{-1} at –120 mV, so $[B]k_{+B} = 200$ sec^{-1} at –60 mV and 400 sec^{-1} at –120 mV. Dividing these numbers by the [B] gives $k_{+B} = 2 \times 10^7$ M^{-1} sec^{-1} at -60 mV and 4×10^7 M^{-1} sec^{-1} at -120 mV. The equilibrium constant is, therefore, 50 μM at -60 mV and 12.5 μM at -120 mV.

If the voltage dependence of k_{+B} is described by Eq. (6.48), then a plot of $\ln(k_{+B}(V))$ vs. membrane potential (V) will be a straight line of slope $-\delta z F/RT$. In this case, the slope of this plot is -11.6 V^{-1}, and the reciprocal of this indicates an e-fold increase in k_{+B} for every 0.086-V hyperpolarization (86 mV) of the membrane potential. At room temperature (293 K), F/RT = 39.6 V^{-1}; so for a drug with a single positive charge, $\delta = 11.6/39.6 = 0.29$, suggesting that when it is at its binding site, the drug has passed through 29% of the membrane electric field (note that this is probably not the same as 29% of the distance across the membrane, as the membrane electric field is unlikely to fall linearly across the channel protein).

Notice that in this example the slope of the relationship between membrane potential and $\ln(k_{-B})$ is equal in magnitude but opposite in sign to that for k_{+B} and that $\delta = 0.58$ for the voltage dependence of K_B, as expected if the blocker traverses a symmetrical energy barrier (Figure 6.8) when exiting from the channel as when blocking the channel. A voltage dependence for k_{-B} of the same sign as for k_{+B} would suggest that unblocking occurred by permeation of the blocker to the other side of the channel. A difference between the magnitudes of δ for k_{+B} and k_{-B} could mean that the energy barrier for access to and exit from the channel is not symmetrical or it could mean that the drug partly permeates the channel and partly exits back to the outside of the membrane.

Problem 6.2

For part (a), assume that the system is at equilibrium and that the law of mass action holds. Use the procedures described in Chapter 1 to derive an expression for p_{AR*} at equilibrium. At equilibrium, the forward and backward rates for each reaction in the mechanism must be equal. The forward and backward rates are defined using the law of mass action:

$$p_R[A]k_{+1} = p_{AR}k_{-1}, \quad p_{AR}k_{+2} = p_{AR*}k_{-2}, \quad p_{AR*}[A]k_{+3} = p_{ARA}k_{-3} \tag{6.54}$$

Each expression is rearranged to give an expression in p_{AR*}:

$$p_{AR} = \frac{k_{-2}}{k_{+2}} p_{AR*}, \quad p_R = \frac{k_{-1}}{k_{+1}[A]} \frac{k_{-2}}{k_{+2}} p_{AR*}, \quad p_{ARA} = \frac{k_{+3}[A]}{k_{-3}} p_{AR*} \tag{6.55}$$

The proportions of the receptor in each state must add up to 1:

$$p_R + p_{AR} + p_{AR*} + p_{ARA} = 1 \tag{6.56}$$

Substituting into this equation and then rearranging the result gives the desired expression:

$$p_{AR*} = \frac{[A]}{\dfrac{k_{-1}k_{-2}}{k_{+1}k_{+2}} + [A]\left(1 + \dfrac{k_{-2}}{k_{+2}} + \dfrac{[A]k_{+3}}{k_{-3}}\right)} \tag{6.57}$$

For part (b),

$$\tau_o = \frac{1}{k_{-2} + [A]k_{+3}}, \quad \tau_b = \frac{1}{k_{-3}} \tag{6.58}$$

For part (c), $1/\tau_o = 5000$ sec^{-1} when [ACh] = 300 μM and $1/\tau_o = 10000$ sec^{-1} when [ACh] = 800 μM. From the answer to part (b), we know that $1/\tau_o = (k_{-2} + [A]k_{+3})$. This has the form of a straight line of slope k_{+3} and intercept k_{-2} when $1/\tau_o$ is plotted against [A]. Thus, the slope is k_{+3} = (10000 – 5000 sec^{-1})/(800 – 300 μM) = 10^7 M^{-1} sec^{-1}. The intercept is k_{-2} = 2000 sec^{-1}. The dissociation rate for the blocker is k_{-3} = 1/40 μsec = 25,000 sec^{-1}. The equilibrium constant for block of the channel is, therefore, $K_3 = k_{-3}/k_{+3}$ = 2.5 mM.

For part (d), substituting into Eq. (6.55) allows the equilibrium occupancy of AR* to be calculated at 300 and 800 μM ACh. The results are 0.503 and 0.565, respectively. Therefore, at 300 μM, the calculated p_{AR*} is close to that observed experimentally. However, at 800 μM, the calculated p_{AR*} is higher than observed. Reasons for this result include the possibility that desensitization is affecting the p_{open} at higher [A]. In addition, the mechanism used to derive Eq. (6.55) may not be correct (as would be the case if a desensitized state must be added to the mechanism).

Problem 6.3

For part (a), the derivation of an expression for p_{AR} in the presence of antagonist, B, is achieved using standard procedures. The result is given in Eq. (6.59):

$$p_{AR} = \frac{[A]}{[A] + \dfrac{k_{-A}}{k_{+A}}\left(1 + \dfrac{[B]k_{+B}}{k_{-B}}\right)} \tag{6.59}$$

For part (b), a plot of the reciprocal of τ_{on} vs. [B] will be a straight line of slope $p_{free}k_{+B}$ and y-axis intercept k_{-B}. Using the data in the table, the slope is found to be 2×10^5 M^{-1} sec^{-1} and intercept 1 sec^{-1}. p_{free} is $1 - p_{AR}$ in the absence of antagonist. Thus, $p_{free} = K_A/([A] + K_A) = 0.1$. As $p_{free}k_{+B}$ = slope, k_{+B} = slope/p_{free} = 2×10^6 M^{-1} sec^{-1} The equilibrium constant $K_B = k_{-B}/k_{+B} = 0.5 \times 10^{-6}$ M. Finally, calculate p_{AR} in the absence of antagonist and then in the presence of each [B] and then use these results to calculate the percentage block produced at equilibrium by each antagonist concentration. When [A] = 100 μM, K_A = 11 μM; p_{AR} = 0.9 in the absence of antagonist, with K_B = 0.5 μM and [B] = 7.5 μM; and p_{AR} = 0.36. The percent block is equal to (0.9 – 0.36)/0.9 × 100 = 60%. When [B] = 20 μM, p_{AR} = 0.191 and the percent block is 79%. When [B] = 45 μM, p_{AR} = 0.098 and the percent block is 89%.

The calculated values for percent block are close to those observed at low blocker concentrations, but at higher concentrations the observed block is greater than predicted. Possible reasons for this may lie in the measurement of the onset time constants or in the assumption about the agonist equilibrating much faster than the antagonist, or the mechanism may be wrong, perhaps because the receptor has more than one binding site or binding of the antagonist promotes desensitization of the receptor.

7 G-Proteins

David A. Brown

CONTENTS

G-proteins are trimeric, signal-transducing, guanine nucleotide-binding proteins. They constitute the first step in transducing the agonist-induced activation of a G-protein-coupled receptor (see Chapter 2) to a cellular response.

7.1 THE DISCOVERY OF G-PROTEINS

G-proteins were discovered as a result of some experiments by Martin Rodbell in 1971 on the stimulation of adenylate cyclase by glucagon, in which he found that the addition of guanosine triphosphate (GTP) was necessary to drive the reaction. Using terminology derived from cybernetic information theory, he envisaged a guanine nucleotide regulatory protein, then called an "N (nucleotide-binding)-protein," acting as an intermediary transducer between the *discriminator* (receptor) and *amplifier* (effector; i.e., adenylate cyclase) (Figure 7.1). He subsequently found that adenylate cyclase was activated strongly and irreversibly by a GTP analog, 5′-guanylylimidophosphate, or [Gpp(NH)-p]′. Because Gpp(NH)-p is resistant to hydrolysis, Rodbell suggested that GTP is "hydrolysed at the activation site;" that is, the transducer acts as a GTPase. This was subsequently shown directly by Cassell and Selinger in 1976. The presence of a separate GTP-binding protein, distinct from the adenylate cyclase enzyme, was established by Alfred Gilman and colleagues who were able to reconstitute Gpp(NH)-p-stimulated adenylate cyclase activity in membranes from a mutant lymphoma cell line (*cyc–*) that contained adenylate cyclase but lacked the G-protein by adding a separately purified 40-kDa GTP-binding factor. In 1980, Howlett and Gilman reported that persistent activation of this cyclase-stimulating G-protein (G_s) led to a decrease in the molecular

0-8493-1029-6/03/$0.00+$1.50

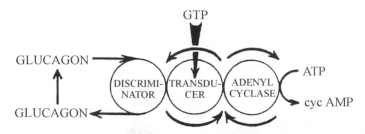

FIGURE 7.1 Martin Rodbell's conception of the role of the G-protein transducer in the activation of adenylate cyclase by glucagon. (From Birnbaumer, L., *FASEB J.*, 4, 3178, 1990. With permission.)

mass of the protein, implying that the G-protein was made up of dissociable subunits. The trimeric nature of G-proteins was then established by Stryer and colleagues. Using the photoreceptor G-protein transducin (G_t), they showed that activation of G_t by Gpp(NH)-p and light led to the dissociation of the trimeric $\alpha\beta\gamma$ complex into Gpp(NH)-p-bound α_t and $\beta\gamma$, and that α_t was responsible for phosphodiesterase stimulation. In 1985, α-transducin was cloned by four groups led by Numa, Bourne, Khorana, and Simon; the α subunit of G_s was cloned by Gilman's group in 1986. Rodbell and Gilman were jointly awarded the Nobel Prize in 1994.

7.2 STRUCTURE OF G-PROTEINS

G-proteins are made up of three subunits: an α subunit of molecular mass ~39–45 kDa, a β subunit (~37 kDa), and a smaller γ subunit (~8 kDa). Some 20 different gene products encode various α subunits, 6 different β subunits, and 12 different γ subunits (see below). In their native trimeric state, the G-proteins are attached to the inner face of the cell membrane through lipophilic tails on the α and γ subunits (myristoyl and palmitoyl on the α, farnesyl or geranylgeranyl on the γ) (Figure 7.2). The β and γ subunits are enjoined rather firmly through a coiled–coil interaction to form a $\beta\gamma$-dimer; the β subunit of this dimer is then attached to the α subunit through complementary peptide-binding sites on the two proteins and through interaction of the lipophilic tails. When the G-protein is activated, this α–β subunit interaction is disrupted, and the trimer dissociates into a monomeric α subunit and a dimeric $\beta\gamma$ subunit (see below). Both α and $\beta\gamma$ subunits remain attached to the membrane but are free to move.

The α subunit has two other important functional domains in addition to the β-binding domain. First, the α subunit interacts with the receptor through a domain that includes the last five amino acids of the C-terminus (Figure 7.3). Second, it bears the guanine nucleotide binding pocket and

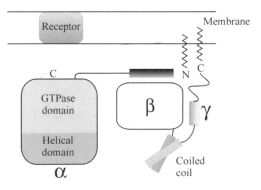

FIGURE 7.2 Diagram to show G-protein α, β, and γ subunits attached to the outer cell membrane. (Adapted from Clapham, D. E., *Nature*, 379, 297, 1996. With permission.)

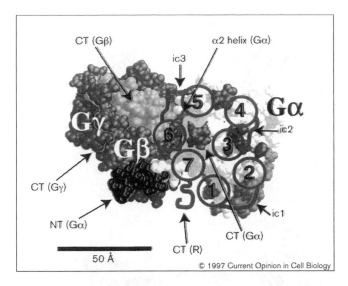

FIGURE 7.3 Superposition of the seven transmembrane helices (numbered 1–7) of a GPCR on the outer surface of a G-protein. Abbreviations: CT, C-terminus; NT, N-terminus; ic1, ic2, and ic3, first, second, and third intracellular loops of the GPCR. (From Bourne, H. R., *Curr. Opin. Cell. Biol.*, 9, 134, 1997. With permission.)

is responsible for the GTPase activity of the G-protein. On the other hand, both α and βγ subunits can interact with the effector.

7.3 G-PROTEIN CYCLE

The cycle of events following receptor activation are summarized in Figure 7.4. The sequence is as follows:

1. In the ground state, the G-protein exists in the trimeric (αβγ) form, with guanosine diphosphate (GDP) bound at the nucleotide-binding site of the α subunit. It is close to, but probably not precoupled to, the receptor. On average, there are more G-proteins than receptors, so one might envisage a single receptor surrounded by a ring of nearby G-proteins, providing for multiple sequential receptor–G-protein interaction.
2. The agonist induces a rapid (<1 msec) conformational change in the receptor, resulting in a realignment and opening up of the transmembrane helices, probably through rotation of helix 6 and separation of helices 3, 6, and 7.
3. The inner face of the activated receptor binds to the C-terminus of the G-protein α subunit (see Figure 7.3). Inner loop 3 (ic3) between transmembrane helices 5 and 6 of the receptor plays a critical role in this interaction. Note, however, that although the α subunit bears the primary binding site for the receptor, attachment of the βγ-dimer to the α subunit is essential for this interaction to occur.
4. Binding of the receptor induces a rapid conformational change (switch) in the G-protein trimer. This is transmitted to the nucleotide binding site, about 3 nm away, and results in a dissociation of bound GDP.
5. The GDP is replaced at the nucleotide-binding site by guanosine triphosphate (GTP), which is present in a three to fourfold excess (50–300 μM) in the cytosol.
6. Binding of GTP promotes a disordering of the carboxyl- and amino-termini of the G-protein α subunit, with two parallel consequences: the GTP-bound α subunit dissociates

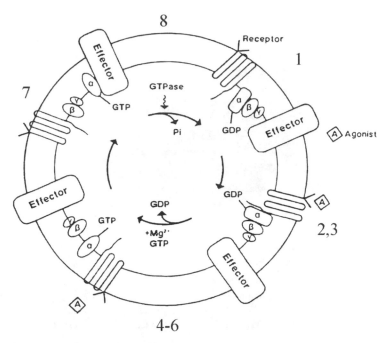

FIGURE 7.4 Diagram of G-protein cycle with (in this case) activation of the effector by the GTP-bound α subunit. See text for letters. (Adapted from Neer and Clapham, *Nature*, 333, 129, 1988. With permission.)

both from the receptor and from the βγ-dimer, releasing free Gα-GTP and free Gβγ. The conformation of Gβγ is not changed on dissociation from the α subunit.

7. Either free Gα-GTP or free Gβγ (or sometimes both) interacts with the effector molecule to activate or inhibit it (see below for examples). This activation is persistent unless reversed by step 8.

8. The terminal (γ) phosphate of GTP is hydrolyzed by the GTPase activity of the G-protein α subunit, leaving GDP bound instead. This reverses the conformational change in step 5 and allows the α subunit to dissociate from the effector and reassociate with the βγ subunit. The reassociation will also reverse βγ-effector interaction because Gα-GDP effectively competes with the effector for βγ-binding. Though of fairly high affinity (e.g., $K_D \sim 50$ nM for GIRK [G-protein-activated inwardly rectifying K+ channel] activation) and persistent in the absence of competing Gα-GDP, βγ-effector binding is not irreversible.

The effect of receptor stimulation is thus to catalyze a reaction cycle. This leads to considerable amplification of the initial signal. For example, in the process of visual excitation, the photoisomerization of one rhodopsin molecule leads to the activation of approximately 500 to 1000 transducin (G_t) molecules, each of which in turn catalyzes the hydrolysis of many hundreds of cyclic guanosine monophosphate (cGMP) molecules by phosphodiesterase. Amplification in the adenylate cyclase cascade is less but still substantial; each ligand-bound β-adrenoceptor activates approximately 10 to 20 G_s molecules, each of which in turn catalyzes the production of hundreds of cyclic adenosine monophosphate (cAMP) molecules by adenylate cyclase.

The duration of receptor-mediated responses depends, in the first instance, on the rate of the GTPase reaction of the α subunit. In solution, these rates are rather slow (time-constants, 10–60 sec), far too slow to account for the off rate of many G-protein-coupled receptor (GPCR)-induced effects. For example, retinal light responses and cardiac responses to vagal stimulation last less than a second. However, in the intact cell, the GTPase reaction is accelerated 10- to 100-fold by GTPase-activating proteins (GAPs). In some cases, the effector itself acts as a GAP; for example,

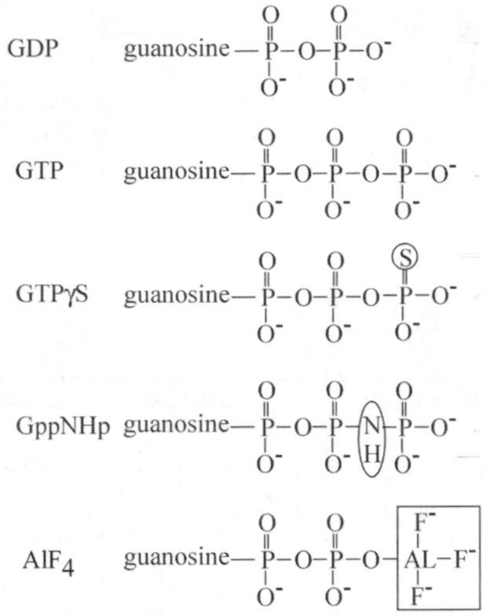

FIGURE 7.5 Some guanosine nucleotides and derivatives. Abbreviations: GDP, guanosine diphosphate; GTP, guanosine triphosphate; GTPγS, guanosine 5'-O-(3-thiotriphosphate); Gpp(NH)-p, 5'-guanylylimidophosphate; AlF$_4$, aluminum fluoride.

phospholipase C accelerates the GTPase activity of the G-protein Gα$_q$. A family of RGS (regulators of G-protein signaling) proteins that accelerates α subunit GTPase activity is discussed further below. Normally (but with the exception of cGMP phosphodiesterase), all three components of the system — receptor, G-protein, and effector — are in the plasma membrane and remain there during all of the steps in the cycle.

7.4 PERTURBING THE G-PROTEIN CYCLE

The G-protein cycle can be perturbed in several ways:

1. Reversal of the cycle depends on hydrolysis of the γ-phosphate of GTP. This is prevented if a nonhydrolyzable, or slowly hydrolyzable, analog of GTP is substituted, for example, 5'-guanylylimidophosphate (Gpp(NH)-p) or guanosine 5'-O-(3-thiotriphosphate) (GTPγS), or by adding AlF$_4$, which forms a third "pseudo" phosphate on GDP in Gα-GDP (Figure 7.5). Under these conditions, effector activation becomes virtually irreversible following brief activation of the receptor (see Figure 7.6 for an example). The effect of receptor activation is essentially to catalyze the G-protein cycle, accelerating it 100- or 1000-fold. Even in the absence of receptor activation by a ligand, a slow basal cycling occurs. This may be due to the fact that a small proportion of receptors exist in the "active" conformation, even in the absence of ligand, as expected from the two-state model of receptors (see Chapter 1). As a result, substitution of Gpp(NH)-p or GTPγS for GTP or the addition of AlF$_4$ can itself induce an effector response in the absence of a receptor ligand, and, indeed, these techniques were used for this purpose in early experiments on adenylate cyclase; however, onset is much slower than that seen for co-addition of ligand.

2. The cycle may be slowed by adding an excess of GDP or, more commonly, guanosine 5'-O-(2-thiodiphosphate) (GDPβS), a more stable analog. Unlike GTPγS, GDPβS is not bound irreversibly and so only competes with GTP; hence, it is only effective when present in a large (tenfold) excess.

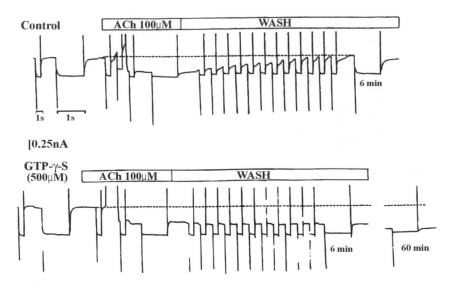

FIGURE 7.6 Irreversible effect of a GTPγS-bound G-protein α subunit. Records show the inhibition of a potassium current in M_1 muscarinic acetylcholine-receptor-expressing neuroblastoma hybrid cells by acetylcholine. The potassium current was recorded as a sustained outward current at a holding potential of –30 mV (dashed line) and was deactivated for 1 sec every 30 sec by hyperpolarizing the cell to –60 mV. In the control cell (upper trace), a brief application of 100 μM acetylcholine (ACh) temporarily inhibited the potassium current, but this recovered about 6 min after removing acetylcholine from the bathing fluid. However, in another cell patched with an electrode containing 500 μM GTPγS (lower trace), the effect of acetylcholine persisted after washout; indeed, the current continued to decline over the next hour, probably reflecting the slow turnover of the G-protein cycle in the absence of GPCR activation. Note that this effect of acetylcholine is probably mediated by $G\alpha_q$, via an unknown second-messenger pathway. (From Robbins et al., *J. Physiol.*, 469, 153, 1993. With permission.)

3. In the presence of NAD^+, the G-protein α subunit can be ADP-ribosylated by two bacterial proteins. *Pertussis* (whooping-cough) toxin (PTx) ADP-ribosylates a cysteine residue in the C-terminus of G-proteins of the G_i and G_o group (Figure 7.7; see below). As a result it prevents receptor–G-protein coupling and blocks responses to GPCR activation. *N*-ethyl-maleimide (NEM) alkylates cysteines and has the same effect. *Cholera* toxin (CTx) ADP-ribosylates an arginine in G-proteins of the G_s (adenylate cyclase-stimulating) class, near the catalytic site of the GTPase domain; consequently, it blocks GTPase activity and produces persistent G_s/adenylate cyclase activation. Transducin and gustducin (the visual and taste-transducing G-proteins; see below) are ADP-ribosylated by both toxins. This reaction has been very helpful in isolating and purifying G-proteins that can be ADP-ribosylated.

7.5 EXPERIMENTAL EVIDENCE FOR G-PROTEIN COUPLING IN RECEPTOR ACTION

7.5.1 GTP Dependence

A G-protein-mediated effect has an absolute requirement for GTP. Reference has already been made to the requirement for GTP in reconstituting hormone-stimulated adenylate cyclase activity. A similar requirement can be demonstrated when the effector is an ion channel, such as the cardiac atrial inward-rectifier K^+ channel which is activated following stimulation of the M_2 muscarinic acetylcholine receptor. Thus, in the experiment illustrated in Figure 7.8, the channel recorded with a cell-

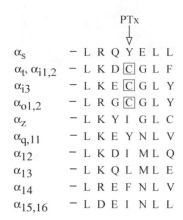

FIGURE 7.7 C-terminal residues of G-protein α subunits. The cysteine ADP-ribosylated by *Pertussis* toxin (PTx) is boxed.

attached patch pipette from an intact atrial cell is tonically activated when acetylcholine (or adenosine) is present in the patch pipette. This activity is lost when the patch is excised (in inside-out configuration) but is then restored on adding GTP to the solution bathing the inside face of the patch.

Even in the absence of an effector, the linkage of an activated receptor to a G-protein can be detected in a receptor-binding assay by the so-called GTP-shift. The apparent affinity of the agonist (but *not* the antagonist), measured either directly or by displacement of agonist with antagonist, is reduced on adding GTP (or a stable analog, such as GTPγS, or even GDP) to the solution (Figure 7.9). This is because a trimeric G-protein, with the guanine nucleotide binding site unoccupied forms a stable complex with the activated receptor such as to slow the dissociation of agonist. The agonist then has a high affinity for the G-protein. Addition of nucleotide breaks this complex to form a dissociated GDP-bound trimer or GTP-bound α subunit; the agonist can then dissociate more rapidly from the receptor, conferring low affinity.

7.5.2 Use of GTP Analogs and Toxins

Stable analogs of GTP and GDP can be used to study the role of the G-protein, as indicated above. Thus, stable GTP analogs enhance agonist-induced receptor-mediated effects and slow their reversal, as shown in Figure 7.6. *Pertussis* and *cholera* toxins can also be used to inhibit or activate certain G-proteins, as indicated.

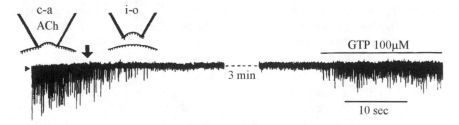

FIGURE 7.8 Requirement for GTP in the activation of inwardly rectifying potassium channels in guinea-pig atrial cell membranes by acetylcholine. The recording started when a pipette containing acetylcholine was attached to an intact atrial cell (c-a). This produced sustained opening of up to three potassium channels (recorded as inward current deflections at –60 mV because the pipette contained 145 mM K⁺). On excision of the membrane patch in inside-out mode (i-o) into the bathing solution (containing 140 mM [K⁺]), the activity stopped, but was resurrected by adding 100 μM GTP to the solution, bathing the inner face of the membrane patch. (From Kurachi et al., *Am. J. Physiol.*, 251, H681, 1986. With permission.)

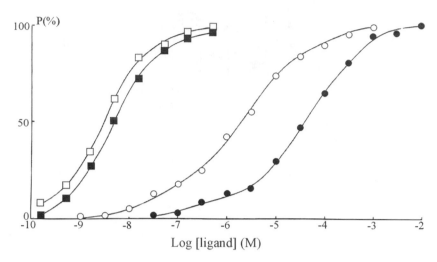

FIGURE 7.9 The GTP shift of agonist binding to a GPCR. Graphs show the binding of carbachol (circles) and atropine (squares) to rat heart homogenates in the absence (open symbols) and presence (closed symbols) of 1 mM GTP. Axes: receptor occupancy (P) and log-molar concentration of ligand. (Adapted from Hulme et al., in *Drug Receptors and Their Effectors*, Birdsall, N. J. M., Ed., Macmillan, New York, 1981, p. 23. With permission.)

7.6 MEASUREMENT OF G-PROTEIN ACTIVATION

The most direct way of measuring activation by a receptor is to measure the rate of hydrolysis of GTP in a broken cell or membrane preparation following receptor activation. Unfortunately, this is not always very easy in practice because of the high background rate (reflecting the basal activity of all the G-proteins in the membrane plus other enzymatic reactions), which may mask the response of the particular G-protein activated by the receptor, and because some G-proteins such as G_s have a slow GTPase rate in such preparations. The method works best for members of the G_o/G_i family, which are abundant, high-turnover G-proteins. An alternative and widely used method is to measure the rate of GTPγS binding, which does not depend on GTPase activity, only on the rate of G-protein activation and GDP dissociation. Methods for measuring fluorescence changes during G-protein activation have also been described.

7.7 TYPES OF G-PROTEIN

Traditionally, G-proteins have been classified in terms of the effector coupling of the α subunit. In spite of the facts that (1) this predates information on primary and secondary structure from cloning work, and (2) the βγ subunits are also involved in effector coupling, this classification is still quite useful.

The first G-protein α subunit to be identified was G_s. The α subunit of G_s (α_s) is responsible for stimulating adenylate cyclase (hence, the subscript "s") and is ADP-ribosylated and activated by CTx. G_s has at least four molecular variants. Some evidence exists that α_s can also enhance the activity of cardiac L-type Ca^{2+} channels, independently of their phosphorylation by cAMP-stimulated protein kinase A. G_{olf} is a cyclase-stimulating homolog in the olfactory epithelium, activated by the large family of olfactory receptors.

G_i is the G-protein responsible for inhibiting adenylate cyclase. The inhibition is mediated by the α subunit. Unlike G_s, G_i is not affected by CTx but instead is ADP-ribosylated (and inhibited) by PTx. Of the three isoforms of G_i (G_{i1-3}), α_{i1} is the most potent inhibitor of cyclase. G_i also activates inward-rectifier (Kir3.1/3.2 and Kir 3.1/3.4) K^+ channels (GIRK channels), and this activation is mediated by released βγ subunits (see below).

G_o was isolated as an other PTx-ribosylated G-protein which co-purifies with G_i but which does not inhibit adenylate cyclase. There are two main isoforms (G_{o1} and G_{o2}), with additional splice-variants. G_o is particularly abundant in the nervous system, comprising up to 1% of membrane proteins. Its main function is to reduce the opening probability of those voltage-gated Ca^{2+} channels (N- and P/Q-type) involved in neurotransmitter release. Hence, it is largely responsible for the widespread auto-inhibition of transmitter secretion by presynaptic receptors and this effect is mediated through released $\beta\gamma$ subunits.

G_t (transducin) is the retinal G-protein responsible (through the α subunit) for stimulating phosphodiesterase (PDE) following light activation of rhodopsin. There are two subtypes, in rods and cones, respectively. G_{gust} (gustducin) is a PDE-stimulating homolog in tongue taste buds involved in bitter-taste reception. Activation of G_{gust} also stimulates phospholipase C (PLC), possibly via the $\beta\gamma$ subunits. G_t and G_{gust} are ADP-ribosylated by both PTx and CTx.

G_q and G_{11} are two closely related and widely distributed G-proteins whose α subunits stimulate PLC. They are not ADP-ribosylated by either PTx or CTx, so they are probably responsible for many instances of PTx-insensitive PLC stimulation. G_{14} and G_{15} are two more distantly related PTx-insensitive G-proteins that can stimulate PLC. G_{12} and G_{13} are other PTx-insensitive G-proteins related to G_q, while G_z is more closely related to G_i; the precise functions of these G-proteins are not yet clear. Though of restricted distribution (to hemopoietic-derived cells), G_{16} is interesting because it lacks receptor specificity and so acts as a universal PLC transducer.

7.8 RECEPTOR–G-PROTEIN COUPLING

The interaction between the receptor and the G-protein is transient and rapidly reversible. This is indicated, for example, by the fact that a single light-activated rhodopsin molecule may activate 500 to 1000 transducin molecules during its 1 to 3 sec lifetime. Hence, the interaction should, in the endpoint, be governed by the normal laws of chemical interaction and expressible in terms of association and dissociation rate constants and binding affinity. The question then arises as to whether the affinity of different receptors for different G-proteins varies. That is, is there specificity in receptor–G-protein coupling, and, if so, what determines this?

Ideally, it might be thought that this question could best be approached by measuring the activation of individual recombinant G-protein trimers (using GTPase reactions, GTPγS binding, or fluorescence methods) by individual recombinant receptors (both in known concentrations) in artificial lipid membranes; however, this is a daunting task. Rubinstein and colleagues have accomplished a near-approach by measuring the GTPase activity of several recombinant α subunits reconstituted with purified β adrenoreceptors and purified bovine G-protein $\beta\gamma$ subunits in phospholipid vesicles. Using a single concentration (10 μM) of isoprenaline, with varying receptor concentrations, they found that the GDP/GTP exchange was stimulated most effectively using α_s, about one third as effectively using α_{i1} or α_{i3}, one tenth with α_{i2}, and negligibly with α_o. A more frequent approach is to assess the interaction of recombinant receptors with recombinant or endogenous G-proteins in cell lines, using GTPase measurements or GTPγS binding in membrane fractions or some downstream effector function as endpoints. This has yielded considerable information regarding what might best be termed "preferences" in regard to individual receptor–G-protein interactions, and, through the use of point-mutations and chimeras, has been particularly useful in delineating some of the structural features of receptors and G-proteins that determine such preferences. From such work, it is clear that the major determinants are the C-terminal sequence of the α subunit, on the one hand (see Figure 7.3), and the third and second inner loops (i3, i2) of the receptor, on the other hand, although other domains of the α subunit and of the β and γ subunits are also involved in the overall interaction.

Such "reconstitutional" approaches suffer from two problems, however. First, the selectivity of receptor–G-protein coupling in their native cell environment depends not only on the relative affinities of the receptor for different G-proteins, but also on the relative proportions and availability of receptors and G-proteins. Thus, some examples of apparent "promiscuity" in receptor–G-protein coupling can undoubtedly be attributed to receptor overexpression. Second, the response of a G-protein to the receptor can be affected by ancillary factors: for example, the presence of particular RGS proteins (see below) that may be cell specific. The question then arises as to how the receptor–G-protein coupling selectivity can best be deduced in the normal cell. Several approaches have been used. A simple one is to test whether the response to activating the receptor is prevented by PTx, thus defining the responsive G-protein as a member of the G_i/G_o family. If so, then this may be followed up by trying to "rescue" the response by applying or expressing individual exogenous α subunits in which the ADP-ribosylated cysteine is substituted by some other amino acid such as isoleucine. Another approach is to disrupt coupling to individual G-protein α subunits using antibodies directed against the C-terminal sequences or using competing short-peptide sequences. This will permit discrimination between, say, $G_{i1/2}$ and G_{i3} or G_o, between G_{oA} and G_{oB}, or between $G_{i/o}$ and $G_{q/11}$, but not between G_{i1} and G_{i2} or between G_q and G_{11}, because the C-terminal sequences for these pairs are the same (see Figure 7.7). Greater selectivity may be obtained by deleting individual G-protein subunits using gene knockouts or, more rapidly and less expensively (but less completely), by reducing protein expression with antisense constructs.

Two general points emerge from such work. First, different approaches do not always give concordant results. For example, antisense-depletion suggests that the activation of GIRK channels by the action of noradrenaline on α_2-adrenoceptors in native sympathetic neurons is mediated selectively by G_i-proteins, rather than G_o-proteins, but activation can be equally well rescued in PTx-treated cells by PTx-resistant forms of both α_o and α_i (Figure 7.10). Conversely, inhibition of the N-type Ca^{2+} current in these same cells by noradrenaline can be rescued after PTx treatment by PTx-resistant α_i even though antisense depletion suggests that inhibition is normally mediated by native G_o proteins, rather than G_i proteins. Thus, rescue experiments, like other expression approaches, tend to show what coupling pathways are possible and do not necessarily define what pathway normally operates. Second, and following from this, a rather surprising degree of specificity in receptor–G-protein coupling in native cells has emerged from some of the antisense-depletion studies, extending not only to closely related α subunits but also to associated β and γ subunits. For example, the inhibition of Ca^{2+} currents in GH_3 pituitary tumor cells by somatostatin appears to be preferentially mediated by the combination $\alpha_{o1}\beta_1\gamma_3$, whereas the very similar effect of acetylcholine, via muscarinic M_4 receptors, is most effectively obtunded by antisense depletion of $\alpha_{o1}\beta_3\gamma_4$. One reason for high *in situ* specificity not predictable from reconstitution experiments may be that, in the normal cell, receptors and cognate G-proteins are not randomly distributed in the cell membrane but are co-localized in "microdomains."

On the other hand, some receptors are truly "promiscuous" in that they can activate two or more G-proteins from quite different classes, even in their normal cellular environment. For example, similar concentrations of thyroid-stimulating hormone (TSH; 0.1–100 U/ml) can stimulate the incorporation of ^{32}P-GTP into α_i, α_o, α_{12}, α_{13}, α_s, and $\alpha_{q/11}$ through activation of the thyrotropin receptor in membranes from human thyroid gland. TRH activation of Ca^{2+} currents in GH_3 cells is obtunded equally by antisense-depletion of α_{i2}, α_{i3}, and $\alpha_{q/11}$, but not of α_o. Some individual genotypic $P2_y$ nucleotide receptors can also couple with equal affinity to PTx-sensitive and PTx-insensitive G-proteins in sympathetic neurons. The degree, or otherwise, of such "promiscuity" is presumably determined by the structure of the receptor protein itself.

More interestingly, some evidence suggests that the degree of preference that one receptor shows for one or another G-protein may depend on the agonist used. Thus, activation of the *Drosophila* octopamine receptor expressed in Chinese hamster ovary (CHO) cells inhibits adenylate cyclase and raises intracellular Ca^{2+} through activation of two different G-proteins: PTx-sensitive and insensitive, respectively. Tyramine and octopamine have been shown to raise Ca^{2+} with similar potencies, but tyramine was considerably more potent in inhibiting cyclase than octopamine. This is in agreement with previous experiments showing that mutations of the highly conserved aspartate involved in amine agonist binding to nearly all receptors affect G-protein coupling in an agonist-

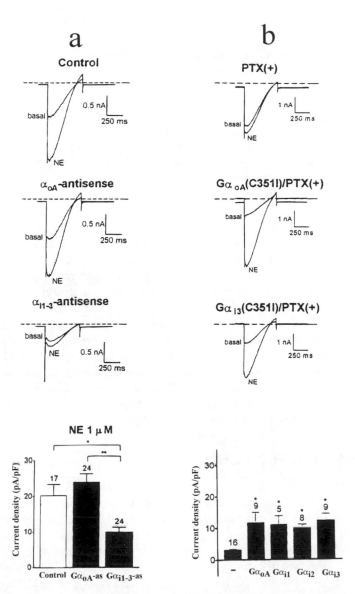

FIGURE 7.10 Contrasting information yielded by antisense depletion and α subunit reconstitution regarding the species of G-protein responsible for adrenergic inhibition of inward rectifier GIRK currents in rat sympathetic neurons. Records show inwardly rectifying GIRK currents generated in cells previously transfected with cDNAs coding for Kir3.1 and Kir.3.2 potassium channels by a voltage ramp from –140 to –40 mV, recorded in the absence (basal) and presence (NE) of 10 μM noradrenaline (norepinephrine). Note that in (a) co-expression of antisense cDNA directed against $G\alpha_{oA}$ had no effect on the activation of current by noradrenaline, whereas co-expression of an antisense directed against the common coding sequences of $G\alpha_{i1-3}$ reduced the response to noradrenaline by about half (as shown in the bar chart below). In (b), a different approach was used, in which the native α subunit was inactivated with *Pertussis* toxin (PTx), thereby inhibiting the effect of noradrenaline (top panel), and an attempt was made to rescue the response by co-transfecting cDNAs coding for different α subunits mutated to remove the PTx-responsive cysteine (see Figure 7.7). In this case, the response was rescued to equal extents by all of the expressed α subunits. (Adapted from Fernandez–Fernandez et al., *Eur. J. Neurosci.*, 2001.)

TABLE 7.1
Some Principal Receptor–G-Protein Coupling Preferences

G-Protein	Receptors
G_s	β-Adrenoceptor; dopamine $D_{1,5}$; histamine H_2; 5-hydroxytryptamine $5HT_{4,6,7}$; glucagon; vasopressin V_2; VIP/PACAP ($VPAC_{1-3}$); prostanoid DP, IP; $CRF_{1,2}$; calcitonin/amylin/CGRP
G_i/G_o	$α_2$-Adrenoceptor; $M_{2/4}$ muscarinic acetylcholine; dopamine D_{2-4}; $5HT_1$; opioid δ, μ, κ, OFQ; somatostatin sst_{1-5}; $GABA_B$; $mGlu_{2-4}$; cannabinoid $CB_{1,2}$
G_q/G_{11}	$α_1$-Adrenoceptor; $M_{1,3,5}$ muscarinic; histamine H_1; $5HT_2$; $mGlu_{1,5}$; nucleotide $P2_Y$; vasopressin V_1; tachykinin NK_{1-3}; bradykinin $B_{1,2}$; neurotensin $NTS_{1,2}$; endothelin $ET_{1,2}$; TRH; cholecystokinin CCK_2; prostanoid FP, TP

dependent manner. One interpretation of this is that different agonists produce different active states of the receptor, or a different distribution of active states, with different affinities for various G-proteins; however, there is no direct information on whether or not ligand-occupied receptors can form multiple active states. Light-activated rhodopsin goes through multiple conformational states before forming the active-state metarhodopsin-II, but none of the intermediate states has more than ~1/10,000th of the affinity of metarhodopsin-II for transducin. In the absence of direct evidence to the contrary, it seems wisest to interpret such phenomena as agonist-dependent variations in coupling efficiency on the assumption that a given receptor can normally form only one active state.

Notwithstanding the various considerations and caveats regarding receptor–G-protein coupling specificity outlined above, and ignoring variations between coupling to different members of the same class of G-proteins, Table 7.1 may be helpful in providing a broad operational summary of the principal receptor–G-protein-coupling preferences. More detailed information is given below in the Further Reading section (see Guderman et al., 1996).

7.9   G-PROTEIN–EFFECTOR COUPLING

The "effector" in this sense is the direct target protein of the activated G-protein subunit(s). Although initially characterized in terms of effector activation by the GTP-bound α subunit, for example, of adenylate cyclase by $α_s$, it is now clear that the freed βγ subunits also act as independent transducers (see Table 7.2). While allowance has to be made in intact systems for an indirect effect of Gβγ through binding to, and inactivation of, Gα-GTP, a direct interaction of Gβγ with the effector protein has been established for the β-adrenergic receptor kinase (βARK), adenylate cyclase, phospholipase C-β1,2,3, phosducin, GIRK K⁺ channels, and N-type ($α_{1B}$) Ca^{2+} channels. Binding to these effectors appears to be principally via a site on the β subunit that overlaps with the site through which βγ binds to the α subunit; hence, the free α subunit acts as a competitor with the effector for βγ binding (see below). Complementary binding sites for βγ on the C-terminus of βARK protein, on the I–II linker of the $α_{1B}$ Ca^{2+} channel (overlapping the binding site for the channel β subunit) and on both N- and C-termini of the GIRK channel have been identified. Some effectors are targets for both α and βγ subunits (e.g., PLCβ1–3; some adenylate cyclase isoforms). In these cases, the two subunits have independent and additive effects. Activation of these enzymes by βγ released from PTx-sensitive α subunits may account for the many instances of PTx-sensitive cyclase or PLC responses to receptor activation.

The question then arises as to how, in an unknown system, one can identify which subunit (α or βγ) carries the message. Two main approaches are available for identifying a βγ-mediated response: *replication* (and occlusion) by expressed or applied βγ subunits and *antagonism* by expressed or applied βγ-binding peptides such as a C-terminus peptide from βARK-1 or α-transducin, which, in essence, compete with the target for free βγ subunits. Positive identification

TABLE 7.2
Types of G-Protein

Subscript ($G_{subscript}$)	Toxin Sensitivity		Effectors	
	PTx	CTx	α Subunit	βγ Subunits
s	−	+	Adenylate cyclase ↑	βARK translocation; $I_{Ca(N)}$ ↓
olf	−	+	Adenylate cyclase ↑	—
t	+	+	Phosphodiesterase ↑	Phospholipase A_2 ↑
gust	+	+	Phosphodiesterase ↑	PLC ↑
i	+	−	Adenylate cyclase ↓	GIRK ↑
o	+	−	—	Ca(N, P, Q) ↓
z	−	−	—	Ca(N)↓, GIRK ↑
q	−	−	PLC ↑	PLC ↑
11	−	−	PLC ↑	—
12	−	−	?	—
13	−	−	?	—
14	−	−	PLC ↑	—
15	−	−	PLC ↑	—
16	−	−	PLC ↑	—

Abbreviations: βARK1, β-adrenergic receptor kinase 1; PLC, phospholipase C; GIRK, G-protein-activated inwardly rectifying potassium channel; Ca(N, P, Q), N-type, P-type, or Q-type calcium channel.

of α-mediated effects is more difficult, because G_α antagonists such as PTx or C-terminus antibodies also prevent release of free Gβγ, and the effects resulting from antisense depletion of α subunits might be attributable to excess unbound Gβγ. Replication by GTPase-deficient α subunits in the absence of positive evidence for the involvement of βγ subunits can be useful.

As an example of dual α- and βγ-mediated effects, one might consider the inhibition of N-type Ca^{2+} currents in sympathetic neurons by acetylcholine (Figures 7.11 and 7.12; see also Hille, 1994). Acetylcholine inhibits these currents through two different muscarinic receptors (M_1 and M_4), using two different G-protein pathways.

Stimulation of M_4 receptors produces a rapid inhibition that is characterized by its voltage dependence. That is, the opening of the channels during a depolarizing voltage step is delayed (so the onset of the current is slowed), and this is temporarily reversed by a strong depolarizing pre-pulse (Figure 7.11a). Such an effect is prevented by PTx and is mediated by a member of the G_i/G_o family which can be narrowed down specifically to G_{oA}, as it is (1) antagonized by injecting an antibody to the C-terminal domain of $G\alpha_o$ but not to C-terminal $G\alpha_{i1/2}$ (Figure 7.11a), and (2) reduced on expressing antisense RNA to $G\alpha_{oA}$ (Figure 7.11b). The final transducer is the βγ-dimer released from the $\alpha_{oA}\beta\gamma$-trimer because (1) the effect of M_4 receptor stimulation is replicated and occluded by overexpression of a common βγ combination ($\beta_1\gamma_2$; Figure 7.11c), and (2), the action of the agonist is prevented by overexpressing the C-terminal peptide domain of βARK-1, which binds and sequesters free βγ subunits (Figure 7.11d). The small, residual voltage-independent inhibition probably results from an additional effect of the α_{oA-GTP} monomer. The effect of the βγ subunits on these channels may be interpreted as follows. A free βγ molecule binds directly to the channel protein at one or more sites, including a site on the I–II linker that contains a binding motif (QXXER) that corresponds to a similar motif in the βARK-1 peptide, hence the competition. This binding leads to a retardation in Ca^{2+} channel opening during a voltage step. Strong depolarization causes the temporary dissociation of this bound βγ molecule and so reverses the inhibition. On repolarization, the dissociated βγ molecule rebinds and inhibition is restored. Rebinding (reinhibi-

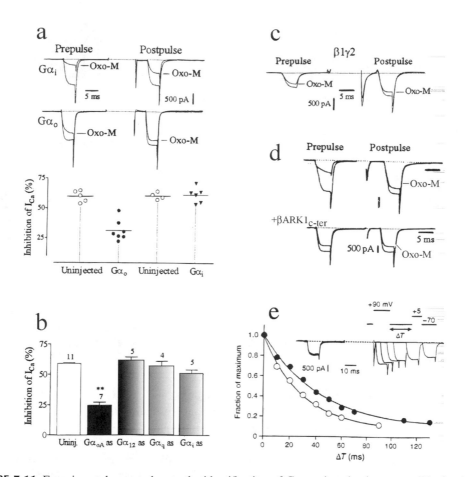

FIGURE 7.11 Experimental approaches to the identification of G-protein subunits responsible for the inhibition of calcium currents in rat sympathetic neurons on stimulating M_4 muscarinic acetylcholine receptors with the muscarinic agonist, oxotremorine-M (Oxo-M). The currents (evoked by 5-msec depolarizing steps to 0 mV from –60 mV) were recorded from dissociated ganglion cells patched with open-tip electrodes containing 20 mM BAPTA; this eliminates the component of inhibition produced by stimulating M_1 receptors (see Bernheim et al., 1991; Beech et al., 1992). As shown in the upper left traces, Oxo-M produced ~60% inhibition of the current, which was transiently and partly reversed by a 10-msec depolarizing step to +90 mV. Preinjection of an antibody directed against the C-terminus of $G\alpha_o$, but not $G\alpha_{i1/2}$, reduced the inhibition (a), suggesting that $G\alpha_o$ was the receiving α subunit for this effect. This was confirmed and narrowed down to the $G\alpha_{oA}$ isoform by expressing antisense cDNA constructs to deplete individual α subunits (b). Overexpression of $\beta_1\gamma_2$ subunits (by cDNA transfection) also inhibited the current and occluded the action of Oxo-M (c), while overexpression of the C-terminal fragment of βARK-1 (which acts as a βγ-binding agent) prevented the voltage-dependent inhibition by Oxo-M (d), implying that inhibition was mediated by βγ subunits freed from the activated G_{oA-abg} trimer. The freed βγ subunits interact directly with the calcium channel in a voltage-dependent manner: depolarization causes the dissociation of the subunits, which then reassociate with an average time-constant of 37 msec on repolarization (e; open circles); overexpression of βARK-1$_{C-ter}$ reduced the effective concentration of free βγ subunits and lengthened the time-constant for reassociation to 51 msec. Note that noradrenaline, instead of Oxo-M, was used to inhibit the current in (e). (Records (a) to (d) are adapted from Delmas et al., *Eur. J. Neurosci.*, 10, 1654–1666, 1998; record (e) is from Delmas et al., *J. Physiol.*, 506, 319–329, 1998.)

tion) follows an exponential time-course, the rate-constant of which is dependent on the concentration of available free $G\beta\gamma$ [$\beta\gamma$], according to the equation $k_{obs} = k_1[\beta\gamma] + k_2$, where k_1 and k_2 are the forward and backward rate constants for the reversible binding of one molecule of $\beta\gamma$ with one channel protein molecule (C): $C + \beta\gamma = C\beta\gamma$. Thus, the rate of reinhibition is accelerated by increasing the concentration of agonist or by applying increasing concentrations of $\beta\gamma$ and is slowed by reducing the amount of available $\beta\gamma$ using βARK-1 peptide (Figure 7.11e). Whereas only one molecule of $G\beta\gamma$ appears to bind to each Ca^{2+} channel molecule, inward rectifier K^+ channels, which are activated by $G\beta\gamma$, are made up of four separate subunits, each of which can bind one molecule of $G\beta\gamma$.

Stimulation of M_1 receptors produces a slower inhibition that is not voltage sensitive and that persists in the presence of PTx (Figure 7.12a). As expected from its resistance to PTx, this is not affected by antisense-depletion of α_{oA} but, instead, is reduced by antisense-depletion of α_q (Figure 7.12b) and is lost in neurons from $G\alpha_q$ knockout mice (Figure 7.12c). Unlike the voltage-sensitive inhibition produced by stimulating M_4 receptors, it is not mediated by $\beta\gamma$-dimers released from stimulated $\alpha_q\beta\gamma$ trimers because (1) it is not affected by the βARK-1 peptide (Figure 7.12d), and (2) agonist inhibition persists after overexpressing free $\beta_1\gamma_2$ subunits (Figure 7.12e). Instead, the effect of the agonist is replicated and occluded by overexpressing a GTPase-deficient (and therefore permanently active, GTP-bound) form of $G\alpha_q$ (Figure 7.12f). This action of $G\alpha_q$-GTP is unlikely to result from a direct interaction of the α subunit with the Ca^{2+} channel but instead probably involves the production and action of another messenger that can diffuse through the cytoplasm to affect Ca^{2+} channels some way away from the site of formation of $G\alpha_q$-GTP, as Ca^{2+} channel activity recorded in a patch pipette attached to the cell membrane can be inhibited by stimulating muscarinic receptors on other parts of the cell membrane outside the patch (Figure 7.12g; also see below and Figure 7.18).

What is the functional significance of these different modes of Ca^{2+} current inhibition? The $\beta\gamma$-mediated inhibition by acetylcholine, or by other transmitters such as noradrenaline and γ-aminobutyric acid (GABA), and the consequential reduction of Ca^{2+} influx in nerve terminals probably provide an important component of the presynaptic autoinhibitory action of transmitters on their own release in both peripheral and central nervous systems, though other effects beyond the step of Ca^{2+} entry may also contribute to the reduced transmitter release. On the other hand, the more remote α-mediated inhibition appears to be restricted to the somatic membrane. Here, its main effect is to reduce the amount of Ca^{2+} available for opening Ca^{2+}-dependent K^+ channels; this enhances somatic excitability, allowing the neuron to fire longer and more rapid trains of action potentials during continuous or high-frequency excitation.

One problem that arises in connection with $\beta\gamma$-mediated responses is how the specificity of receptor–effector coupling is maintained. Thus, most $\beta\gamma$-mediated effects, on ion channels at least, are inhibited by PTx, implying that they result from activation of G_i or G_o. There are exceptions; for instance, $\beta\gamma$-mediated inhibition of Ca^{2+} currents and activation of GIRK currents in sympathetic neurons can also be induced by vasoactive intestinal peptide (VIP), acting through G_s. However, these are exceptions and, generally speaking, voltage-dependent Ca^{2+} current inhibition or GIRK activation in native cells is restricted to receptors that couple to PTx-sensitive G-proteins such as α_2-adrenoceptors or muscarinic M_2 or M_4 receptors. Adrenoceptors that couple through G_s or $G_{q/11}$ or muscarinic receptors that couple through $G_{q/11}$ do not normally induce these $\beta\gamma$-mediated effects. In contrast, while there are differences in relative affinity between different $\beta\gamma$ combinations, both GIRK channels and Ca^{2+} channels appear to respond to a wide variety of $\beta\gamma$ subunit combinations when directly applied or expressed, including those that normally associate with PTx-insensitive α subunits. Hence, specificity is clearly conferred by the α subunit. How this is translated to specificity of effector response is not yet clear.

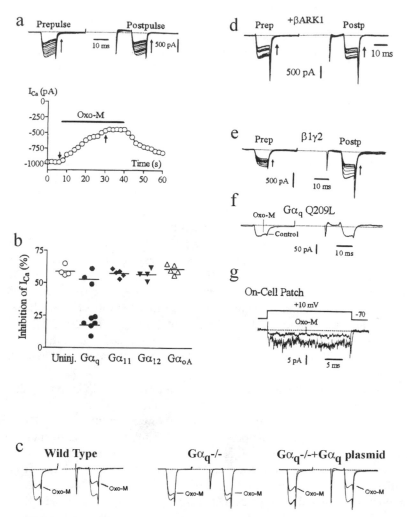

FIGURE 7.12 Experimental approaches to the identification of G-protein subunits responsible for the inhibition of calcium currents in rat sympathetic neurons on stimulating M_1 muscarinic acetylcholine receptors with the muscarinic agonist, oxotremorine-M (Oxo-M). In these experiments, the $M_4/G_o/\beta\gamma$-mediated inhibition illustrated in Figure 7.11 has been blocked by prior treatment with *Pertussis* toxin, and the calcium currents were recorded using the perforated-patch variant of the patch-clamp method (which preserves normal cytoplasmic constituents). Under these conditions, oxotremorine-M produces a slowly developing inhibition that is not reversed by strong depolarization (a). This form of inhibition is not affected by expressing antisense to $G\alpha_{oA}$, but instead is selectively reduced by antisense depletion of $G\alpha_q$ (b). In confirmation of this, inhibition is strongly reduced in ganglion cells from transgenic mice deficient in $G\alpha_q$ ($G\alpha_q$ −/−), and inhibition is restored in these cells by expressing free $G\alpha_q$ (c). Unlike M_4-mediated inhibition (Figure 7.11), this form of inhibition is not affected by overexpressing the βARK-1 peptide (d) and persists after overexpressing free $\beta_1\gamma_2$ subunits (e). Instead, the inhibition is replicated and occluded by overexpressing a GTPase-deficient α subunit of G_q (f), suggesting that it is mediated by the GTP-bound α_q subunit. This probably does not interact directly with the calcium channel but instead triggers an enzyme cascade that produces some messenger substance that diffuses through the cytoplasm to affect the channels, as full inhibition is seen when a cluster of channels is recorded with a cell-attached patch pipette and Oxo-M is added to the bathing solution in contact with the cell membrane outside the patch (g). (Records (a), (b), and (d) through (g) are adapted from Delmas et al., *Eur. J. Neurosci.*, 10, 1654–1666, 1998; record (c) is adapted from Haley et al., *J. Neurosci.*, 20, 3973–3979, 2000.)

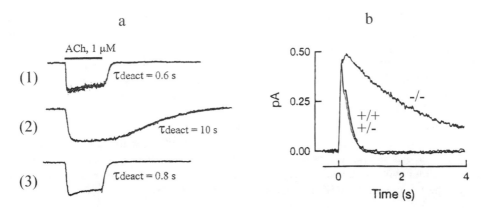

FIGURE 7.13 Role of RGS proteins in accelerating the offset of G-protein-mediated effects. (a) Inwardly rectifying GIRK potassium currents activated by stimulating M_2 muscarinic acetylcholine receptors with acetylcholine (ACh), recorded (1) from a rat atrial myocyte, (2) from a CHO cell cotransfected with the cardiac GIRK channels (Kir3.1 + Kir3.2) plus the M_2 receptor, and (3) from a CHO cell transfected as in (2) but also with RGS protein RGS4. Note that the response in the CHO cell (2) is slower to reach a steady state and much slower to deactivate compared to the atrial cell, but it replicates the response of the atrial cell following transfection of RGS4 (3). (b) Average single-photon responses of retinal rod photoreceptors taken from normal (+/+) mice and from heterozygote (+/–) and homozygote (–/–) RGS9 knockout mice. The light flash was delivered at time = 0 seconds. (Record (a) is adapted from Doupnik et al., *Proc. Natl. Acad. Sci. USA*, 94, 10461–10466, 1997; record (b) is from Chen et al., *Nature*, 403, 557–560, 2000. With permission.)

7.10 REGULATION OF G-PROTEIN SIGNALING

7.10.1 RGS PROTEINS

(See Vries et al., 2000, in the Further Reading section.) RGS proteins are members of a large (20 or more) family of loosely related proteins that have in common a 130-amino-acid RGS domain that allows them to bind to G-protein α subunits. They have (to varying extents) two main actions on G-protein signaling as a consequence of this binding. First, and most importantly, they act as GAPs (GTPase-activating proteins); that is, they accelerate the hydrolysis of GTP by the activated G-protein and hence accelerate recovery of the effector from activation by $G\alpha_{GTP}$ or by $G\beta\gamma$. They do not affect the rate of GDP–GTP exchange and do not alter the rate of G-protein activation by the receptor. Second, they can also reduce binding of $G\alpha_{GTP}$ to the effector, probably by physically blocking the interaction. This may be independent of their GAP activity, which should also reduce the effector response to a given degree of G-protein activation (see below), as it can be seen when the α subunit is activated by nonhydrolyzable GTPγS. For example, the RGS protein, RGS4, inhibits the response of PLC-β1 to GTPγS-activated G_q.

Figure 7.13a shows an example of the effects of an RGS protein on the activation of GIRK channels by stimulating M_2 muscarinic acetylcholine receptors with acetylcholine. This is the K^+ channel in the cardiac pacemaker cells that is opened by acetylcholine released following vagal stimulation and is responsible for the hyperpolarization and slowing of the pacemaker (see below). However, when only GIRK channels and M_2 receptors are reconstituted in oocytes or mammalian noncardiac cells, the channels take several seconds to close down again after removing acetylcholine; whereas, in the heart, the current recovers in less than a second. As shown in Figure 7.13a, the off rate for GIRK deactivation following acetylcholine removal in the reconstituted system is accelerated more than 10 times by co-expressing RGS4 and now matches the off rate for the native atrial current.

The large number of RGS proteins have varying degrees of selectivity for different α subunits and varying effects on different effector systems (see Vries et al., 2000). These properties are usually assessed in reconstituted expression systems. What is less clear at present is the role that individual RGS proteins play in native cells. One interesting approach to this question makes use of the fact that coupling of RGS proteins to the α subunit can be disrupted by a point mutation in the α subunit without any other disruption to Gα function. By combining such a mutation with another mutation to eliminate PTx sensitivity (see Figure 7.10), it has been established that an endogenous RGS protein is involved in the inhibition of Ca^{2+} currents in sympathetic neurons by noradrenaline-activated G_o, as replacement of the endogenous $G_o\alpha$ with the mutated $G_o\alpha$ has been shown to reduce the sensitivity to noradrenaline by about tenfold and to slow the rate of onset and recovery of inhibition. However, even this involves a degree of reconstitution, with the consequent problems addressed earlier. An alternative approach is genetic deletion. Thus, there is a dramatic (greater than tenfold) slowing of the recovery of the photoresponse of isolated retinal rods in knockout mice deficient in the retina-specific RGS protein RGS-9 (Figure 7.13b).

7.10.2 EFFECTORS AS GTPASE-ACTIVATING PROTEINS

Some enzyme effectors also act as GAPs, accelerating the hydrolysis of GTP and hence promoting the rapid turnoff of the G-protein-activated enzyme itself. For example, the GTPase activity of pure $G\alpha_q$-GTP is very slow (10 to 60 sec) when measured in solution but is increased 50-fold on adding its effector target PLC-β1, to a more physiological half-life of 1 sec. Likewise, addition of phosphodiesterase shortens the half-life of GTP-bound α-transducin from 20 sec to 5 sec. This accelerating effect of the phosphodiesterase effector is synergistic with the effect of the visual RGS protein RGS9 mentioned above. Whether ion-channel effectors also act as GAPs in the absence of RGS proteins is unclear.

7.11 KINETICS OF GPCR-MEDIATED SIGNALS

Effects mediated by G-protein coupled receptors (GPCRs) are very much slower than those mediated by, for example, ligand-gated ion channels, primarily because more steps are involved between activation of the receptor and the final response. For example, even in a simple, three-step, G-protein-mediated effect, such as the opening of atrial GIRK channels following the activation of M_2 muscarinic receptors by acetylcholine, which follows the scheme:

$$ACh + R \rightarrow R\text{-}ACh + G_{\alpha\beta\gamma} \rightarrow [\alpha_{GTP}] + \beta\gamma + GIRK_{closed} \rightarrow \beta\gamma\text{-}GIRK_{open}$$

the minimum latency to the development of the GIRK current and consequent membrane hyperpolarization, following a pulse-application of acetylcholine, is about 30 msec (Figure 7.14). This contrasts with the <1-msec latency of the opening of nicotinic channels following application of acetylcholine to muscle endplate nicotinic receptors. By analogy with the response of rhodopsin to a flash of light, it is likely that the initial binding of acetylcholine to the muscarinic receptor and subsequent conformational change take no more than a millisecond or so; the extra time is required for the diffusion and docking of the activated receptor to the G-protein, the exchange of GTP for GDP, and dissociation of the G-protein, as well as the diffusion and docking of the freed βγ subunits with the potassium channel. Following its peak, the current then declines over a period of several hundreds of milliseconds; this is determined by the rate of GTP hydrolysis and consequent dissociation of the α subunit from the effector or recapture of the βγ subunit from the effector by the newly formed GDP-bound α subunit (see above and Figure 7.13).

The effect of stimulation of cardiac adrenoceptors is even more leisurely because several more steps follow activation of the G_s protein by the β-adrenoceptor. For example, to increase the force of cardiac contraction, we have (1) activation of adenylate cyclase by $G\alpha_S$-GTP, (2) formation of cAMP, (3) activation of protein kinase A by the cAMP, then (4) phosphorylation of the calcium channel protein by the kinase. As a result, it takes about 5 to 6 sec from the time the receptors are

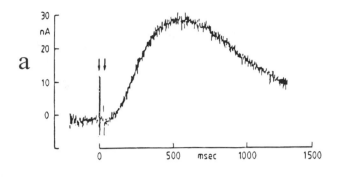

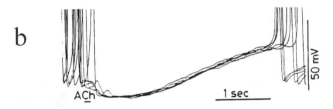

FIGURE 7.14 Time-course of G-protein-mediated activation of GIRK potassium channels in rabbit sino-atrial node cells. (a). Outward current evoked by a 33-msec, 50-nA iontophoretic pulse of acetylcholine (between arrows). (b). Response of the unclamped cell to an iontophoretic pulse of acetylcholine (ACh). (Record (a) is adapted with permission from Trautwein et al., in *Drug Receptors and Their Effectors*, Birdsall, N. J. M., Ed., Macmillan, New York, 1980, pp. 5–22; record (b) is adapted with permission from Noma, in *Electrophysiology of Single Cardiac Cells*, Noble, D. and Powell, T., Eds., Academic Press, San Diego, CA, 1987, pp. 223–246.)

activated to the first increase in calcium current amplitude (Figure 7.15a). Most of this time is taken up with the steps leading to the generation of a sufficient amount of cAMP (adenylate cyclase is a relatively slow-acting enzyme), as the latency is reduced to around 150 msec on applying a concentration jump of cAMP by flash photolysis of an intracellularly accumulated photolabile cAMP precursor (Figure 7.15b).

However, latency alone is not a good guide to the number of steps in the G-protein-mediated cascade; geometry and packing density are also important. Thus, the (almost) equally complex cascade reaction involved in the response of photoreceptors to a light flash (in which rhodopsin activates the G-protein transducin, which in turn activates phosphodiesterase, which reduces the concentration of cGMP and so shuts cGMP-gated cation channels) is very fast, with a minimum latency of around 10 msec at the highest intensity flashes (Figure 7.16). The reason for this is the very high density of receptors, G-proteins, and phosphodiesterase in the rod discs. Also, phosphodiesterase has a much higher (substrate-diffusion-limited) turnover rate than adenylate cyclase. As a rule of thumb, the usual ratio of receptors to G-proteins to ion-channel effectors is probably around 1:10:0.1; because most ion channels seem to have a density of around 1 per square micrometer, this gives about 10 receptors and about 100 G-proteins per square micrometer. In contrast, there are about 2500 transducin molecules and about 167 effector (phosphodiesterase) molecules per square micrometer of rod disc membrane. Conversely, even the direct activation, or inhibition, of an ion channel might be very slow at low densities of channels and G-proteins (Figure 7.17).

For ion-channel effectors, Figures 7.8 and 7.12 illustrate another way of deciding whether the activated G-protein subunits interact directly with the channel or indirectly through a cascade reaction leading to a cytoplasmic messenger, using the patch-clamp technique shown; the GIRK potassium channels recorded in a cell-attached patch in Figure 7.8 are activated by acetylcholine

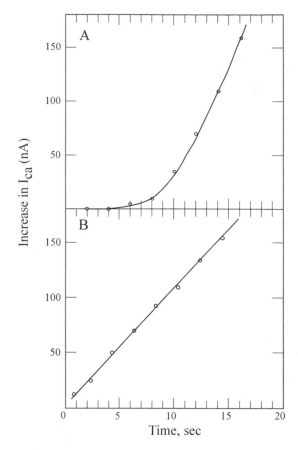

FIGURE 7.15 Time-course of the increases in amplitude of the calcium current recorded from bullfrog atrial trabeculae following (A) rapid application of the β-adrenoceptor agonist isoprenaline (3 μM), and (B) rapid intracellular release of cAMP by flash-photolysis of *o*-nitrobenzyl cAMP. Applications/flashes were made at time zero. (From Nargeot et al., *Proc. Natl. Acad. Sci. USA*, 80, 2395–2399, 1983. With permission.)

in the patch pipette but not on adding acetylcholine to the bathing solution outside the patch, implying a local effect of the receptor-activated G-protein on the channel. In contrast, the calcium channels in Figure 7.12 are closed by adding a muscarinic receptor agonist to the extra-patch membrane via the bathing solution, implying that some diffusible messenger is produced to carry the message through the cytoplasm from the receptor-activated G-proteins to the patch-enclosed channels. Another example of such a remote signaling pathway carrying the message from muscarinic receptor-activated G-proteins to another type of potassium channel is illustrated in Figure 7.18.

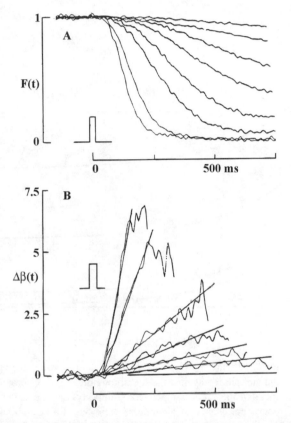

FIGURE 7.16 (A) Photocurrents of salamander rod cells following light flashes giving between 10 and 2000 rhodopsin molecule isomerizations. (B) Calculated increments in phosphodiesterase hydrolytic rate constant. (From Lamb, T. D. and Pugh, Jr., E. N., *Trends Neurosci.*, 15, 291–299, 1992. With permission.)

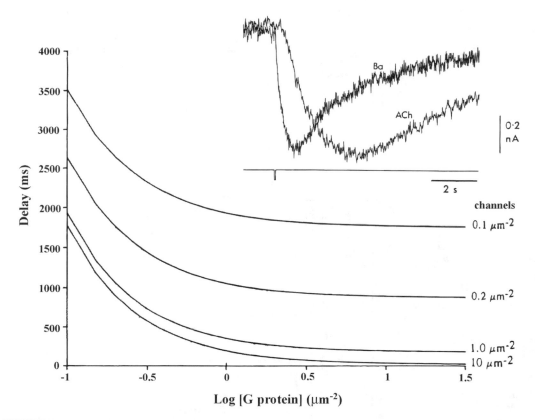

FIGURE 7.17 Calculated latency (delay) between activation of a muscarinic acetylcholine receptor and the closure of a potassium M-channel plotted against the membrane density of G-proteins (in logarithmic units) for different potassium channel densities. It is assumed (for simplicity) that the activated GTP-bound α subunit interacts directly with the potassium channel. Calculations were based on Lamb and Pugh (1992), with the following diffusion coefficients: receptor, 0.7 μm/sec; Gαβγ, 1.2 μm/sec; Gα, 1.5 μm/sec; channel, 0.4 μm/sec. Inset: Observed latencies to current inhibition at 35°C in a neuroblastoma hybrid cell expressing M_1 muscarinic acetylcholine receptors following 100-msec pressure application of barium ions (Ba, which directly plugs the channels) and acetylcholine (ACh). The mean latency difference (ACh − Ba) was ~272 msec. At estimated channel and G-protein densities of 1 and 25/μm², the direct-hit G-protein–channel interaction would predict a latency of ~180 msec. (Adapted from Robbins, J. et al., *J. Physiol.*, 469, 153–178, 1993; additional unpublished material from J. Robbins.)

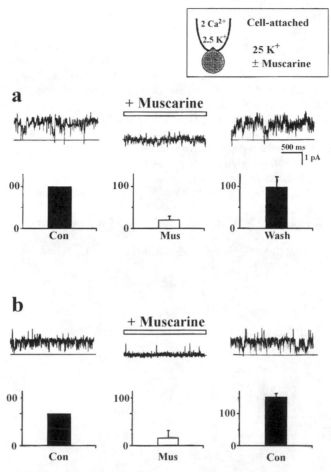

FIGURE 7.18 An example of remote G-protein–effector interaction. Records show M-type potassium channel activity recorded from rat sympathetic neurons in cell-attached patch pipettes held at ~0 mV. Activity is suppressed when the muscarinic acetylcholine receptor agonist, muscarine (10 μM), is applied to the cell membrane outside the patch electrode. (The bathing solution contained 25 mM [K+] to set the membrane potential at E_K (~–30 mV) and prevent depolarization by muscarine.) The fact that muscarine cannot diffuse through the tight seal between the pipette glass and the membrane (and diffusion of an activated G-protein through the membrane to a channel inside the electrode patch would be very slow) implies that some diffusible substance is produced to carry the message from activated receptors and G-proteins outside the patch to the channel inside the patch. The record and bar chart in (b) were obtained using patch pipettes already filled with muscarine solution. In spite of this, channels were active and could still be closed by adding muscarine to the extra-patch membrane. This suggests that channels could not be closed by a local (direct) interaction of the activated G-protein with the channel (also, that not enough receptors were present in the patched membrane to generate a sufficient amount of messenger to close the channels). (Adapted from Selyanko et al., *Proc. Roy. Soc. London Ser. B*, 250, 119–125, 1992.)

7.12 FURTHER READING

Beech et al., *Neuron*, 8, 97–106, 1992.

Bernheim et al., *Neuron*, 6, 859–867, 1991.

Birnbaumer, L., Transduction of receptor signal into modulation of effector activity by G-proteins: the first 20 years or so, *FASEB J.*, 4, 3068–3078, 1990.

Bourne, H. R., How receptors talk to trimeric G-proteins, *Curr. Opin. Cell. Biol.*, 9, 134–142, 1997.

Clapham, D. E., The G-protein nanomachine, *Nature*, 379, 297–300, 1996.

Clapham, D. E. and Neer, E., G-protein βγ subunits, *Annu. Rev. Pharmacol. Toxicol.*, 37, 167–203, 1997.

Gudermann, T., Kalkbrenner, F., and Schultz, G., Diversity and selectivity of receptor–G-protein interaction, *Annu. Rev. Pharmacol. Toxicol.*, 36, 429–459, 1996.

Hille, B., Modulation of ion channel function by G-protein-coupled receptors, *Trends Neurosci.*, 17, 531–536, 1994.

Ikeda, S. R. and Dunlap, K., Voltage-dependent modulation of N-type calcium channels: role of G-protein subunits, *Adv. Second Messenger Phosphoprotein Res.*, 33, 131–151, 1999.

Lamb, T. D. and Pugh, Jr., E. N., G-protein cascades: gains and kinetics, *Trends Neurosci.*, 15, 291–299, 1992.

Rodbell, M., The role of hormone receptors and GTP-regulatory proteins in membrane transduction, *Nature*, 284, 17–22, 1974.

Vries, L. D., Zheng, B., Fischer, T., Elenko, E., and Farquhar, M., The regulator of G-protein signaling family, *Annu. Rev. Pharmacol. Toxicol.*, 40, 235–271, 2000.

Wickman, K. D. and Clapham, D. E., G-protein regulation of ion channels, *Curr. Opin. Neurobiol.*, 5, 278–285, 1995.

8 Signal Transduction through Protein Tyrosine Kinases

IJsbrand Kramer

CONTENTS

0-8493-1029-6/03/$0.00+$1.50

8.1   INTRODUCTION

8.1.1   Phosphorylation as a Switch in Cellular Functioning

Phosphorylation of protein was discovered in the era of "allosteric regulation." Regulation of enzyme activity could be explained by the concentration of substrates, the presence of cofactors, and the concentration of the end product (allosteric effectors). One of the pathways thus analyzed was the glycolytic pathway. The first step in this pathway is the conversion of glycogen to glucose-1-phosphate which is mediated by an enzyme called *glycogen phosphorylase*. Enzyme activity was found to be regulated through allosteric interactions by adenosine 5′-monophosphate (stimulatory) and glucose-6-phosphate (inhibitory). Glycogen phosphorylase could be isolated in two forms: an active form (designated with an *a*) and a less active form (designated with a *b*). In 1956, Krebs and Fischer discovered that phosphorylase *b* could incorporate one organic phosphate molecule on a serine residue, a process that accompanies an increase in its activity. Through incorporation of a phosphate, phosphorylase *b* obtained the characteristics of phosphorylase *a*, being less sensitive to the inhibitory action of glucose-6-phosphate and more sensitive to the stimulatory action of adenosine 5′-monophospate. Thus, apart from allosteric regulation, a covalent modification such as phosphorylation could also affect enzyme activity. The phosphorylation is catalyzed by a protein kinase, phosphorylase kinase. Later it was discovered that a phosphorylase phosphatase catalyzed dephosphorylation, which brings the enzyme back into the phosphorylase *b* state. By 1970, it was clear that almost all enzymes were regulated by phosphorylation/dephosphorylation, and investigators began to question why it was necessary to have two broad systems for controlling enzyme activity: allosteric regulation and phosphorylation. Moreover, in the case of phosphorylase and another enzyme, glycogen synthase, it was clear that allosteric and covalent regulation probably worked through similar conformational changes. A basic difference between these two modes of action became apparent when it was found that hormone receptors, through the release of intracellular second messengers, in turn controlled the phosphorylase kinase activity. While allosteric control generally reflects intracellular conditions, phosphorylation occurs in response to extracellular signals. Phosphorylation allows the organism to control metabolism in individual cells. Phosphorylation and dephosphorylation reactions, as will be seen in the following paragraphs, are always part of a cascade of reactions. Cascade systems allow for an enormous amplification as well as fine modulation of an original signal. While the field of serine/threonine protein kinases exploded, a new type of protein kinase entered the arena in 1978 with the discovery that the Rous sarcoma virus contained a protein kinase, named v-src, that phosphorylated protein on a tyrosine residue. It was then discovered that growth factor receptors contain protein tyrosine kinases, and a new field of research rapidly developed.

8.1.2   GROWTH FACTORS, INTERLEUKINS, INTERFERONS, AND CYTOKINES

Research on tyrosine-kinase-containing receptors was initiated in the area of cell biology. Factors that could support growth of cells in culture were isolated and named after (1) the cells they were isolated from, (2) the cells they stimulated, or (3) the principle action they performed. For example, platelet-derived growth factor (PDGF), epidermal growth factor (EGF), or transforming growth factor (TGF). In the area of immunology, factors were studied that directed maturation and proliferation of white blood cells. The factors discovered were named interleukins or colony-stimulating factors. In virology, factors were studied that interfered with viral infection: interferons. And, in cancer research, factors were studied that could influence the growth of solid tumors — for example, tumor necrosis factor (TNF). Each area of research believed that the factors functioned by and large only in the category in which they came to light. It was also believed that each factor had a set of additional actions that were related to each other in some obvious way. With progress, it became apparent that growth factors also acted on cells of the immune system and had totally unrelated actions. Moreover, it was shown that the context in which the cells were studied (e.g., presence of other factors, presence of other cells, attached or in suspension, type of substrate) also determined the outcome of the cellular response. A good example is TGF-β, a factor initially shown to enhance cell transformation, hence its name. Later it was found that this factor was a strong growth inhibitor of transformed epithelial cell lines and that it was a very potent chemotactic factor for neutrophils. It has been proposed that a common name for these factors should be *cytokines*, defined as follows:

> A cytokine is a soluble (glyco)protein, nonimmunoglobulin in nature, released by living cells of the host, which acts nonenzymatically in picomolar to nanomolar concentrations to regulate host cell function.

This information is not directly relevant for understanding the action of protein tyrosine kinases, but it illustrates that various areas of research are coming together and introducing new insights into cell functioning. It also illustrates that tyrosine phosphorylation is not limited to growth-inducing cytokines. Tyrosine phosphorylation has been shown to regulate cell–cell and cell–matrix interactions through integrin receptors and focal adhesion sites. It is also involved in stimulation of the respiratory burst in neutrophils. Occupation of the B-cell immunoglobulin M (IgM) and high-affinity IgE receptor as well as occupation of the T-cell and interleukin-2 (IL-2) receptor results in tyrosine phosphorylation. Finally, tyrosine phosphorylation is also involved in selection of transmitter responses induced by neuronal contact.

Only a fraction of what is known about the role of protein tyrosine kinases in cellular functioning will be dealt with in this chapter, but it nevertheless should reveal some principles that allow the reader to better understand current literature on the subject. The chapter is divided into two broad sections: one dealing with receptors that contain protein tyrosine kinases as an integral part of the molecule (receptor protein tyrosine kinases, or PTKs) and one dealing with receptors that associate with cytosolic protein tyrosine kinases (nonreceptor PTKs). Because studies with genetically accessible organisms such as *Drosophila* and *Caenorhabditis elegans* have made important contributions to the discovery of signal-transduction pathways, we will illustrate some of the analogies between the various species in an appendix to this chapter. Knowledge of these will also facilitate your understanding of the signal-transduction nomenclature.

8.2 RECEPTORS CONTAINING PROTEIN TYROSINE KINASES

8.2.1 CROSS-LINKING OF RECEPTORS CAUSES ACTIVATION

This section focuses on the signal-transduction pathway initiated by binding of growth factors to their receptors. We will restrict the subject to a number of principles that generally apply for tyrosine-kinase-containing receptors, with the EGF, PDGF, and nerve growth factor (NGF) receptors as examples. EGF and PDGF are true growth factors, inducing proliferation of epithelial cells and fibroblasts, whereas the main role of NGF is to ensure survival of neurons and/or neurite outgrowth, not proliferation.

Tyrosine-kinase-containing receptors come in several different forms, unified by the presence of a single membrane-spanning domain and an intracellular protein tyrosine kinase catalytic domain (receptor PTK). The extracellular chains vary considerably, as illustrated in Figure 8.1. Many growth factor receptors contain immunoglobulin domains, which play a role in ligand binding; therefore, they are part of the immunoglobulin superfamily. A general feature is that ligand binding results in dimerization of the receptors. Cross-linking of receptors by growth factors can be achieved in a number of ways. PDGF and NGF are disulfide-linked dimeric ligands that cross-link their

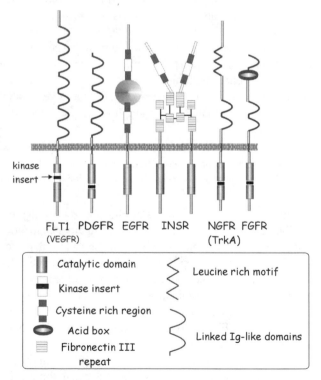

FIGURE 8.1 Classification of protein tyrosine kinase (PTK)-containing receptors. All of these receptors possess a single-membrane-spanning segment and all of them incorporate a kinase catalytic domain, in some cases interrupted by an insert. The extracellular domains vary as indicated, but many contain an immunoglobulin motif that acts as ligand binding site. Some of these receptors exist in various isoforms. FLT1, Fms-related tyrosine kinase (receptor for vascular endothelial growth factor [VEGF]); PDGFR, platelet-derived growth factor receptor; EGFR, epidermal growth factor receptor; INSR, insulin receptor; NGFR, nerve growth factor receptor (also known as TrkA); FGFR, fibroblast growth factor receptor. (Adapted from Heldin, p.4.)

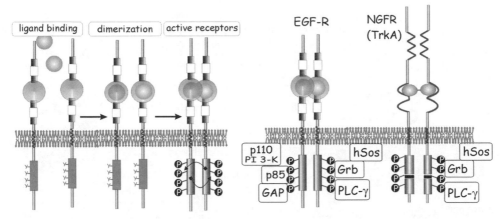

receptor signalling complex

FIGURE 8.2 Activation and receptor signaling complex formation. On occupation by its ligand, protein tyrosine kinase (PTK)-containing receptors form a dimer, which induces a change in the conformation of the cytoplasmic domain that reveals its latent PTK activity. This phosphorylates the tyrosine residues on the linked receptor molecule (interphosphorylation). The dimerized, phosphorylated molecule constitutes the catalytically active receptor. Activated EGF, PDGF, or NGF receptors (EGF-R, PDGF-R, or NGF-R, respectively) associate with effectors, including enzymes (e.g., PLCγ, GAP) or adaptor proteins that recruit enzymes (e.g., Gab-1, p85 PI_3-kinase, Grb2), to form receptor signaling complexes.

receptors upon binding. When they bind to their receptors, cross-linking is automatic. EGF, a monomeric ligand, changes the receptor conformation in the extracellular domain, allowing the occupied monomers to recognize each other. The activation signal is, of course, more complicated than this. For activation of all the receptor functions, not only must the receptor molecules be brought together as dimers, but they must also be oriented correctly in relation to each other.

Dimerization allows the kinase activity of both intracellular chains to encounter target sequences on the other, linked receptor molecule. This enables the intermolecular cross-phosphorylation of several tyrosine residues (Figure 8.2). The phosphorylated dimer then constitutes the active receptor. It possesses an array of phosphotyrosines that enable it to bind proteins to form *receptor signaling complexes*. Additionally, the dimerized and phosphorylated receptor has the potential of phosphorylating its targets.

8.2.2 Src and PTB Homology Domains and the Formation of Receptor Signaling Complexes

Once the formation of receptor signaling complexes was established, it was important to establish how these proteins interact with the tyrosine phosphorylated receptor. Sequence analysis of proteins that bind has shown that many, but not all of them, contain domains also present in the cytoplasmic protein tyrosine kinase Src, hence the name *SH2 domains*. Others contain domains that were previously identified as phosphotyrosine-binding domains (PTB). Evidence for a role of SH2 domains in transmitting the signals due to receptor PTKs came from the finding that deletion of the SH2 domains abolished the interaction with the receptors and cellular response. Further evidence came from the finding that only the γ isoforms of phospholipase C (PLC) are directly activated by these receptors. Significantly, PLCγ, but not the β and δ isoforms, possess SH2 domains. In conclusion, the assembly of signaling complexes depends on the recruitment by tyrosine-phosphorylated receptors of proteins having an SH2 or PTB domain. Many proteins containing SH2 domains associate with receptor PTKs in the formation of signaling complexes, and a selection of these is illustrated in Figure 8.3. Some of these proteins themselves become phosphorylated as a result of

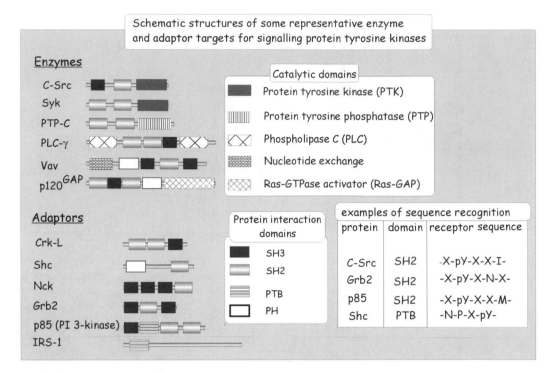

FIGURE 8.3 Domain organization of proteins that associate with phosphorylated tyrosine kinase (PTK)-containing receptors. Proteins that associate with tyrosine-phosphorylated receptors contain SH2 or PTB domains, which recognize specific amino-acid stretches in the vicinity of phosphorylated tyrosine residues. Unlike the enzymes, the adaptors lack intrinsic catalytic activity but serve to link phosphorylated receptors with other effector proteins. Some of the proteins presented in this figure are discussed in this chapter.

this association, although it is not clear whether or not this process is always necessary for their activation. In the case of PLCγ, phosphorylation is certainly necessary.

Of the variety of adaptors and enzymes that interact with EGF, PDGF, or NGF receptors, some appear to bind more tightly than others, exhibiting sensitivity to the amino-acid residues in the immediate vicinity of the phosphotyrosines (Figure 8.3). Thus, a particular receptor might transmit its signal through a panel of SH2- or PTB-containing proteins. It remains unclear, however, if two or more intracellular proteins can bind to a single receptor molecule simultaneously.

8.2.3 BRANCHING OF THE SIGNALING PATHWAY

A number of signal-transduction pathways branch out from the receptor signaling complex. Five such branches are described in the following text (see Figure 8.4).

8.2.3.1 The Ras Signaling Pathway

8.2.3.1.1 Ras and Cell Transformation

Infection of rats with murine leukemia viruses can provoke the formation of a sarcoma. A major advance was the discovery that the Harvey murine sarcoma virus encodes a persistently activated form of the H-ras gene, a monomeric guanosine triphosphate (GTP)-binding protein, or GTPase, in which valine is substituted for glycine at position 12. GTP-binding proteins act as monostable switches. They are "on" in the GTP-bound state and "off" in the guanosine diphosphate (GDP)-bound state. Binding of GTP occurs through the dissociation of GDP (exchange reaction), and GTP is subsequently lost through hydrolysis (GTPase reaction). The state of activation is kinetically

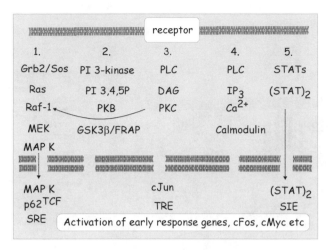

FIGURE 8.4 Branching of the signal-transduction pathways. Following activation of receptor PTK, several signal-transduction pathways can be activated, five of which are indicated here (see text for further details).

regulated, positively by the initial rate of GDP dissociation and subsequent association of GTP and then negatively by the rate at which the GTP is hydrolyzed (Figure 8.5). The valine-to-glycine substitution prevents hydrolysis of GTP, resulting in a constitutive active Ras (also referred to as a gain-of-function mutation). Expression of this mutant in quiescent rodent fibroblasts resulted in altered cell morphology, stimulation of DNA synthesis, and cell proliferation. When overexpressed, normal H-c-Ras also induces oncogenic transformation as does microinjection of the mutant protein. Conversely, injection of neutralizing antibodies to inhibit normal Ras function reverses cell transformation. Finally, stimulation of quiescent cells with serum or with purified growth factors causes the activation of Ras, through promotion of the exchange of GDP for GTP. It became apparent that Ras is an important component in the signaling pathways regulating cell proliferation, but how Ras would fit into the known pathways emanating from growth factor receptors remained unclear for a considerable time.

8.2.3.1.2 Regulation of Ras in Vertebrates

The activated growth factor receptor binds Grb2, an adaptor protein, through its SH2 domain, and this action recruits the guanine nucleotide exchanger hSos to the plasma membrane, bringing it in the vicinity of Ras. The activated hSos now exchanges GDP for GTP and brings Ras to its activated state, ready to signal into the cell through interaction with its effector molecules.

The Ras–GTPase activating protein p120[GAP] contains two SH2 domains (Figure 8.3). It also binds to phosphotyrosines on activated receptors, and it is a component of the signaling complex that assembles on activated PDGF receptors (Figure 8.2). It is unclear what role the association of GAP plays in signal transduction. For instance, cells that express a mutant of the PDGF receptor that fails to bind GAP manifest normal activation of Ras.

8.2.3.1.3 From Ras to MAP Kinase and Activation of Transcription

The events following the activation of Ras ultimately led to the activation of MAP kinase,* followed by activation of expression of immediate-early response genes. Activation of MAP kinase requires two intermediate steps, both of which involve a phosphorylation (Figure 8.5). The immediate activator of MAP kinase is MAP-kinase-kinase (also called MAP kinase–ERK kinase, or MEK), a most unusual enzyme that phosphorylates MAP kinase on both a threonine (T) and a tyrosine (Y) residue. These are in the target-sequence seven residues (LTEYVATRWYRAPE) (Table 8.1)

---

* Mitogen-activated protein kinase; since cloning, referred to as ERK, extracellular-signal-regulated kinase (ERK).

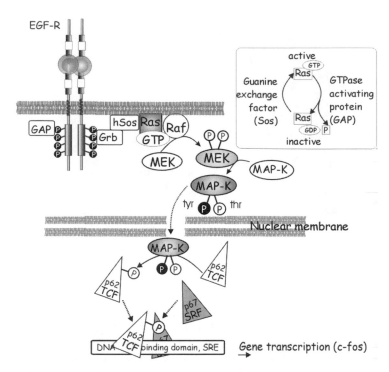

FIGURE 8.5 Regulation of the ras–MAP kinase pathway by receptor protein tyrosine kinases. The adaptor protein Grb2, in association with the guanine exchange factor Sos, attaches to the tyrosine-phosphorylated receptor through its SH2 domain. This brings the Grb2/hSos complex into the vicinity of the membrane, where it catalyzes the guanine nucleotide exchange on Ras. The activated Ras associates with the serine/threonine protein kinase Raf-1. Its localization at the membrane results in activation and subsequent phosphorylation of the dual-specificity kinase MEK. This causes double phosphorylation of MAP kinase (tyrosine and threonine residues) and exposes a signal peptide that allows MAP kinase to interact with proteins that guide it into the nucleus (translocation). Inside the nucleus, MAP kinase phosphorylates $p62^{TCF}$, which then associates with $p67^{SRF}$ to form an active transcription factor complex that binds to DNA at the serum-response element (SRE).

on the N-terminal side of the conserved motif APE, present in the catalytic center of the kinase. Phosphorylation at these sites renders the protein kinase catalytically competent. To date, MAP kinase appears to be the unique substrate for phosphorylation by MEK, indicating a particularly high level of specificity.

Moving further upstream, the first kinase downstream of Ras is Raf-1 (also known as MAP-kinase-kinase-kinase, or MAPKKK) This kinase was initially identified as an oncogene product causing fibrosarcoma in the rat. The subsequent finding that activated Ras recruits Raf-1 to the membrane and consequently brings about kinase activation links MAP kinase with the Ras pathway. In the activation of Raf-1, it is its recruitment to the plasma membrane, not its actual association with activated Ras, that is necessary. Of course, the association with Ras is essential under normal conditions; however, a mutant form of Raf-1 possessing a C-terminal–Caax box that acts as a site for prenylation (and which is therefore permanently associated with the plasma membrane) insti-gates the downstream events independently of Ras. Accordingly, the role of Ras in the physiological situation can be regarded as that of a membrane-located recruiting sergeant.

8.2.3.1.4 Beyond MAP Kinase: Activation of Gene Expression

The activated MAP kinase exposes a signal peptide that enables it to interact with proteins that promote its translocation into the nucleus. Inside, it catalyzes the phosphorylation of its substrates on Ser–Pro and Thr–Pro motifs. In the case of stimulation by EGF and PDGF, the activation of

TABLE 8.1
Dual Phosphorylation Sites in MAP Kinase Family Members

	Kinase	Domain VII	Linker L12	Domain VIII (Catalytic Loop)
		TEY Motif		
Human	ERK1	DFGLAR	IADPEHDHTGF	L<u>TEY</u>VATRWYR<u>APE</u>IMLNSK
Rat	ERK1	DFGLAR	IADPEHDHTGF	L<u>TEY</u>VATRWYR<u>APE</u>IMLNSK
Human	ERK2	DFGLAR	VADPHDHTGF	L<u>TEY</u>VATRWYR<u>APE</u>IMLNSK
Rat	ERK2	DFGLAR	VADPHDHTGF	L<u>TEY</u>VATRWYR<u>APE</u>IMLNSK
		TGY Motif		
Mouse	p38/HOG	DFGLAR	HTDDE------------------	M<u>TGY</u>VATRWYR<u>APE</u>IMLNWN
		TPY Motif		
Rat	SAPKa	DFGLAR	TACTN-------------FM	M<u>TPY</u>VVTRYYR<u>APE</u>VILGMG
Rat	SAPKb	DFGLAR	TAGTS------------FM	M<u>TPY</u>VVTRYYR<u>APE</u>VILGMG
Rat	SAPKg	DFGLAR	AGTS-------------- FM	M<u>TPY</u>VVTRYYR<u>APE</u>VILGMG
Human	JNK1	DFGLAR	TAGTS------------FM	M<u>TPY</u>VVTRYYR<u>APE</u>VILGMG

MAP kinase is an absolute requirement for cell proliferation. In the case of NGF, its stimulation plays a role in neurite outgrowth and survival. The early response genes become activated within an hour of receptor stimulation. Their activation is transient and can occur under conditions in which protein synthesis is inhibited. Activation of the EGF, PDGF, or NGF receptor results in the rapid induction of the transcription factor c-Fos, one of the first cytokine-inducible transcription factors to be discovered.* It occupies a central position in the regulation of gene expression. Other early response genes include *c-myc*, *junB*, and *c-jun*. The promoter region of the *c-fos* gene contains a serum-response element (SRE), a DNA domain that binds the transcription factors p67[SRF] (serum-response factor) and p62[TCF] (ternary-complex factor).** Phosphorylation of p62[TCF] at residue ser-383 and ser-389 by MAP kinase increases the formation of a complex of both transcription factors with the DNA to promote transcription of the *c-fos* gene (Figure 8.5). Activation of the MAP kinase pathway enhances transcription of early response genes, such as *c-fos*, which in turn must be implicated in the expression of a large number of genes given the presence of 12-*O*-tetrade-canoylphorbol-13-acetate (TPA)-responsive element (TRE) in the promoter region of many genes.

8.2.3.1.5   Other Ras Activators and Effectors

Guanine nucleotide exchange factors other than hSos have also been found to activate Ras, as have other effectors (see Table 8.2). These may interact with unique sequences in the effector loop. The question remains, however, as to how many different effectors can attach to activated Ras and what determines the level of their priority.

8.2.3.1.6   A Family of MAP Kinases

Once it was cloned, it was apparent that MAP kinase is a member of a substantial family of proteins that may be classified into three main functional groups. The first of these mediate mitogenic and differentiation signals, and the other two are associated with cellular responses to stress and inflammatory cytokines. Members of GTPases homologous to Ras (rho family of GTPases), in particular Cdc42 and Rac, play a role in the initiation of these cascades. The MAP kinase family members operate in three pathways (Figure 8.6):

---

* *c-fos*, from feline osteosarcoma virus, is an oncogene that acts as transcription factor.
** p62[TCF] was first identified as part of a complex of three components, together with p67[SRF] and DNA. It was therefore referred to as *ternary-complex factor*. p62[TCF] is also known as Elk-1.

TABLE 8.2
Some of the Many Influences of, by, and for Ras

Activators (Guanine Nucleotide Exchanger)	Inhibitors (GTPase)	Effectors
hSos	GAP	Raf
CrkL	Neurofibromin	PI$_3$-kinase
ras GRP	—	Ral GDS
Ras GRF2	—	—
Smg GDS	—	—

1. *ERK pathway.* ERK1 and ERK2 are the prototypic MAP kinases described in the previous text. The ERK (extracellular-signal-regulated kinase) family has seven members; however, most of the higher numbered isoforms do not appear to function in the mitogenic pathway.
2. *SAPK/JNK pathway.* Within the SAPK (stress-activated protein kinase) class, the Jun N-terminal kinases (JNKs) form a subfamily (SAPK/JNK1–3).
3. *p38/HOG pathway.* High-osmolarity glycerol (HOG) induced by osmotic stress in yeast (*Saccharomyces cerevisiae*), resulting in the activation of this 38 kDa protein kinase. The p38 MAP kinases form another subfamily of four members.

Each of these pathways involves a kinase cascade resulting in the phosphorylation and activation of the MAP kinase family member. Each contains a dual phosphorylation site (TEY, TPY, or TGY) and the central residue in the motif characteristic of the class, as shown in Table 8.1. It is evident that cells are endowed with parallel signal-transduction pathways and that they may operate individually or in combination to initiate specific patterns of gene expression. Additionally, crosstalk between the pathways undoubtedly occurs. None of these pathways has a unique function; it is more likely that the combination of pathways that are activated (or silenced) together with the

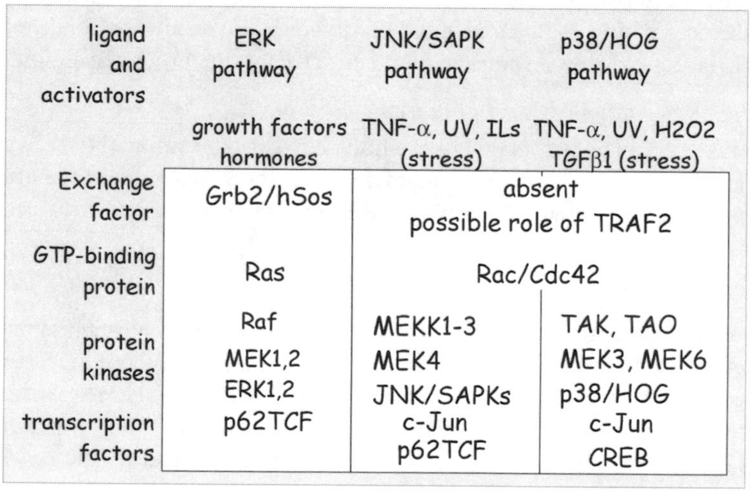

	ERK pathway	JNK/SAPK pathway	p38/HOG pathway
ligand and activators			
	growth factors hormones	TNF-α, UV, ILs (stress)	TNF-α, UV, H2O2 TGFβ1 (stress)
Exchange factor	Grb2/hSos	absent possible role of TRAF2	
GTP-binding protein	Ras	Rac/Cdc42	
protein kinases	Raf MEK1,2 ERK1,2	MEKK1-3 MEK4 JNK/SAPKs	TAK, TAO MEK3, MEK6 p38/HOG
transcription factors	p62TCF	c-Jun p62TCF	c-Jun CREB

FIGURE 8.6 Parallel pathways to transcription and the MAP kinase family. The MAP kinases can be classified into three groups, based on the identity of the intermediate residue in their dual phosphorylation motifs (TEY, TGY, or TPY). This classification also defines three distinct signal-transduction pathways indicated as the ERK, the JNK/SAPK, and the p38/HOG pathway, each having unique protein kinases acting upstream.

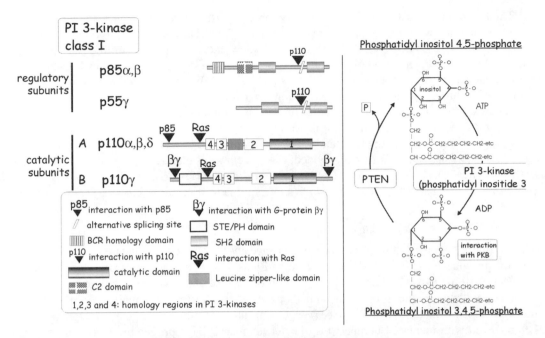

FIGURE 8.7 Classification of phosphatidylinositol-3 kinases (PI-3 kinases). (Left) The enzymes are classified into three groups based on the molecular structure of the subunit that contains the kinase domain. Class I is subdivided into group A and B. Group A contains α, β, and γ, which interact with the regulatory subunits, p85 or p55. Group B has one member, p110γ, regulated by G-protein βγ subunits. It is also found associated with a p101 protein of unknown identity. (Right) The PI-3 kinases phosphorylate the 3OH position in the inositol ring of the phosphatidylinositol lipids. The PH domain of PKB interacts preferentially with the PI-3,4,5-P product. PTEN is an inositol 3-phosphate phosphatase and counteracts the phosphorylation by PI₃-kinase. (Adapted from Vanhaesebroeck et al., *TIBS*, 22, 267–272, 1997.)

cellular context decides the outcome of the response, including proliferation, differentiation, invasion of tissue, or cell death.

8.2.3.2 The PKB Signaling Pathway

The tyrosine phosphorylated growth factor receptors recruit p85$^{PI_3-kinase}$, an adaptor molecule that associates with p110$^{PI_3-kinase}$, and together they form a lipid kinase called phosphatidylinositol-3 kinase (PI₃-kinase). This protein kinase plays an important role in a number of cellular processes: regulation of glycogenesis (in response to insulin), regulation of cell size, migration, survival, and proliferation. In this chapter, we will focus on its role in cellular proliferation (EGF, PDGF) through regulation of protein synthesis and its role in apoptosis (NGF) through inactivation of BAD and caspase-9 and inhibition of nuclear translocation of the transcription factor FKHRL-1.

8.2.3.2.1 PI-3 Kinase

The PI-3 kinases comprise a family of enzymes subdivided in three classes. They have distinct substrates and various forms of regulation. They all have four homologous regions, the kinase domain being most conserved (Figure 8.7). Uniquely, the class I enzymes activate protein kinase B and therefore will be discussed in this chapter. This class of phospholipid kinases phosphorylate PI, PI-4-P, and PI-4,5-P2 (the preferred substrate) at the 3 position of the inositol ring (Figure 8.7). These enzymes have two subunits: regulatory (p55 or p85) and catalytic (p110), each existing in various forms.

The multidomain structure of the regulatory subunit, particularly p85, suggests that they should be able to interact with a number of signaling proteins. The SH2 domains enable them to bind to phosphotyrosine residues, and the SH3 domains allow interaction with proline-rich sequences present, for instance, in the adaptor molecule Shc, the GTPase-activating protein Cdc42GAP, or the regulator of T-lymphocyte receptor (TCR) signaling, Cbl. In addition, the p85 subunit contains a breakpoint cluster region (BCR) homology domain that interacts with members of the Rho family of GTPases, Rac and Cdc42, providing yet further opportunities for regulation.

The catalytic p110 subunit has four isoforms, all of which contain a kinase domain and a Ras interaction site. In addition, the α, β, and γ isoforms possess an interaction site for the p85 subunit. The class I enzymes can be further subdivided; class IA enzymes interact through their SH2 domains with phosphotyrosines present on either protein tyrosine kinases or to docking proteins such as insulin-receptor substrates (IRSs; GAB-1) or linkers for activation of T cells (LATs; in the case of T cells).

8.2.3.2.2 Phosphatidyl Inositol Phosphatases

The phosphorylation of inositol can be counteracted by two lipid phosphatases: SH2-containing inositol phosphatase (SHIP) and phosphatase and tensin homolog deleted from chromosome 10 (PTEN). SHIP dephosphorylates at the 5 position of inositol and was discovered as a protein that associates with the adaptor protein Shc in hemopoietic cells. SHIP plays a major role in modulating the signaling of hemopoietic cell-surface receptors. Its absence, through targeted disruption in mice, is associated with increased numbers of granulocyte–macrophage progenitors and with excessive infiltration of tissues by these cells. PTEN was discovered as a tumor suppresser because inactivating mutations were detected in glioblastomas, melanomas, and breast, prostate, and endometrial carcinomas. Its sequence reveals the characteristics of a dual-specificity protein phosphatase but its favorite substrates are phosphoinositides. It dephosphorylates at the 3 position of the inositol ring, counteracting the phosphorylation by PI$_3$-kinase (Figure 8.7). Ectopic expression in PTEN-deficient tumor cells results in arrest of the cell cycle in the G$_1$ phase eventually followed by apoptosis. It also reduces cell migration, a finding that may explain why the loss of the gene product is frequently associated with late-stage metastatic tumors.

8.2.3.2.3 Activation of PI-3 Kinase

The EGF and PDGF receptors directly bind the p85-adaptor subunit of PI$_3$-kinase through the interaction of their phosphorylated tyrosine residues with the SH2 domain of the adaptor. This recruitment is most likely enforced by a simultaneous binding of activated Ras to the p110-catalytic domain of the lipid kinase. In the case of NGF, the situation is different. Activation of the NGF receptor (TrkA) causes the phosphorylation of a "docking protein" at a number of tyrosine residues. This docking protein, named Grb2-associated binder 1 (Gab-1) resembles one of the main substrates of the insulin receptors, IRS-1, a protein with a similar function. The SH2 domain of the p85-adaptor protein now binds to Gab-1. Binding of PI$_3$-kinase to the activated receptor or docking protein recruits it to the membrane and brings it into contact with the phospholipids (its substrate), which constitutes its activation. Importantly, the subsequent generation of PI-3,4,5-P3 results in activation of a serine/threonine protein kinase B (PKB).

8.2.3.2.4 Protein Kinase B and Activation through PI-3,4,5-P3

Protein kinase B, or Akt, was discovered as the product of an oncogene of the acutely transforming retrovirus AKT8, causing T-cell lymphomas in mice. It encodes a fusion product of a cellular serine/threonine protein kinase and the viral structural protein Gag. This kinase is similar to both protein kinase Cϵ (PKCϵ; 73% identity to the catalytic domain) and protein kinase A (PKA; 68%). It differs from other protein kinases in that it contains a pleckstrin homology (PH) domain, which allows it to bind to polyphosphoinositide head groups (and also to G-protein $\beta\gamma$ subunits). To date, three subtypes have been identified: α, β, and γ, all of which show a broad tissue distribution. It

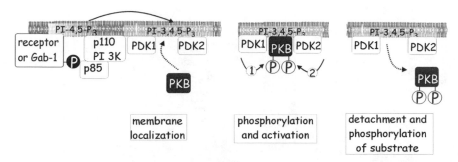

FIGURE 8.8 Mechanism of activation of protein kinase B (PKB). PI$_3$-kinase is recruited to the membrane via direct association with the receptor PTK or via association with the docking protein Gab-1. It catalyzes the generation of phosphatidyl-3,4,5-inositolphosphate, which serves as a membrane-recruitment signal for PKB. Associated with the membrane, it is first phosphorylated in its catalytic domain by PDK1 and then by PDK2 in the hydrophobic motif. The activated PKB then detaches from the membrane.

was found that PI-3 kinase, through the production of PI-3,4,5-P3 is the activator of PKB. The mechanism of this activation has turned out a multistep process, with the phospholipid playing two distinct roles. One of these is direct, recruiting PKB to the membrane through binding of the lipid head-group to the PH domain in the N-terminal segment. The other interaction is indirect, involving the recruitment of two soluble protein kinases, PDK1 and PDK2 (3-phosphoinositide-dependent protein kinase 1 and 2), also endowed with a PH domain. Binding of PI-3,4,5-P3 is crucial, as it enables PDK1, PDK2, and PKB to come together (Figure 8.8). PDK1 phosphorylates PKB in its catalytic loop, but the full activation signal requires a second phosphorylation in the C-terminal domain. This reaction is dependent on PDK2, which has yet to be properly identified. Double phosphorylation of PKB causes its detachment from the membrane, and this enables it to interact with its substrates elsewhere in the cell. The viral oncogene product, v-Akt, has a lipid anchor (myristoyl group), which means that the protein kinase is already located at the membrane, which may facilitate its activation.

8.2.3.2.5 PKB and Regulation of Protein Synthesis

The PI$_3$-kinase/PKB pathway regulates protein synthesis through activation of the eukaryotic translation initiator factor-4E (eIF-4E) and the ribosomal protein kinase p70 S6-kinase. eIF-4E is the limiting initiation factor of protein synthesis in most cells, and its activity plays a principal role in determining global translation rates. It is regulated by phosphorylation (for instance, through the MAP kinase pathway) but also by binding to translational repressor proteins, 4E-BPs. These repressors are inactivated by phosphorylation. The S6 protein is a component of the 40S ribosome subunit, and its phosphorylation increases the rate of translation, resulting in enhanced protein synthesis. The S6 component is phosphorylated by S6 kinase, for which several isoforms have been identified, one of which is p70-S6 kinase. Their activities are regulated by insulin, growth factors, or glucagon. Both 4E-BP1 and p70-S6 kinase are under the control of PKB, but this is indirect, involving yet another protein kinase, FKBP-rapamycin-associated protein (FRAP)/mTOR, a human homolog of the yeast TOR gene (Figure 8.9). This protein kinase was initially recognized as the target of rapamycin, an immunosuppressant and inhibitor of protein synthesis. FRAP/mTOR phosphorylates 4E-BP1, which causes the release of eIF-4E, which can now participate in initiation of protein synthesis. It also phosphorylates p70-S6 kinase, which has a stimulatory effect on protein translation.

8.2.3.2.6 Activation of PKB and Regulation of cyclinD Expression

Another substrate of PKB is glycogen synthase kinase 3β (GSK3β), whose phosphorylation causes its inactivation. As its name indicates, this protein kinase was originally discovered as a regulator

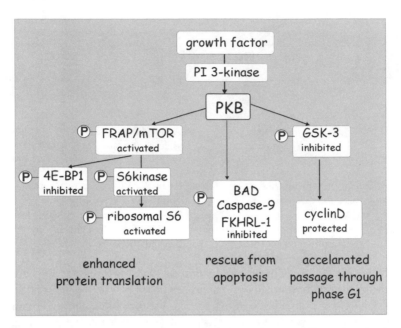

FIGURE 8.9 Regulation of protein synthesis, cell cycle, and survival. (A) Through activation of PKB, PI-3 kinase controls initiation and translation in protein synthesis. Activated PKB phosphorylates and activates the protein kinase FRAP, which phosphorylates 4E-BP1, an inhibitor of the initiation factor eIF-4E. The liberated eIF-4E attaches to the cap structure of mRNA and, by ironing out a hairpin, facilitates the association of eIF-2GTP and the 40S ribosomal subunit. FRAP also phosphorylates and activates p70S6 kinase which in turn phosphorylates the S6 protein of the 40S ribosomal subunit. Phosphorylated S6 increases the efficiency of protein translation. (B) PKB controls the stability of cyclinD1 at two levels. It phosphorylates and inactivates GSK3β, thereby preventing the phosphorylation of cyclinD1 and hence its ubiquitin-mediated destruction. PKB also phosphorylates and activates FRAP through which it regulates stability of cyclinD1 mRNA and the protein itself by an as yet unclear pathway (not shown). (C) PKB controls cell survival through sequestration of FKHRL in the cytosol and inactivation of BAD and caspase-9.

of glycogen synthase. GSK3β also plays an important role in the destruction of protein mediated via the ubiquitination pathway. When cyclinD1 is phosphorylated by GSK3β, it becomes ubiquitinated, a process that involves the addition of a number of small ubiquitin peptides in sequence, which serve as a recognition signal for the 26S proteosome cellular-protein-destruction machinery. Phosphorylation and inhibition of GSK3β by PKB, therefore, prevents destruction of cyclinD1 (Figure 8.9).

In addition, activation of PKB also enhances transcription of the cyclinD1 gene, although the signal-transduction pathway causing this effect has not yet been revealed. The combination of an increased expression and a reduced destruction causes accumulation in the cell of the cyclinD1 protein. CyclinD1, associated with its catalytic subunit, cyclin-dependent kinase 4 or 6 (CDK4 or 6) is the driving force of the cell cycle during the G_1 phase; therefore, it is one of the most important cyclins in regulating cellular proliferation.

8.2.3.2.7 PKB and Cellular Survival

As mentioned earlier, NGF is not considered a true growth factor; on the contrary, its presence causes neurite outgrowth in PC12 cells, a sign of cellular differentiation. It also has an important role in neuronal survival. Neurons starved of NGF initiate a process of programmed cell death, apoptosis. The presence of NGF must somehow maintain an intracellular survival signal, and PKB plays an important role in this event because it induces a number of phosphorylations that rescue cells from apoptosis. PKB promotes rescue through at least two pathways (Figure 8.9). One is through direct phosphorylation and inactivation of components of the apoptotic machinery, including BAD and caspase-9. BAD, a member of the Bcl-2 family of regulators of apoptosis, promotes dimerization and activation of the initiator caspases (those that initiate the process of apoptosis). Caspases are proteases that contain a cysteine in their catalytic site and cleave protein at an asparate residue, hence their name (cysteine-asparate proteases). Caspase-9 is one such initiator caspase, and its role is to cleave and activate other so-called effector caspases, those that destroy vital components of the cell (inhibitors of DNA nucleases, DNA repair enzymes, and components of the cytoskeleton). PKB can also directly phosphorylate caspase-9, rendering the enzyme less sensitive to activation. The other type of protection is offered by phosphorylation of FKHR-L1, a transcription factor (member of the *Drosophila* forkhead/winged-helix family AFX, FKHR, and FKHR-L1, which are orthologs of DAF-16, a forkhead factor that regulates longevity in *Caenorhabditis elegans*). When phosphorylated, FKHRL1 is retained in the cytosol and is prevented from activating genes critical for induction of factors that promote cell death such as Fas ligand. Once expressed, Fas ligand will bind to the cell-surface receptor and induce receptor trimerization, resulting in the activation of initiator caspases. This event will inevitably result in cell death.

8.2.3.3 The PLCγ and Protein Kinase C Signal-Transduction Pathway

8.2.3.3.1 PKC, a Family of Protein Kinases

Among the activities set in motion by activation of the EGF and PDGF receptors is the generation of diacylglycerol (DAG) and inositol-1,4,5-phosphate (IP$_3$) by PLCγ. The DAG remains in the membrane and acts as a stimulus for PKC. The consequence is the transformation of a phosphotyrosine signal through activation of PLCγ into a phosphoserine/phosphothreonine signal. One of the first substrates of PKC is the EGF receptor itself. This becomes phosphorylated on a serine residue very close to the transmembrane domain and has the effect of inactivating the receptor. The mammalian PKCs comprise a family of 12 distinct members which can be subdivided into three subfamilies classified on the basis of sequence similarities and their modes of activation. The subfamilies are conventional PKCs (cPKCs), including α, β$_1$, β$_2$, and γ; novel PKCs (nPKCs), including δ, ε, η, and θ; and atypical PKCs (aPKCs), including λ, ι, ζ, and μ (PKD). Some of their characteristics are presented in Table 8.3.

The majority of these members are a receptor for phorbol esters, the tumor-promoting products obtained from croton oil. One of them, 12-*O*-tetradecanoylphorbol-13-acetate (TPA), is a potent

---

TABLE 8.3
Some Characteristics of the Different Members of the Protein Kinase C (PKC) Family

	Conventional PKC	Novel PKC	Atypical PKC
Requirement for Activation			
DAG	Yes	Yes	No
Ca^{2+}	Yes	No	No
Phospholipid	Yes	Yes	Yes
Conserved Domains			
Pseudo substrate	Yes	Yes	Yes
C1, DAG binding	Yes	Yes	Yes
C2, Ca^{2+} binding	Yes	Yes	No
C3, catalytic	Yes	Yes	Yes
C4, catalytic	Yes	Yes	Yes

activator of PKC. With the aim of understanding the mechanisms of action of PKC that underlie tumor promotion by phorbol esters, two independent experimental strategies have been applied. One involves searching for transcriptional control elements that mediate the phorbol-ester-induced alterations in gene expression and then working backwards to identify the transcription factors that bind these elements and finally the signal-transduction pathway that regulates their activation. The second approach has been to overexpress various isoforms of PKC and to study changes in cell phenotype. Despite an immense effort, the role of PKC in tumor promotion remains far from clear, and PKC has failed to qualify as a true oncogene.

8.2.3.3.2 PKC and Activation of TRE and SRE by Phorbol Ester

Analysis of the promoter regions of TPA-inducible genes (for instance, collagenase, metallothionein IIA, and stromelysin) revealed a conserved seven-base-pair palindromic motif (TGACTCA). This TPA-responsive element (TRE) is recognized by activator protein 1 (AP-1). At that time, it was understood that AP-1 is at the receiving end of a complex pathway that transmits the effects of phorbol ester tumor promoters from the plasma membrane to the transcriptional machinery, possibly involving protein kinase C. AP-1 encompasses a group of dimeric transcription factor complexes composed of Jun–Jun, Jun–Fos, or Jun–ATF,* known oncogenes linked by a protein–protein inter-action motif known as a leucine zipper. The oncogenic variants of these transcription factors have increased half-lives and show enhanced transcriptional activity as a consequence of partial deletions.

It was found that activation of PKC causes the dephosphorylation of c-Jun only in the basic region where it binds DNA. Phosphorylation of this segment can also be achieved (in the test tube) by glycogen synthase kinase 3β (GSK-3β), so it was postulated that PKC stimulates the binding of c-Jun DNA through the inhibition of GSK-3β (Figure 8.10). This would result in the dephos-phorylation of the basic region. Consistent with this idea is that activation of PKC (α, β_1, β_2, and γ) causes phosphorylation and thus deactivation of GSK-3β. However, a molecular interaction between GSK-3β and c-Jun has not been demonstrated nor is it clear which phosphatase strips the phosphate residues from c-Jun. That this cannot be the whole story became clear from the finding that phosphorylation at the N-terminus is also crucial for both transcriptional activity and cell transformation by c-Jun.

The discovery of a Jun N-terminal protein kinase (JNK-1) that phosphorylates c-Jun through interaction with a specific kinase docking site drew the field away from PKC and TRE and focused attention on the serum-response element (SRE) and the newly emerging family of MAP kinases. In addition to its role in regulating serum-mediated expression of the transcription factor c-fos, the SRE is also involved in the cellular response to phorbol ester. As already mentioned, the SRE binds two transcription factors: the serum-response factor (SRF) and the ternary-complex factor p62^{TCF} (Elk-1). Growth factors regulate the transcriptional activity through phosphorylation of p62^{TCF}, a mode of activation that also applies for phorbol ester.

8.2.3.3.3 PKC and Modulation of the MAP Kinase Signal-Transduction Pathways

As the signal-transduction pathway emanating from growth-factor receptors that activate the SRE was gradually resolved and found to involve Ras and members of the MAP kinase family, the role of PKC remained obscure. PKCϵ was found to activate the Ras-activated kinase c-Raf, and the two enzymes cooperate in the transformation of NIH3T3 fibroblasts. In rat embryo fibroblasts, activation of Raf-1 is also essential for the transforming effect of PKC. Because all growth factors induce the generation of DAG and hence activate PKC, it follows that PKC enforces the Ras-initiated growth factor signal at the level of Raf-1. However, this does not necessarily result in enhanced

---

* Adenovirus transcription factor (ATF) is a protein activated by the adenovirus protein E2a and has turned out to be CREB (cAMP-responsive, element-binding protein); Jun is named for avian sarcoma virus 17 (I am told that *junana* is 17 in Japanese).

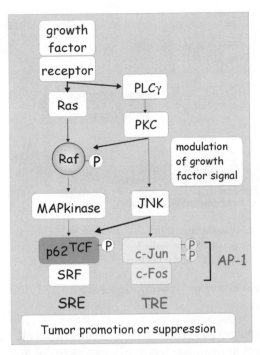

FIGURE 8.10 Protein kinase C (PKC) and activation of the TPA-responsive element (TRE) and serum-response element (SRE). PKC and growth factors were initially thought to activate distinct signal-transduction pathways, resulting in the activation of TRE and SRE, respectively. This notion ended when it was realized that TPA also activates the SRE and that growth factors can activate the TRE through activation of Jun N-terminal kinase (JNK). PKC may have an important role in modulation of both of the different MAP kinase pathways. Its particular effect on GSK3β, resulting in the dephosphorylation of the basic region of c-Jun, may also serve to enhance the action of JNK, a protein kinase that phosphorylates the N-terminal region and promotes dimerization of the transcription factor.

cell proliferation. More recent findings using kinase-dead and constitutively activated mutants confirm that several PKC isoforms can activate the MAP kinase pathway, in some cases leading to the activation of both MAP kinase (ERK) and JNK. This dual signal reintegrates at the level of phosphorylation of p62^{TCF} (Figure 8.10). Activation of JNK could equally result in the phosphorylation of c-Jun, resulting in the activation of AP-1 at a TRE site. Collectively, these studies suggest that PKC acts primarily as a modulator of the Ras signal-transduction pathways that emanate from growth-factor receptors. The commitment, either to promote or to suppress activity, is determined at the level of the MAP kinases.

8.2.3.4 The Ca²⁺/Calmodulin Pathway

The cleavage of phosphatidyl inositol-4,5-phosphate (PIP$_2$) by PLCγ results in the liberation of IP$_3$, which binds to its receptor at the endoplasmic reticulum, thus opening Ca²⁺ channels. The resulting elevation of cytosolic free Ca²⁺ causes the activation of a number of serine/threonine protein kinases, all containing a Ca²⁺-binding regulatory subunit, calmodulin (also present in a number of other enzymes; see Figure 8.11). These include the broad-spectrum Ca²⁺/calmodulin-dependent protein kinase II (CaMKII), myosin light-chain kinase (MLCK), phosphorylase kinase, and elongation factor 2 kinase (EF-2 kinase), in addition to the protein phosphatase calcineurin, an essential player in the activation of T lymphocytes. Clearly, Ca²⁺ is an extremely versatile second messenger modulating numerous intracellular signals, a subject too vast to deal with in a single book chapter.

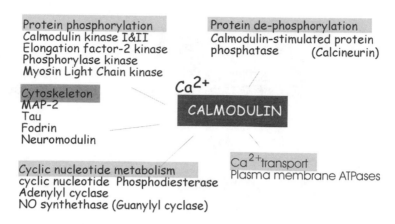

FIGURE 8.11 Multiple signal-transduction pathways initiated by calmodulin. Calmodulin bound to Ca^{2+} interacts and activates many enzymes, opening up a wide range of possible cellular responses. Abbreviations: MAP-2, microtubule-associated protein 2; NO, nitric oxide; Tau, tubulin assembly unit.

8.2.3.5 Direct Phosphorylation of Transcription Factors and Activation of STATs

The simplest way in which a plasma membrane receptor could alter gene expression would be by direct phosphorylation of transcription factors. The activation of transcription by the interferons is an example. Transcription factors known as STATs (signal transducers and activators of transcription) were recognized as targets for interferon receptors, but it is now apparent that they also mediate the signals of EGF and PDGF receptors. The STATs p84[Stat1a] and p91[Stat1b] are recruited to the tyrosine-phosphorylated growth factor receptor via their SH2 domains. Following phosphorylation, they combine, through mutual interaction of their SH2 domains, with the tyrosine phosphates to form a dimeric complex; as a consequence, they translocate to the nucleus, where they promote transcription of early response genes such as *c-fos* (Figure 8.12). The STAT dimer, formed after tyrosine phosphorylation by the PDGF receptor, was originally described as simian-sarcoma-virus-inducible factor (SIF), a transcription factor complex activated by the viral oncogene, v-Sis. This viral oncogene codes for the precursor of PDGF and activates a similar signal-transduction pathway.

8.3 RECEPTORS THAT ASSOCIATE WITH PROTEIN TYROSINE KINASES

8.3.1 Family of Nonreceptor Protein Tyrosine Kinases

This section deals with an important family of receptors that have no intrinsic catalytic activity but nevertheless induce responses similar to those of the receptor tyrosine kinases. The question of how they signal was resolved with the finding that many of these receptors recruit catalytic subunits from within the cell in the form of one or more nonreceptor protein tyrosine kinases (nonreceptor PTKs). These can be divided into nine families: Abl, Fes/Fer, Syk/Zap70, Jak, Tec, Fak, Ack, Src, and Csk. Four additional nonreceptor PTKs (Rlk/Txk, Srm, Rak/Frk, and Brk/Sik) do not appear to belong to any of the defined families (Figure 8.13). These proteins exist within the cytosol as soluble components, or they may be membrane associated through farnesylation (C15 isoprenoid) or palmitoylation (C16) of the C-terminal region (Src, Fyn, Lyn, or Yes) or through the presence of a PH domain (Btk/Tec family members). A large number of vertebrate genes encode for nonreceptor PTKs (a minimum of 33). Recruitment of nonreceptor PTKs and the consequent tyrosine phosphorylations are usually the first steps in the assembly of a substantial signaling complex consisting of a dozen or more proteins that bind and interact with each other.

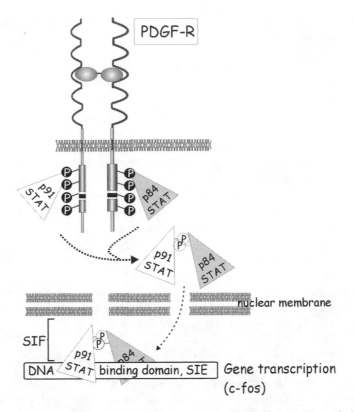

FIGURE 8.12 Direct phosphorylation of the STAT class of transcription factors. Through their SH2 domains, the p84$^{\text{Stat1a}}$ and p91$^{\text{Stat1b}}$ associate with the receptor and become phosphorylated on tyrosine residues. They form a dimer (called the Sis-inducible factor, or SIF) that translocates to the nucleus, where it binds to a Sis-inducible element (SIE) and activates transcription of, for example, the *c-fos* gene.

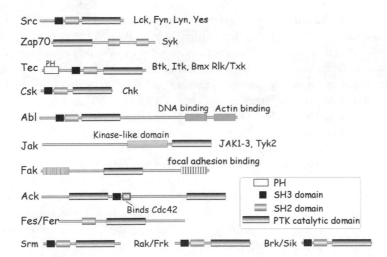

FIGURE 8.13 Nonreceptor PTKs. These protein kinases form a large family, and most of them contain SH2 and SH3 domains. Several were originally discovered as transforming genes of a viral genome, hence names such as src or abl, derived from Rous sarcoma virus or Abelson murine leukemia virus, respectively. (Adapted from Hunter, T., *Biochem. Soc. Trans.*, 24(2), 307–327, 1996.)

Examples of the class of receptors that recruit nonreceptor PTKs include those that mediate immune and inflammatory responses:

- The T-lymphocyte receptor (TCR) is involved in detection of foreign antigens, presented together with the major histocompatibility complex (MHC). Subsequently, it regulates the clonal expansion of T cells.
- The B lymphocyte receptor for antigen is important in the first line of defense against infection by microorganisms.
- The interleukin-2 receptor (IL-2R) is important in that the cytokine IL-2, secreted by a subset of T-helper cells, enhances the proliferation of activated T and B cells and increases the cytolytic activity of natural killer (NK) cells and the secretion of IgG.
- Immunoglobulin receptors, such as the high affinity receptor for IgE, are present on mast cells and bloodborne basophils. These receptors play an important role in hypersensitivity and the initiation of acute inflammatory responses.

For other cells, such as endothelial or epithelial cells:

- Integrins present in focal adhesion complexes cause the recruitment of two types of protein tyrosine kinases to the plasma membrane: focal adhesion kinase (FAK) and Src. They play a role in cell survival and proliferation.

8.3.2 MODE OF ACTIVATION OF NONRECEPTOR PROTEIN TYROSINE KINASES

The nonreceptor PTKs are a large group of signaling proteins that have diverse roles in the control of cell proliferation, differentiation, and death. Some are widely expressed; others are restricted to particular tissues. Their early classification was dominated by the discovery of pp60^{src}, to the extent that the major group of kinases were simply known as the Src family. There are at least ten known subfamilies of nonreceptor PTKs.

The Src family kinases share a similar structure. A unique domain at the N-terminus is followed by an SH2 domain and an SH3 domain (prototypes of the domains that are widely expressed). The SH3 domain is then attached by a linking region to a kinase domain and finally a C-terminal tail (see Figure 8.13). Many of these kinases function by becoming associated with macromolecular signaling complexes assembled at membrane sites. Membrane association may be promoted by the unique N-terminal domain. Within the Src family, Src itself (pp60^{c-src}), Fyn, Lyn, and Yes are N-terminal myristoylated. This 14-carbon aliphatic chain provides the opportunity for membrane attachment that may be strengthened by palmitoylation at a nearby cysteine. Similarly, members of the Btk/Tec family may become membrane associated through their PH domains, which can bind polyphosphoinositide lipids. Other nonreceptor PTKs are recruited to their sites of action through the association of their SH2 domains with phosphotyrosine residues on their targets.

Regardless of their location, most Src family kinases are generally inactive. They are commonly held in this state by a crucial phosphorylated tyrosine (in pp60^{c-Src}, Y527 in the C-terminus) which engages N-terminal SH2 domain. Furthermore, a sequence in the linker takes on a structure that resembles a proline-rich region, so that it binds to the SH3 domain. These interactions cause the molecule to adopt a compact structure. The bending of the carboxyl tail causes a rotation of the smaller lobe of the kinase domain, which distorts the active site. Activation therefore requires removal of the C-terminal phosphate, made possible because the sequence of amino acids immediately adjacent to the phosphotyrosine is not optimal for tight binding to the SH2 domain. SH2 domains bind phosphotyrosines most effectively when they reside in a pYEEI motif. An equivalent sequence in the Src C-terminus lacks the isoleucine at pY+3 and is not so tightly bound. This gives the opportunity for access by a phosphatase (such as CD45 in lymphocytes) (Figure 8.14). Having lost the carboxyl-tail phosphate, the activation loop at the edge of the catalytic site can then become

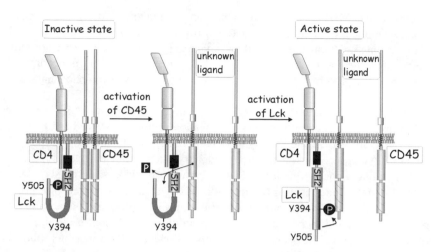

FIGURE 8.14 Activation of nonreceptor PTKs. Lck is held in an inaccessible compact state through phosphorylation of residue Y505, which interacts with the intramolecular SH2 domain. Upon activation of CD45 (ligand unknown), the pY505 is removed and the molecule opens up. Autophosphorylation at the Y-394 residue in the catalytic domain constitutes the activation of the PTK.

phosphorylated, greatly increasing the catalytic activity. Activation of Src family kinases therefore requires first a dephosphorylation and then a phosphorylation.

8.3.3 T CELL RECEPTOR SIGNALING

8.3.3.1 Activation of T Lymphocytes and Interaction between TCR and MHC

T lymphocytes have a central role in cell-mediated immunity. When activated, they proliferate and differentiate to become either cytotoxic (NK) or helper (Th) T cells. Cytotoxic T cells kill specific targets, most commonly virus-infected cells, while helper T cells assist other cells of the immune system, such as B lymphocytes (to induce the production of antibodies) and macrophages (to augment the release of inflammatory cytokines that enables an effective host defense). T lymphocytes are activated through interaction with cells that present antigen in the context of a major histocompatibility complex (MHC). The cell–cell interaction occurs in the following manner. The selective event is the recognition of an antigen placed in the groove of the MHC by the T-cell receptor (TCR). In the case of an intracellular or viral antigen, protein fragments (antigens) are presented by MHC class I; in case of a microbial infection antigens, they are presented by MHC class II. Before the lymphocyte becomes fully activated, the interaction between the antigen-presenting cell and the T lymphocyte has to be enforced by a number of other interactions, such as CD4 (or CD8) interacting with MHC and B7 with CD28 (among others). The full response comprises induction of expression of IL-2 and its receptor followed by autocrine stimulation, resulting in cell proliferation, an event also referred to as clonal expansion.

8.3.3.2 Signal Transduction Downstream of TCRs

In spite of having no intrinsic catalytic domains, activation of T lymphocytes commences with tyrosine phosphorylations, activation of PLC-γ with production of IP_3 and DAG, and elevation of cytosolic free Ca^{2+}. Thus, the consequences of receptor ligation are not dissimilar from those induced by the receptors for EGF or PDGF. An early study trying to explain the induction of tyrosine kinase activity resulted in the discovery of the nonreceptor protein tyrosine kinase Lck (p56[lck]), a T-cell-specific member of the Src family. Lck is associated with the cytosolic tail of CD4 (in helper T cells) or CD8 (in cytotoxic T cells) (Figure 8.14). As mentioned, the extracellular domains of these molecules bind to the MHC protein, which not only strengthens the rather weak interaction established between the TCR and antigen but also brings CD4 (or CD8) into the vicinity of the TCR complex, leading Lck to its targets on the ?–chains. However, as with other Src family kinases, Lck is inactive until specific residues have been dephosphorylated. This is accomplished by yet another transmembrane protein, CD45, which possesses protein tyrosine phosphatase activity (see Figure 8.14)

Activation of Lck results in the phosphorylation of the ζ-chains of the TCR. The target tyrosines are confined to immunoreceptor tyrosine-based activation motifs (ITAMs). ITAMs are also present in the α, δ, and ε chains of CD3 and are targets of another Src family kinase, Fyn (p59^{fyn}) associated with the ε chain. Fyn is also activated by dephosphorylation. Both Fyn and Lck are needed for efficient TCR signaling. Phosphorylation of ITAMs provides docking sites for SH2 domain-bearing molecules, and the immediate result is the recruitment of yet another nonreceptor protein tyrosine kinase, ZAP-70 (ζ-chain-associated protein tyrosine kinase of 70 kDa). Once bound, this in turn becomes phosphorylated and thereby activated, causing phosphorylation of multiple substrates. As with growth factor receptors, the sequence of events follows a pattern in which phosphotyrosines bind SH2-domain-containing (or PTB-) proteins that may themselves be PTKs and can phosphorylate other proteins in succession. At each stage, there is the opportunity for branching, through a range of effectors. By successive recruitment, an extensive signaling complex is assembled that includes multiple effector enzymes (Figure 8.15). An important branch-point is offered by the

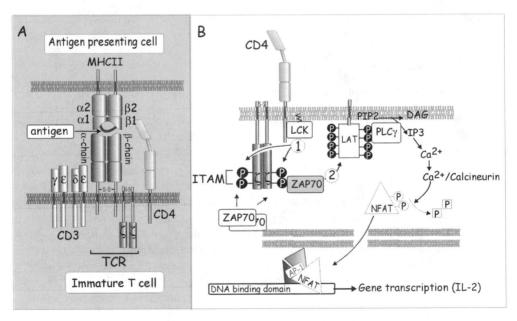

FIGURE 8.15 Clonal expansion of naïve T lymphocytes through signaling from the TCR. (A) The TCR possesses a disulfide-linked heterodimer of α and β chains. These have hypervariable regions that detect the antigen, presented as a short peptide in the groove of an MHC molecule. This heterodimer along with two ?-chains, forms a complex with four polypeptides (γε and γδ) of the CD3 molecule. CD4 and CD8 molecules are also associated with the TCR in helper and cytotoxic T cells, respectively. These molecules bind to the MHC and bring Lck, a nonreceptor PTK, into the vicinity of the ζ-chains. (B) The TCR activates Lck, which phosphorylates the two ζ-chains in the ITAM motif. The phosphotyrosine residues form a docking site for the SH2 domain of ZAP70, another cytosolic PTK, which, in turn, phosphorylates several (maximally nine) tyrosine residues on the transmembrane adaptor protein LAT. Various proteins attach to LAT, including the guanine exchange factor Vav, the adaptor Grb2, the adaptor subunit of PI-3 kinase, and PLC-γ. All of these play important roles in the activation of the IL-2 gene. The elevation of intracellular Ca^{2+} activates calcineurin, which dephosphorylates NF-AT (nuclear factor of activated T cells). Together with the AP-1 complex, NF-AT drives the transcription of the IL-2 gene.

integral membrane protein LAT (linker for activation of T cells), which presents no less than nine substrate tyrosine residues. When phosphorylated, these recruit a broad range of signaling molecules, all through interaction with SH2 domains. These include the adaptor proteins Grb2, SLP76 (SH2-domain-containing leukocyte protein of 76 kDa, an adaptor protein), the enzymes PLC-γ PI$_3$-kinase (through its p85 regulatory subunit), and the guanine nucleotide exchange factors Dbl and Vav.

The signaling complex formed around the TCR and the branching pathways that emanate from it resemble the mechanisms used by the growth factors. However, the destinations of these pathways are not all clear. The PLC-γ pathway (DAG, IP$_3$, and elevation of intracellular free Ca^{2+}) leads to activation of the phosphatase calcineurin, which activates the transcription factor NF-AT (nuclear factor of activated T cells). This is essential for clonal expansion of T cells because of its pivotal role in the induction of IL-2 expression. NF-AT requires the assistance of the activator protein 1 (AP-1) complex in order to drive expression of IL-2.

8.3.3.3 The IgE Receptor and a Signal for Exocytosis

Tissue mast cells and circulating basophils are of hematopoietic lineage. Best known for their roles in allergy, they mediate both immediate and delayed hypersensitivity reactions. They also help to defend the body against bacterial and parasitic infections and take part in inflammatory responses. Their immunological stimulus is provided by polyvalent antigen that binds and cross-links IgE, which itself is bound to a high-affinity immunoglobulin receptor, IgE-R (specifically, FcεRI). Initially, the signaling mechanism has similarities with that of lymphocytes in that it involves the successive recruitment of tyrosine kinases and SH2-domain-containing proteins (adaptors and effectors).

The IgE-receptor aggregation sets in motion a series of events. The immediate consequence is the secretion of preformed products stored in secretory granules which takes place within a few minutes. The released substances include vasoactive agents and mediators of inflammation (histamine, proteoglycans, neutral proteases, acid hydrolases). Then, over minutes to hours, the cells synthesize and secrete cytokines (among others, IL-2 and IL-6) and arachidonate-derived inflammatory mediators, such as the leukotriene LTB$_4$. The formation of new granules and recovery of cell morphology then continues over a period extending from hours to weeks.

The initial events that follow receptor aggregation involve the recruitment of Src-family tyrosine kinases, including Lyn and Syk. Like the T cell receptor, the IgE-R is located together with the scaffold protein LAT in a lipid raft (microdomain). Phosphorylation of LAT by Syk provides a docking site for a number of SH2 domain-containing proteins (Figure 8.16). Of these, Vav is of importance because it regulates activation of members of the Rho family of GTPases. Vav is endowed with numerous domains that enable it to integrate diverse incoming and outgoing signals. These include one SH2 domain, two SH3 domains, a Dbl homology (DH) domain, a pleckstrin homology (PH) domain, a leucine-rich region, and a cysteine-rich region. The DH domain, in particular, is characteristic of the guanine nucleotide exchange factors that catalyze GTP/GDP exchange on Rho-family GTPases. These mediate diverse cellular responses, including the reorganization of the cytoskeleton and the regulation of the Jun N-terminal kinases. In mast cells, Cdc42 and Rac play two important roles. Their activation is the key determining step committing cells to undergo exocytosis. The steps linking these GTPases to the proteins that regulate membrane fusion remain unknown. Second, they are involved in the regulation of interleukin release, a response that involves activation of JNK.

A second pathway of activation in mast cells is triggered by agents such as the wasp venom peptide mastoparan. Rather than interacting with cell-surface receptors, such "receptor-mimetic" agents are able to insert into the membrane to cause direct activation of heterotrimeric G-proteins of the Gi class. Here, it is the β subunits of the G-protein that provide the signal for exocytosis. As in the pathway from the IgE-R, it is possible that Vav participates in the integration of these signals, as it possesses a PH domain (binds β subunits) and has guanine nucleotide exchange activity.

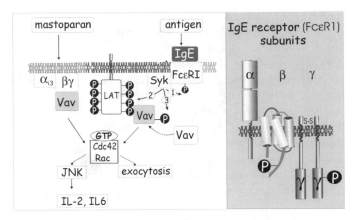

FIGURE 8.16 The role of nonreceptor PTK in IgE-mediated exocytosis in mast cells. Binding of IgE to its receptor FcεRI results in activation of the nonreceptor PTK syk, which phosphorylates three targets: the receptor itself, the docking protein LAT, and the exchange factor Dbl. The exchange factor activates the GTPases Cdc42 and Rac, both of which play a role in the immediate exocytosis of the vesicles that contain inflammatory mediators and in the long-term release of cytokines, an event that requires activation of JNK.

8.3.3.4 Integrin Signaling

8.3.3.4.1 The Role of FAK in Rescue from Apoptosis

The survival of endothelial and epithelial cells depends critically upon the contacts with each other and with the extracellular matrix. Without contact, they die through the controlled process of cell death, apoptosis. In the case of cell detachment, the situation provoking programmed cell death has been called *anoikis*, meaning homelessness. This mechanism protects the organism against dysplastic growth (meaning wrongly formed), preventing stray cells from colonizing inappropriate locations. Cells have an intrinsic drive to self-destruct but are normally prevented from doing this by signals emanating from specific rescue pathways. One such signal (outside-in) follows from the attachment of the integrin $\alpha_5\beta_1$ to the extracellular matrix.

When fibroblasts spread on fibronectin, an abundant component of the extracellular matrix, members of the integrin family of adhesion molecules, mainly $\alpha_5\beta_1$ and $\alpha_V\beta_3$, form multimeric clusters that attach to the cytoskeleton at focal adhesion sites. These are composed of a number of proteins, some having structural roles, others signaling. Together they form a focal adhesion complex as depicted in Figure 8.17. The important structural components vinculin and talin form a binding site for the actin cytoskeleton and thus direct the formation of stress fibers and actin structures within the cortical region of the cell. Talin also forms the site of attachment for the tyrosine kinase FAK (focal adhesion kinase). Attachment resulting in activation and autophosphorylation (at Tyr-397) enables FAK to act as a docking site for the SH2 domain of the p85-regulatory subunit of PI-3 kinase, leading to the generation of phosphatidyl inositide 3-phosphate lipids.

Downstream in the pathway of rescue, PKB effects a number of phosphorylations that prevent apoptosis (Figure 8.17) (see Section 8.2.3.2). It is of interest to note that both growth factor receptors, such as TrkA, and adhesion molecules generate rescue signals through activation of protein tyrosine kinases, and apparently cells require both attachment to extracellular matrix and the presence of a particular growth factor in order not to die.

The importance of FAK is underlined by the finding that cells expressing a constitutively active form survive in suspension even though they are "homeless." Here, the protein kinase is active regardless of the failure to make contact with an extracellular matrix. Rescue from apoptosis also occurs when cells express constitutively activated oncogenic forms of Ras or Src and thus activate PI$_3$-kinase and the MAP kinase pathway. Unlike FAK, these not only prevent apoptosis but also promote proliferative signals that result in tumor formation.

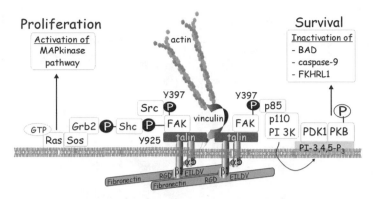

FIGURE 8.17 Survival and proliferation. The focal adhesion site promotes cell survival signals through activation of protein kinase B (PKB). As tissue cells spread out on an extracellular matrix, focal adhesion sites are formed. These are composed of clustered β_1 integrins associated with talin, vinculin, and the actin cytoskeleton. The focal adhesion kinase (FAK) attaches to talin, autophosphorylates on a tyrosine residue (Y397), and provides the activation signal for PI-3 kinase. Production of PI-3,4,5-P3, which acts as a binding site for the PH domains of PDK1 and PKB, follows. PKB is phosphorylated on two serine/threonine residues and detaches from the membrane to phosphorylate and inactivate substrates that would otherwise sensitize the cells to apoptosis. These include BAD, caspase-9, and the transcription factor FKHRL-1. The focal adhesion site promotes cell proliferation signals through activation of Ras. Autophosphorylation of FAK (Y397) also generates a docking site for Src, which phosphorylates FAK at a second tyrosine residue, Y925, which acts as the docking site for the adaptor Shc, which itself becomes phosphorylated and binds Grb2. This initiates the activation of the Ras–MAP kinase pathway, necessary for initiation of the cell cycle.

8.3.3.4.2 The Role of FAK and Src in Cell Proliferation

The formation of focal adhesion sites not only rescues cells from apoptosis but is also an essential requirement for the proliferation of tissue cells, driven by growth factors. If, for instance, EGF or PDGF are added to suspended fibroblasts, the activation of the MAP kinase pathway is merely transient, and the cells fail to proliferate (and in the long run die through apoptosis). Proliferation only proceeds under the influence of two independent stimuli, one due to a growth factor and the other from adhesion molecules. The integrin clusters allow the binding of FAK, which undergoes autophosphorylation (at Tyr-397) and then recruits Src (or Fyn) kinases to cause further phosphorylation (at Tyr-925) and the formation of an activated PTK complex (Figure 8.17). The phosphorylated FAK, residue Tyr-925, now binds the adaptor protein Shc, which binds Grb-2 and activates the Ras pathway (see Section 8.2.3.1). This may serve to augment the signal from the growth factor receptor and results in prolonged activation of MAP kinase (ERK). The sustained signal ensures progression from G_o to G_1 and entry into the cell cycle.

8.4 APPENDIX

8.4.1 HOMOLOGOUS PATHWAYS IN *DROSOPHILA*, *CAENORHABDITIS ELEGANS*, AND MAMMALS

This section explains how genetic studies with *Drosophila* and *Caenorhabditis elegans* have contributed to the discovery of the Ras signal-transduction pathway operative in mammalian cells.

8.4.1.1 Photoreceptor Development in the Fruit Fly *Drosophila melanogaster*

The compound eyes of insects are formed of a hexagonal array of small units, or *ommatidia* (in the case of the fruit fly, approximately 800 "small eyes"). Each is composed of eight photoreceptor cells

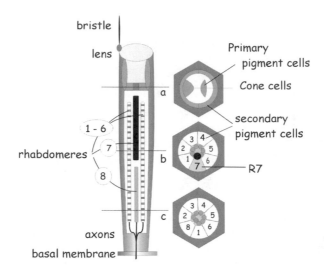

FIGURE 8.18 The *sevenless* mutation in fly eyes. The events leading to the development of cell R7 in eyes of *Drosophila* have provided a key to understanding the pathway downstream of receptor PTKs. Genes acting downstream of the *sevenless* receptor were revealed by screening for mutations that affect the development of cell R7. The eye is built up of ommatidia, groups of eight photoreceptor cells each covered by a single lens. The drawing illustrates the basic anatomy of a single ommatidial unit in longitudinal section. Sections cut at a, b, and c are shown in transverse section on the right. Because two of the cells, R7 and R8, do not extend the full length of the ommatidial unit, the transverse sections b and c only reveal seven, not all eight, cells. (Adapted from Dickson and Hafen, *Curr. Opin. Genet. Dev.*, 4, 64–70, 1994.)

(R1–R8) and 12 accessory cells. On the basis of their morphology, order of development, axon pattern projection, and spectral sensitivity, the photoreceptor cells can be classified into three functional classes: R8, the first to appear, followed by R1 to R6 and then R7. The photosensitive pigment resides in a microvillus stack of membranes, the rhabdomere. The larger rhabdomeres of cells R1 to R6 are arranged as a trapezoid surrounding the rhabdomeres of cells R7 and R8, the R8 rhabdomere being located below R7 (Figure 8.18). The development of R7 requires the products of two genes, *sevenless* (*sev*) and *bride-of-sevenless* (*boss*). The phenotypes generated by loss-of-function mutations in either of these genes are identical, R7 failing to initiate neuronal development (the fly being "sevenless"). These mutations are readily detected in a behavioral test. Given a choice between a green and an ultraviolet (UV) light, normal (WT) flies will move rapidly toward the UV source. Failure to develop cell R7, the last of the photoreceptor cells to be added to the ommatidial cluster, correlates with the lack of this fast phototactic response, and the flies move toward the green light.

While the *sev* product is required only in the R7 precursor, *boss* function must be expressed in the developing R8. Cloning revealed the *boss* product to be a 100-kDa glycoprotein having seven transmembrane spans and an extended N-terminal extracellular domain. Although ultimately expressed on all of the photoreceptor cells, at the time that R7 is being specified it is only present on the oldest, R8. The product of the *sev* gene is a receptor protein tyrosine kinase. Evidence for direct interaction between the products of these two genes came from the demonstration that cultured cells expressing the *boss* product tend to form aggregates with cells expressing *sev*.

It is now understood that the binding of Boss (the ligand) to Sev (the receptor kinase) leads to the activation of a protein kinase and that this ultimately determines the fate of R7 as a neuronal cell. Because a reduction in the gene dosage of the fly *Ras1* impairs signaling by Sev, and persistent activation of *Ras1* obviates the need for the *boss* and *sev* gene products, it follows that the activation of Ras is an early consequence of Sev activity. Further genetic screens of flies expressing constitutively activated Sev led to the identification of two intermediate components of this pathway: *Drk* (*downstream of receptor kinases*) and *Sos* (*son of sevenless*) (for the sequence of events, see

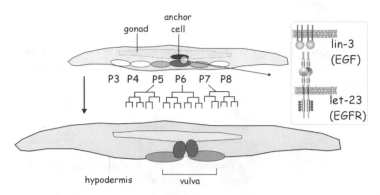

FIGURE 8.19 Vulval development in *Caenorhabditis elegans*. Because it is a relative simple structure, formed from just a few cells, the vulva is well suited for the genetic analysis of cell differentiation during embryological development It is the product of just three cell lineages, the descendants of cells p5.p, p6.p, and p7.p. Development is initiated by a signal from the anchor cell that lies adjacent to p6.p. The ligand, lin-3 (a homolog of EGF), produced by the anchor cell, binds its receptor Let-23 (homologous to the EGF-R) on the surface of cell p6. Cell p6.p, in turn, releases signals to its neighbors, p5.p and p7.p. This initiates a sequence of events involving the MAP kinase pathway that determines the fate of these cells as components of vulval tissue. (Adapted from Kornfeld, K., *Trends Genet.*, 13, 55–61, 1997.)

Table 8.3). The Sos protein shows substantial homology with the yeast CDC25 gene product, a guanine nucleotide exchange catalyst for RAS. While a reduction in the gene dosages of *Drk* and *Sos* impair the signal from constitutively activated Sev, there is no effect on signaling from constitutively activated Ras. In the pathway of activation, this places the functions of the *Drk* and *Sos* products into a position intermediate between Sev and Ras. The *Drk* gene codes for a small protein consisting exclusively of Src homology domains, two SH3 domains flanking a single SH2 domain. Having no catalytic activity of its own, Drk acts as an adaptor. It binds to the tyrosine phosphorylated receptor and links it to the proline-rich domains of Sos.

8.4.1.2 Vulval Cell Development in *Caenorhabditis elegans*

In the nematode *C. elegans*, a similar pathway of activation involving autophosphorylation of a tyrosine kinase receptor leads to activation of the GTPase Let-60, a homolog of Ras. This determines the development of vulval cells. Again, these proteins were first identified from genetic analysis of lethal mutations (*let*, or lethal mutants), morphological changes in vulval development (*sem*, or sex muscle mutants), or alterations in cell lineage (*lin*, or lineage mutants). They constitute the components of a signal-transduction pathway based on a secreted product of the anchor cell (Lin-3, most likely the equivalent of EGF), a tyrosine kinase receptor of the p5.p cell (Let-23), an adaptor having SH2 and SH3 domains (Sem-5) that associates with a (Sos-like) guanine nucleotide exchange protein. This brings about nucleotide exchange on Let-3 (Figure 8.19).

In both worm and fly, the Ras protein acts as a switch that determine cell fate. In *C. elegans*, the activation of Ras determines the formation of vulval as opposed to hypodermal (skin) cells (for sequence of events, see Table 8.4). In *Drosophila* photoreceptors, the activation of Ras determines the development of R7 as a neuronal as opposed to a cone cell. In both cases, Ras proteins operate downstream of receptor tyrosine kinases that are activated by cell–cell interactions.

8.4.1.3 *Drosophila, Caenorhabditis* elegans, and the Discovery of the Ras Pathway in Vertebrates

Elucidation of the Ras pathway in vertebrates was based on the identification of proteins having sequence homologies with those present in *Drosophila* and *C. elegans*. Expression or microinjection

TABLE 8.4
Comparison of Signal-Transduction Pathways Downstream of a Protein Tyrosine Kinase Receptor in Species of Three Separate Phyla

	Species		
	---	---	---
Pathway	*Drosophila melanogaster*	*Caenorhabditis elegans*	Mammals
	Eye Formation	Vulval Induction	Proliferation
Ligand	Boss	Anchorless	Cytokines
RTK	Sev	Let-23	Receptor
SH2 adaptor	Drk	Sem5	Grb2/Shc
Regulation of Ras	Sos GAP1	Gap-1	hSos GAP
Ras	Dras	Let-60	Ras
Raf-1	Draf	Lin-45	Raf-1
MEK	D-MEK	MEK-2	MEK-1
MAP kinase	ERK-A	MPK-1	ERK
Transcription factors	Sina	Lin-31, Lin-1/Ets	p62^{TCF}, *c-jun*

of these proteins (and appropriate reagents such as peptides, antibodies, etc.) were used to restore or modulate the activity of this pathway in cells derived from mammals, flies, or worms and bearing loss-of-function mutations. A vertebrate protein Grb2 (growth-factor receptor binding protein 2), lacking catalytic activities but having SH2 and SH3 domains, was found to be capable of restoring function in Sem-5-deficient mutants. In addition, Grb2 was found to associate with a protein that is recognized by an antibody raised against the *Drosophila* protein, Sos. In this way, the sequence of events became apparent. Grb2 is an adaptor protein, linking the phosphorylated tyrosine kinase receptor to the guanine nucleotide exchanger in vertebrates. The mammalian Sos homolog, hSos, is likewise a guanine nucleotide exchange factor that interacts with Ras. Grb2 is composed exclusively of Src homology domains, one SH2 flanked by two SH3 domains. Because of the nature of the interaction of SH3 with proline-rich sequences, it is likely that Grb2 and Sos remain associated even under nonstimulating conditions. The main effect of receptor activation is to ensure the recruitment of the Grb2/Sos complex to the plasma membrane (for a sequence of events, see Table 8.4).

8.4.1.4 MAP Kinases in Other Organisms

Pathways regulated by MAP kinases are widely distributed and can be found in all eukaryotic organisms. In *Saccharomyces cerevisiae*, physiological processes regulated by MAP kinases include mating, sporulation, maintenance of cell-wall integrity, invasive growth, pseudohyphal growth, and osmoregulation. MAP kinase is a regulator of the immune response and embryonic development in *Drosophila*. It has also been implicated as a regulator in slime molds, plants, and fungi.

8.4.2 ONCOGENES, MALIGNANCY, AND PROTEIN TYROSINE KINASES

8.4.2.1 Viral Oncogenes

Infection by viruses carrying oncogenes can cause malignant cell growth. Although first recognized as causative agents in avian cancers 90 years ago, for much of the twentieth century there was doubt that any human cancers were initiated in this way. Even now, almost all the information in this area refers to nonhuman animals, which presents a number of problems. First, as was already

TABLE 8.5
Components of Tyrosine Kinase Signal Transduction Cascades Are Discovered as Cellular (or Viral) Oncogenes

Receptor Protein Tyrosine Kinase	Nonreceptor Protein Tyrosine Kinase	Serine/Threonin Protein Kinase	SH2/SH3 Adapter	Nucleotide Exchange Factor	GTPase
Bek	Abl	Akt/PKB	Crk	Bcr	H-Ras
Eck	Blk	Cot	Nck	Dbl	K-Ras
Elk	Fgr	Mos	—	Ost	N-Ras
Eph	Fsp	Pim	—	Tiam	—
ErbB	Fyn	Raf	—	Vav	—
Flg	Hck	—	—	—	—
Fms	Lck/Lyn	—	—	—	—
Kit	Src	—	—	—	—
Met	Yes	—	—	—	—
Neu	—	—	—	—	—
Ret	—	—	—	—	—
TrkA	—	—	—	—	—
TrkB	—	—	—	—	—
TrkC	—	—	—	—	—

apparent in the first decade of the last century, demonstration of a viral mode of transmission depends on the induction of disease by transfer of tissue filtrates from animal to animal. Some viruses only become oncogenic as a consequence of multiple passages and through different animal species. Second, while many human cancers are certainly associated with viral infection, it is far from certain in most cases whether the virus has initiated the condition or whether it is merely conducive to induction by another agent, such as a chemical carcinogen. In general, the transforming products of the viral oncogenes behave as persistently activated mutants of endogenous cellular proteins having key regulatory roles in mitogenesis.

8.4.2.2 Nonviral Oncogenes

Tumors not caused by viral infection (e.g., by chemical carcinogens) also express persistently activated products, such as oncogenic Ras. As an example of the role of oncogenes in cell transformation, mutated forms of Ras are found in 40% of all human cancers and in more than in 90% of pancreatic carcinomas. In general, these oncogenes represent gain-of-function mutations of normal cellular genes involved in signal transduction and gene transcription. A number of these mutated proteins operate in the early stages of tyrosine kinase signal-transduction pathways. Cells may be transformed as a consequence of hypersecretion of growth factors, expression of a variant form of a receptor tyrosine kinase or a nonreceptor tyrosine kinase, overexpression of SH2/SH3-containing adaptor proteins, overexpression of serine/threonine protein kinases, or expression of variants of the small GTPases or their accessory proteins. At the downstream end of the signal-transduction pathway, variants of transcription factors also act as potent cell transformers. Although tyrosine kinase phosphorylation accounts for only about 5% of total cellular phosphorylation activity, it has a key position in many signal-transduction pathways, and it is probably for this reason that the incidence of these genes in malignancy is so high. Some examples are given in Table 8.5.

8.5 ABBREVIATIONS

4E-BP	eukaryotic initiation factor 4E-binding protein
AKT	acutely transforming retrovirus (AKT8)
AP-1	activator protein 1
ATF	adenovirus transcription factor (= CREB)
BCR	breakpoint cluster region, a GTPase
CD4	cluster of differentiation 4 (antigen typing on leukocytes)
Cdc	cycle-deficient cell
CDK	cyclin-dependent kinase
Boss	bride-of-sevenless
CaMK	calmodulin-dependent kinase
Cbl	Cas NS-1 B-cell lymphoma
CREB	cAMP-responsive, element-binding protein
Crk	CT10 regulator of kinase
DAF-16	dauer phenotype
DAG	diacylglycerol
Dbl	diffuse B-cell lymphoma
Drk	downstream of receptor tyrosine kinase
EF-2	elongation factor 2
EGF	epidermal growth factor
EIF-4E	eukaryotic initiation factor 4E
ERK	extracellular signal regulated kinase
EST	expressed sequence tag
FAK	focal adhesion complex kinase
FKHRL	forkhead related-L (forkhead gene promotes terminal as opposed to segmental development in the *Drosophila*)
Fos	feline osteosarcoma
FRAP	FKBP-rapamycin-associated protein
Gab-1	Grb2-associated binder 1
GAP	GTPase-activating protein
GRB	growth-factor-receptor bound
GSK-3β	glycogen synthase kinase 3β
HOG	high-osmolarity glycerol
IL-2	interleukin-2
IRS-1	insulin receptor substrate 1
ITAM	immunoreceptor tyrosine-based activation motif
JAK	janus kinase
JNK	Jun N-terminal kinase
Jun	avian sarcoma virus 17 (*junana*, 17 in Japanese)
LAT	linker of activated T cells
Lck	lymphocyte kinase from murine lymphoma LSTRA cells
Let	lethal mutant
Lin	lineage mutant
MAP kinase	mitogen-activated protein kinase
MAPKAP	MAPK-activated protein kinase
MEK	MAP kinase–ERK kinase

MEKK	MEK kinase
MHCII	major histocompatibility complex II
MKP	MAP kinase phosphatase
MLCK	Myosin light-chain kinase
Myc	myelocytomatosis virus MC29
NGF	nerve growth factor
NK	natural killer cell
nrPTK	nonreceptor protein tyrosine kinase
PAK	P21-activated protein kinase
PDGF	Platelet-derived growth factor
PDK1	phosphatidyl inositol-dependent kinase 1
PI-3 kinase	phosphatidylinositol-3 kinase
PIP2	phosphatidylinositol-4,5-phosphate
PH	pleckstrin homology domain
PLC	phospholipase C
PKB	protein kinase B
PKC	protein kinase C
PTB	phosphotyrosine-binding domain
PTEN	tensin homolog deleted from chromosome 10
PTK	protein tyrosine kinase
PYK2	proline-rich protein tyrosine kinase 2
Rac	Ras-like C3 substrate (however, it turns out Rac is not a C3 substrate; some Rho contamination was present in the Rac protein preparations being studied)
Raf	rat fibrosarcoma
Ras	rat sarcoma
RBD	Ras-binding domain
RGD	arginine–glycine–aspartic acid
Rho	Ras homologs
SAPK	Stress-activated protein kinase
Sem	sex muscle mutant
Sev	sevenless
Shc	Src homology collagen-like
SH2	Src homology 2
SHIP	SH2-domain-containing inositol phosphatase
SIF	v-Sis-inducible factor
Sina	seven in absentia
v-Sis	simian sarcoma virus gene
SLP76	SH2-domain containing leukocyte protein with a molecular weight of 76 kDa
Sos	son of sevenless
Src	sarcoma
SRE	serum-response element
SRF	serum-response factor
STAT	Signal transducer and activator of transcription
TAK1	TGF-β_1-activated kinase 1
TAM	tyrosine-based activation motif
TCF	ternary complex factor
TCR	T-cell receptor

TRE   TPA-responsive element
TrkA   tyrosine receptor kinase A
TPA   12-*O*-tetradecanoylphorbol-13-acetate
Vav   sixth letter in the Hebrew alphabet
ZAP70   zeta-associated protein 70

8.6 FURTHER READING

Bos, J. L., *ras* oncogenes in human cancer: a review, *Cancer Res.,* 49, 4682–4689, 1989.

Cantrell, D. A., T cell receptor signal transduction pathways, *Annu. Rev. Immunol.,* 14, 259–274, 1996.

Collins, T. L., Deckert, M., and Altman, A., Views on Vav, *Immunol. Today*, 18, 221–225, 1997.

Cooper, J. A. and Howell, B., The when and how of Src regulation, *Cell*, 73, 1051–1054, 1993.

Corvera, S. and Czech, M. P., Direct targets of phosphoinositide 3-kinase products in membrane traffic and signal transduction [review], *Trends Cell. Biol.,* 8, 442–6, 1998.

Downward, J., How BAD phosphorylation is good for survival, *Nat. Cell. Biol.,* 1, E33–E35, 1999.

Deller, M. C. and Jones, E. Y., Cell surface receptors, *Curr. Opin. Struc. Biol.,* 10, 213–219, 2000.

Giancotti, F. G., Integrin signaling: specificity and control of cell survival and cell cycle progression, *Curr. Opin. Cell. Biol.,* 9, 691–700, 1997.

Gomperts, B., Kramer, I., and Tathan, P., *Signal Transduction,* Academic Press/Elsevier, 2002.

Hunter, T., Tyrosine phosphorylation: past, present and future, *Biochem. Soc. Trans.,* 24(2), 307–327, 1996.

Kane, L. P., Lin, J., and Weiss, A., Signal transduction by the TCR for antigen, *Curr. Opin. Immunol.,* 12, 242–249, 2000.

Kaplan, D. R. and Miller, F. D., Signal transduction by the neurotrophin receptors, *Curr. Opin. Cell. Biol.,* 9, 213–212, 1997.

Karin, M., Liu, Z. G., and Zandi, E., AP-1 function and regulation, *Curr. Opin. Cell. Biol.,* 9, 240–246, 1997.

Kornfeld, K., Vulval development in *Caenorhabditis elegans*, *Trends Genet.,* 13, 55–61, 1997.

Metzger, H., The receptor with high affinity for IgE, *Immunol. Rev.,* 125, 37–48, 1992.

Nishizuka, Y., Protein kinase C and lipid signaling for sustained cellular responses. *FASEB J.,* 7, 484–496, 1995.

Raff, M., Cell suicide for beginners, *Nature*, 96, 119–122, 1998.

Roovers, K. and Assoian, R. K., Integrating the MAP kinase signal into the G_1 phase cell cycle machinery, *Bioessays*, 22, 818–826, 2000.

Treisman, R., Regulation of transcription by MAP kinase cascades, *Curr. Opin. Cell. Biol.,* 8, 205–215, 1996.

Wymann, M. P. and Pirola, L., Structure and function of phosphoinositide 3-kinases, *Biochim. Biophys. Acta,* 1436, 127–150, 1998.

Section V

Receptors as Pharmaceutical Targets

9 Receptors as Pharmaceutical Targets

James W. Black

CONTENTS

9.1 HORMONE RECEPTORS

The objective of pharmaceutical research is to discover and develop new substances that can be characterized by their selectivity and specificity. Selectivity describes the particular effects on physiological or pathological states that the substance can produce. These descriptions, such as hypnotic, hypoglycemic, hypotensive, and anti-inflammatory, may be wholly empirical; however, this does not impede their therapeutic utility. Thus, the clinical utility of drugs such as morphine and digitalis was established long before we had biochemical explanations for their actions. Specificity, on the other hand, refers to the biochemical hypotheses that claim to explain the selectivity of a substance. Thus, activation of enkephalin receptors is proposed as the mechanism by which morphine acts, and inhibition of Na^+-/K^+-dependent ATPase has been claimed to specify the activity of digitalis. All kinds of biochemical events have been used to specify drug actions. Interactions with enzymes, ion channels, and membrane transporters have been widely used to explain drug actions. However, pharmacological receptors are probably the favorite site of drug action used in explanatory models of their selective activity.

Receptor is a much-used term in biology: sensory receptors, telereceptors, mechanoreceptors, baroreceptors, chemoreceptors, T-cell receptors, and so on. Plainly, *receptor* requires an adjective or prefix to be informative. As used here, a receptor is the site of action of hormones, neurotransmitters, modulators of various kinds, and autocoids. As yet, no class name has been agreed upon for the receptors associated with these agents; however, all of these agents fulfill the role of intercellular messengers. As this was the concept behind Bayliss and Starling's invention of the term *hormone*, it is convenient to think that a class of molecules (e.g., hormone receptors) has common features in the same way as a class of enzymes has common features. Thus, enzymes induce chemical changes in substrates without themselves being permanently changed in the process; that is, they are catalysts. By the same token, hormones change the chemical properties of their corresponding receptors without themselves being chemically changed in the process; that is, hormones rather than their receptors are behaving like catalysts. Thus, the hormone receptor both recognizes and responds to its conjugate messenger. For ease of writing, this is the collective sense in which receptors will be referred to in this chapter.

Hormones, broadly defined in this way as chemical messengers, can all be characterized by their selectivity and specificity. The selectivity of hormones describes their role in physiological and pathophysiological regulatory processes. The specificity of hormones refers to the evidence that they produce their effects by interacting with identifiable protein receptors. Hormones, then, have drug-like qualities, like a natural, physiological pharmacopoeia. This is the idea that makes hormone–receptor systems so attractive to pharmaceutical researchers. When new-drug researchers use the drug-like qualities of a hormone as the starting point, they are already a long way to the goal of discovering a protodrug with desirable selectivity and specificity.

The selectivity of a hormone always entails the concepts of *affinity*, the likelihood of hormone and receptor interacting with each other, and *efficacy*, the response-generating power of the hormone which derives from activation of the receptors. These concepts are defined by parameters in classical thermodynamic models of hormone–receptor interactions. As these hormone-defining parameters are not readily accessible, even in radioligand-binding studies, the industrial pharmacologist usually settles for the empirical parameters of dose–response curves — namely, the maximum response and the dose required for half-maximal response. Modern pharmaceutical research based on hormone–receptor interaction is founded on measuring and interpreting dose–response curves. The target is the ability to manipulate hormonal efficacy as implied in dose–response curves. A significant fraction of a contemporary pharmacopoeia is about drugs that mimic, enhance, prolong, or abolish the efficacy of hormones.

9.2 PARTIAL AGONISTS: PROBLEMS IN DETECTING CHANGES IN EFFICACY

The author was introduced to the problems of efficacy and its expression in bioassays within months of starting his first project in pharmaceutical research while using isoprenaline, a fully efficacious analog of the hormones noradrenaline and adrenaline, to drive the rate of beating of the isolated guinea-pig heart (the Langendorff preparation) via activation of β-adrenoreceptors. Soon after beginning the project, the dichloro analog of isoprenaline, DCI, was described as an antagonist of isoprenaline on bronchial muscle. However, in our cardiac preparation, we found that DCI was as efficacious as isoprenaline itself. Subsequently, the Langendorff preparation was replaced with the rate-controlled guinea-pig papillary muscle preparation. On the new preparation, DCI had no agonist activity but was now a competitive antagonist of the catecholamines. The subsequent rapid development of β-adrenoreceptor antagonists was based on this observation. The tissue-dependence of the efficacy of DCI was puzzling, so we were not prepared for a second encounter with the phenomenon.

The second encounter occurred several years later when our laboratory switched interests to histamine antagonists. No *in vitro* assays for studying histamine-stimulated gastric acid secretion were known at that time, so we used the anaesthetized rat lumen-perfused stomach preparation (the Ghosh and Schild preparation). The guanidino analog of histamine (IEG) was one of the first compounds tested. For practical purposes, IEG behaved like a fully efficacious agonist. Several frustrating years later, it was found that IEG was not quite as efficacious as histamine. When IEG was dosed during a plateau of a maximal secretory response to histamine, a small degree of inhibition was revealed. The subsequent rapid development of histamine H_2-receptor antagonists was based on this observation. It was eventually found that, had the rat isolated uterus preparation been used for the screening bioassay, it would have immediately shown that IEG was much less efficacious than histamine.

Both DCI and IEG are now classified as partial agonists. Partial agonist, by definition, is a comparative description. When substance B is unable to produce as large a maximum response as substance A in a particular tissue, and when they can be shown to be producing their effects by acting on the same population of receptors, then substance B is defined as a partial agonist. This is a very limited definition, however. These initial observations with DCI and IEG are now generally recognized. The expression of partial agonism is tissue-dependent in a very sensitive way. DCI would have been classified as a full agonist as judged by heart-rate changes and as a simple competitive antagonist as judged by papillary muscle contractions. The variations in the expression of efficacy between closely related analogs of a hormone acting on a particular tissue and the variations in the expression of efficacy by a particular analog acting on different tissues have both practical and theoretical implications.

Kenakin and Beek published a beautiful data set comparing the activities of isoprenaline (classified as a full agonist) with prenalterol (classified as a partial agonist) on six different tissues. Across the tissues, the potency of isoprenaline varied by two orders of magnitude: in tissues where the potency of isoprenaline was very high, the efficacy of prenalterol was also very high, nearly the same as isoprenaline. Where the potency of isoprenaline was low, prenalterol had no detectable agonist activity and, indeed, now behaved like a competitive antagonist. From the point of view of pharmaceutical research the implications are clear. Try to find several tissues that will express the activity of the hormone of interest. The relative potencies of the hormone can point to the likelihood that a particular tissue will expose the efficacy of a partial agonist. In pharmaceutical research, it is necessary in the early stages of a hormone-receptor-based project to be able to detect small changes in the efficacy of hormone analogs. An assay without too much amplification is needed. However, in the later stages of the project (for example, when compounds have been discovered that behave like simple competitive antagonists), high-efficacy amplification systems are required to detect signs of residual agonist activity.

From a theoretical point of view, the efficacy of an agonist in the tissue is dependent on the ratio between the well-understood concept of receptor density and the much more opaque concept of "some kind of coupling factor," the intrinsic ability of bound receptor to generate an intracellular stimulus. The possibility that the same class of receptors might have different coupling efficiencies in different tissues cannot be ignored; however, differences in the density of receptor expression between tissues is now well recognized and is the most attractive way of interpreting the tissue dependence of efficacy. The attractiveness of the concept is not just because of its simplicity but also because it points to a way in which the new technology of controlling the expression of cloned receptor genes can be harnessed to generate new systems to detect and measure efficacy. Although these new receptor expression systems are an interesting extension to the range of bioassays, they are in no sense a replacement for traditional bioassays based on intact, isolated tissues *in vitro*.

9.3 THE VALUE OF BIOASSAYS

The essence of using intact-tissue bioassays in a hormone-related pharmaceutical project is that the hormone can be used to light up its population of conjugate receptors in a conceptually simple biomolecular interaction. If the resulting events are dominated by this initial binding interaction, as described by the Hill equation, rectangular hyperbolic dose–response curves are likely. Simple hyperbolic dose–response curves are certainly found in *in vitro* bioassays, but departures from such simplicity are much more common. We are continuing to understand the different events that can lead to complicated dose–response curves. The receptors themselves can be a source of distortion. The dynamics of receptor expression can introduce variation due to internalization or desensitization. However, the most common receptor-mediated complicating factor occurs when the hormone activates more than one population of receptors. Disclosure of receptor heterogeneity is always interesting and challenging. The problem facing the pharmaceutical researcher is what to do about the discovery. The current climate is that we should always be trying to find more and more specific ligands. However, when a hormone activates more than one set of receptors to produce the same end result, albeit by different processes of transduction, it may be practically more prudent to search for highly nonselective ligands. This may be the best way to reach the goal of desirable selectivity.

The hormone itself can introduce complexity into bioassays. Many hormones must now be seen and understood not as chemical entities but as chemical pathways where hormonal activity is distributed across a number of chemical species. The more we learn about the pharmacological properties of members of a pathway, the more we are realizing that each one has a mix of common and unique properties. The practical point is that we must be careful about which "hormone" we choose to drive our bioassays. A hormonal chemical pathway may contain sinks as well as sources. Metabolism and uptake of a hormone can introduce significant distortions into bioassays. All of these factors leave their fingerprints on dose–response curves, and a pharmaceutical researcher developing a new bioassay has to learn to read the signs.

A particularly exciting challenge to industrial pharmacologists occurs when the cells that synthesize the hormone, with or without storage, are found in the same tissue as their conjugate receptors. For example, these cells can be neurons, mast cells, or enterochromaffin cells. Controlled release of synthesized or stored substances can be achieved by either chemical or electrical stimulation. Intact-tissue bioassay in this mode of indirect agonist offers two exciting opportunities. First, tissue architecture constrains and directs the release of substances to particular cellular targets in a manner that may not be achievable by the hormone diffusing into the tissue uniformly from the organ bath compartment. Second, indirect release may be able of producing a composite of co-released substances that potentially can interact with each other. Both of these phenomena are clearly recognized now and offer opportunities to the pharmaceutical researcher. Potentiating interactions at the post-receptor level occurring between co-released substances offer a particularly important opportunity for the future of drug research.

9.4   ARE BIOASSAYS VALUABLE IN PHARMACEUTICAL RESEARCH?

So far, we have reviewed the various ways in which complex dose–response curves in intact-tissue bioassays can be the result, the pharmacological resultant, of two or more interacting activities. Now, if all that these bioassays achieved was to blur and obscure the underlying activities, they would have to give way to the newer, analytically simpler assays based on chemistry and biochemistry. However, the beauty of intact-tissue bioassays is that they are analytically tractable; by using families of dose–response curves and appropriate mathematical models, the complexity of intact hormone–receptor systems can, indeed, be interpreted. Bioassay allows them to be studied as systems in ways denied to simple biochemical assays.

Are intact-tissue bioassays capable of being a stand-alone, initial technology for discovering new drugs in hormone–receptor-directed pharmaceutical projects? The answer, based on our own experience and much published evidence, must be positive; but without a doubt, *in vitro* bioassays are slow, resource intensive, and expensive and require skilled investigators. The questions today are about whether we can economize on these bioassays or even eliminate them altogether by using more productive chemical screens. Radioligand-binding assays are an obvious example. They have been widely used in the industry for many years but we do not know how their use is optimized in relation to bioassay, even after several years of personal experience observing radioligand-binding assays running alongside bioassays for both gastrin and cholecystokinin receptors. Every compound we have made has been evaluated in both kinds of assay. No doubt, not surprisingly, we have obtained much more information about new compounds using bioassay; however, in retrospect, could we have economized on the bioassays by using binding assays to select out inactive compounds? The judgment at this time is that we would have missed some interesting compounds. To some extent, this is a matter of style more than tactics. In the main, all of the compounds made in our program have been designed to try to answer a question about structure–activity relations. Several thousand dollars will have been spent in making each of them. As a result, a trivial biological evaluation of the binary type, 0 or 1, is inappropriate. At issue is the struggle between biologists and chemists to learn to understand and trust each other. It is not too much of a caricature to see that the chemist believes that every molecule he struggles so hard to make will have interesting properties if only the biologist would evaluate it adequately; the biologist, on the other hand, is convinced that his assays will reveal the desired properties of a molecule if only the chemist would make the right compound. Our experience shows it takes at least two years of continuous collaboration before the chemist and biologist really learn mutual trust!

9.5 THE ITERATIVE PROCESS OF DRUG DEVELOPMENT

A medicinal chemist is involved in a new hormone–receptor-targeted drug project right at the start. To get involved, enough of the structure of the hormone needs to be known to allow all the possible shapes of the molecule to be visualized by physical valence-wire models, by space-occupying nuclear models, or, nowadays, by various computerized simulations on a computer. Whatever way is chosen, these chemists, in principle, walk around the molecule in their mind as they carry out imaginative interrogations: what is it about this molecule that interests me as a chemist? Where are the likely sources of noncovalent interactions and the receptor-ionic charges, electron densities on carbonyls and amino groups, pi-electron systems, and so on? Today, chemists may have additional information from the molecular modeler about conformational probabilities. Whatever the input to their imagination, medicinal chemists distill out a single first question, a question which they believe they can try to answer by making a simple analog or derivative of the natural hormone. Of course, the question cannot be answered with surgical precision. Every precise change in the molecule produces many more consequential changes in its conformation, in charge distribution, in electrostatic fields, and so on, which ensure that the chemical question will likely have an opaque biological answer first time around.

Answers to the chemists' questions are provided by bioassays. Because there are questions to be answered, every biological result, including (even especially) that the new molecule is totally inactive, is full of interest. Whatever the result, a new question is raised, a new inquisitorial compound has to be made, a new biological test has to be carried out. This iterative process is, in principle, at the heart of all traditional hormone–receptor pharmaceutical research programs; however, in practice, the process cannot be driven like this as a single logical cycle. Generally speaking, compounds take longer to synthesize than to evaluate in bioassay. On average, a medicinal chemist will produce 15 target compounds per year, so a team of chemists are usually involved, working in parallel on parceled-out parts of the perceived problem. The molecular modelers, who are also part of the iterative loop, also have to work at a different rhythm from either the synthetic chemists or biological analysts; nevertheless, the principle of the interrogative loop is always in play.

During our lifetime, we have witnessed continuous and extraordinary advances in medicinal chemical technology, chemical analytical methods, and chromatography, but the most spectacular changes seen in about 40 years of pharmaceutical research have been in molecular modeling. The pharmaceutical industry has made a huge investment in this runaway technology. I sense, though, a certain amount of industrial disappointment in the yield from this investment and would agree that molecular modeling has not dramatically shortened the number of iterative loops in going from a hormone to a hormone-based compound with potential clinical utility. However, this is to miss the point. Three features of molecular modeling are no longer in doubt. The technology is allowing us to tackle problems, such as the ubiquitous polypeptide hormones, that would have been logically and imaginatively impossible 20 years ago. The technology continues to advance with breathtaking speed, a speed that would have been impossible without the earlier major investments. The technology is making a greater and greater contribution to the synthetic chemist's imagination. As far as molecular modeling is concerned, this author is a junkie.

9.6 ME-TOOISM

The logical, imaginative, and iterative approach to new drugs based on hormone–receptor systems sketched out above stands in marked contrast to the industrial approach we experienced 40 years ago and to the direction in which the industry is now moving compulsively at hectic speed. In the past, industrial research was criticized for its practice of random screening and for its generation of "me-too" drugs. Of course, the biological screening was not random; far from it, as the screening tests were chosen with great care to reflect identified medical needs. Pharmacologists tried to reflect the importance of meeting medical needs by using experimental pathology paradigms for screening tests. Thus, assays were often based on experimentally induced animal pathology such as sterile inflammatory responses to foreign bodies such as cotton-wool, or turpentine, or arthritis induced by antigen–adjutant presentation, or stomach ulcers induced by histamine or aspirin, or convulsions induced by leptazol or electricity, and so on. The compounds screened were not chosen at random, either. They were chosen by working one's way, systematically, through the company's accumulated compound collection, its database, or by systematically ringing the changes of substituents in a lead molecule epitomized by "methyl, ethyl, propyl, butyl, futile"! The intellectual sterility of the process was not because of randomness but because of the lack of a necessary connection between the chemistry and bioassay.

In parentheses, the critical charge of me-tooisms was also, I believe, misplaced. To some extent, I can accept the commercial charge of me-tooism. Premium prices have undoubtedly been asked for compounds with clinically insignificant acute differences, but side effects become recognized on a slow, time-dependent basis. Therefore, inevitably, the older drug has accumulated more reports of side effects on its data sheet and the newer me-too drug can be pedaled by marketing manipulators as "just as good but safer." Personally, I do not have such a cynical view of me-tooism, and there are two reasons for this. Me-too drugs establish the image-challenging thought that compounds having quite different chemical structures can nevertheless have congruent pharmacological properties. The concept of such classes of drugs is the basis of pharmacology. Second, while the different chemical structures have one feature in common, they invariably present often usable and important differences in their pharmacokinetic and toxicological profiles.

9.7 SHORT-TERMISM

As indicated, the development of hormone–receptor-based research programs have changed all that. The logical, imaginative, iterative approach that has been painted has been shown to work regularly and reliably. The record is clear. If you follow John Locke's advice of "steadily intending your mind in a given direction," you will succeed; however, the fact that the number of iterations and years it will take are entirely unpredictable. This has become a significant problem, as the pharmaceutical industry has allowed itself to be pressured into short-termism as an antidote to exponentially escalating costs of research and development, particularly thanks to extensions to the drug regulatory requirements and to development costs. Consequently, the emphasis today is on speed, on what is called *high-throughput screening*. The potential for high-throughput screening is based on the spectacular advances in immunological and molecular biological technology made in the last 10 years or so. A whole range of procedures are now available that include cloned receptor genes co-transfected with reporter genes in cell lines or, with even greater chemical purity, assays such as the scintillation proximity assays, where the pure chemical receptors are bound to beads that house the scintillant, thus solving the distance problem. All of these new assays can be executed robotically, and all of these new assays have the following features in common. They are ingenious. They are fundamentally chemical and not biological assays. They are highly productive but express the absolute minimum of information (presence or absence, 0 or 1). Fundamentally, these are automated assays. Important questions are not being asked, so intelligent analysis is compromised. Nevertheless, do these productive, automated, assays provide a greater, faster yield of chemical leads?

At this moment, the question has yet to be answered, but a vital complementary question also must still be answered. Where are the compounds to come from to feed the assays, which can consume around 2000 or more chemicals per week? The immediately obvious sources are the in-house compound libraries. The major drug-research-based companies now have anywhere between 0.5 and 1 million compounds in their compound libraries. So a research program that can assay about 2000 compounds per week will be kept occupied for at least a few years just working through its own library. The problem with in-house libraries is that they are not an ensemble of randomly structured organic molecules. The distribution is severely lumpy. By that I mean that many of the synthesized molecules will be in closely related groups, having been synthesized for previous programs, successful as well as unsuccessful. Unless one is irredeemably optimistic, this may not be an ideal pool of molecules to trawl for new leads.

9.8 COMBINATORIAL CHEMISTRY

The hunger at the heart of this new passion for high-throughput screening has to be satisfied from some other generous source of new compounds for screening. Swapping by contract or purchasing by corporate takeover or amalgamation are obvious approaches, but they are very expensive, offer limited strategies, and do not avoid the lumpiness problem. Fortunately, advances in chemistry have been as extraordinary as the advances in molecular and genetic biology. Combinatorial chemistry is the name of the new game.

I have no personal experience with combinatorial chemistry, but the technology for making large numbers of molecules coupled to appropriate chemical selection procedures began with laboratory experiments to study molecular evolution in purely chemical systems. Spiegelman and co-workers started with a bacterial phage, one of whose four genes was a replicase enzyme, to make copies of itself. They showed that repeated exposures *in vitro* of viral RNA, the replicase, and supplies of the four nucleotides led to entirely new RNA sequences with a 15-fold increase in replication rate; the mutations arose from errors in replication. Subsequently, combination of methods to induce mutations in RNA or DNA, plus repeated steps of amplification by PCR (polymerase chain reaction), has led to the ability to generate up to 10^{13} sequences of single-strand DNA. These can then be screened on columns on which are bound an appropriate protein. A high-affinity DNA ligand for thrombin was discovered in this way. When organic chemists took over from molecular biologists, they developed the techniques for generating libraries of 10^6 to 10^7 peptide sequences. The reactions and the assays were carried out on beads. The technology has advanced by introducing control of sequence development plus the ability to tag each sequence for ease of identification.

Synthesis of constrained peptide sequences has now been followed by combinations of non-peptide molecules. As greater constraints are introduced, the numerical productivity falls, but presumably the proportion of leads increases.

Combinatorial chemistry is now a rapidly developing activity which, as a technology, is attracting the attention of highly ingenious chemists. At this time, it is impossible to predict where this technology will lead us. We do not know whether some of the basic limitations will be overcome. At this time, all the methods are restricted to binary reactions that take place readily. This is in contrast to the problems facing a synthetic chemist who wants to make a specified molecule. Not only are a number of sequential steps needed, but also many of the stages require demanding conditions for the reactions to occur. Thus, it is difficult to see how combinatorial chemistry can, in the near future, be the basis for the iterative, interrogative approach to hormone–receptor-related ligands.

High-throughput screening of databases plus input from combinatorial chemistry is designed to generate leads. As I understand the process, leads will then be developed using more conventional methods. The assumption seems to be that finding leads is the rate-limiting step in the drug discovery process. Now, I am not convinced that this is so. Developing and optimizing leads into clinically testable new chemical entities (NCEs, as they are termed in the industry) is usually a much slower phase. However, the productivity of the industry, as judged by the discovery of completely new drugs, is limited more by the choice of targets than by the discovery of leads. Care in choosing a target is the most critical decision point in pharmaceutical research.

9.9 SELECTING TARGETS FOR DRUG DEVELOPMENT

My personal approach to choosing targets is to seek answers to six questions:

1. Is the project purged of wishful thinking?
2. Is a chemical starting point identified?
3. Are relevant bioassays available?
4. Will it be possible to confirm laboratory-defined specificity in humans?
5. Is a clinical condition relevant to this specificity?
6. Does the project have a champion?

The wishful-thinking criterion is the most important of all. All drug-discovery projects begin with a desire to prevent illness or treat sickness. Wishful thinking refers to the tenuousness of the perceived relationship between that desire and the means proposed to satisfy it. The most common example today is the claim made again and again: once we know the gene product, then we will be able to find new drugs. So far, no one has shown that this will be likely or even possible. Fortunately, most hormone–receptor-directed projects are relatively free of wishful thinking as far as discovering a ligand is concerned, although the potential utility of the ligand might well be fanciful. Fortunately, again, a hormone–receptor project has a chemical starting point, the hormone itself. We are inclined here to an assumption that we cannot prove; namely, that in seeking new ligands based on the chemistry of the hormone we stand a fair chance of retaining the evolutionarily derived selectivity of the hormone. Hormone–receptor targets also score well on the bioassay criterion. Very often the bioassay expresses an important feature of the selectivity of the hormone. Ideally, efficacy detection offers advantages: for example, in having several bioassays including radioligand-binding assays to choose from. Assays based on different species can be very valuable. Assays based on different species can be very valuable. An important criterion, I believe, is to develop ligands whose activity is not species-dependent — the most reliable predictor for extrapolation to humans.

In choosing a target, it is important to imagine how to investigate the proposed new ligand in humans. Will we be able, in practice as well as in principle, to confirm the selectivity of the ligand as defined in the laboratory experiment? This can be particularly challenging in relation to central nervous system (CNS)-directed compounds. However, most of the hormones, transmitters, and modulators found in the brain are also found in the gut, so perhaps the specificity of a CNS ligand can be evaluated in the periphery. It is also important before choosing a target to imagine what clinical disorder might be explored by the new specific ligand. No commercial judgment should be involved at this point. The only test is feasibility. For drugs with a new, previously unavailable specificity, plenty of evidence shows that prior commercial assessment is rarely valid. When a drug is developed with a specified mode of action, physicians will have the opportunity to explore unanticipated disorders.

The last question usually has an obvious answer: the need for a champion. The need derives from the common experience that drug research programs often go through lengthy periods of stalemate. During these periods, passion and conviction are needed to prevent the faint hearts from quitting.

Index

A

Acetylcholine receptors
  clusters, 190
  desensitization of, 189–190
  muscarinic, 218, 222, 225
  nicotinic, *See* Nicotinic acetylcholine receptors
Acetylcholine-binding protein, 118–119
Activation of receptors
  agonist binding vs., 12
  α-amino-3-hydroxy-5-methyl-4-isoxazole propionate, 119
  conformational changes during, 98–99
  del Castillo–Katz model, 58
  description of, 12
  efficacy of, 30
  insulin-like growth factor I receptor, 147–148
  ion-channel receptors
    analysis of, 192–193
    description of, 184
  partial agonism and, 26–28
  T cell receptor, 257
  ternary complex model, 160
Activator protein 1, 252
Active conformation
  metabotropic glutamate receptors, 96
  mutation shifting of equilibrium toward, 98
Active receptor, 12
Adaptor proteins, 104, 106
Adenosine triphosphate receptors, 112, 127–128
Adenylate cyclase, 82–83
Adrenocorticotrophic hormone, 89
Affinity constant, 12
Agonist(s)
  α-amino-3-hydroxy-5-methyl-4-isoxazole propionate, 119
  binding of, 12, 42
  classification of, 47–48
  concentration of
    Hill coefficient findings, 15
    ligand effects, 65
    P_{open} curve determinations based on, 191–192
    receptor proportion with, 28–30
    tissue response and, relationship between, 6–12
  description of, 22
  desensitization induced by, 107, 160, 189
  dissociation equilibrium constant of
    definition of, 7, 12, 15
    irreversible competitive antagonism for
      determining, 57–59

  efficacy of, 25–26, 273
  full, 22
  G-protein–receptor coupling effects, 222, 224
  intrinsic activity of, 24–26
  inverse, 32–36
  irreversible competitive antagonism effect on response of, 55–57
  nonpeptide, 101, 103
  partial, *See* Partial agonists
  receptor activation by, 98
  tissue response and, 9–10
Agonist–receptor complex, 31
Alkylation, 54–55
Allosteric antagonism, 60, 64, 66, 104
Allotopic antagonism, 60
α-Amino-3-hydroxy-5-methyl-4-isoxazole propionate receptors
  description of, 119
  molecular cloning of, 120
  neurotransmission mediation by, 119
  N-methyl-D-aspartate receptor colocalization with, 119–120
Angiotensin, 100
Antagonism
  allosteric, 60, 64, 66
  allotopic, 60
  chemical, 41–42
  description of, 97
  functional, 41–42
  indirect, 42
  inhibitory sites, 60
  insurmountable
    definition of, 55
    reversible noncompetitive antagonism, 59–60
  ion-channel receptors
    analysis of, 197–198
    bursts, 200, 202
    closed periods caused by, 200
    description of, 197
    dissociation rate constants, 203
    at equilibrium, 199
    frequency, 200
    mechanisms, 197–198
    relaxations, 198–199
    single-channel analysis, 200–202
    time scale of, 202–203
    use dependence, 203
    voltage dependence, 203–205
  irreversible competitive
    agonist response effects, 55–57